HEALTH, ILLNESS, and DISABILITY

HEALTH, ILLNESS, and DISABILITY

A Guide to Books for Children and Young Adults

Pat Azarnoff

R. R. BOWKER COMPANY

NEW YORK and LONDON, 1983

Published by R. R. Bowker Company
205 East Forty-second Street, New York, NY 10017
Copyright © 1983 by Xerox Corporation
All rights reserved
Printed and bound in the United States of America

Library of Congress Cataloging in Publication Data

Azarnoff, Pat.
  Health, illness, and disability.
  Includes indexes.
  1. Medicine — Juvenile literature — Bibliography.
I. Title [DNLM: 1. Book selection.   2. Adolescence —
Bibliography.   3. Child — Bibliography.   4. Health —
Bibliography.   5. Pediatrics — Bibliography.   6. Handicapped —
Bibliography. ZWS 100 A992h]
Z6658.A98   1983   [R130.5]   016.61   83-19743
ISBN 0-8352-1518-0

Contents

Preface   vii

Guide to Use   xi

Bibliographic Guide   1

Directory of Publishers   155

Title Index   165

Subject Guide   189

Subject Index   197

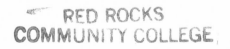

Preface

Health, Illness, and Disability: A Guide to Books for Children and Young Adults provides librarians and information specialists, mental health and health science professionals, educators, child development specialists, and parents and children with a guide that describes books on young people's experiences with their bodies and with disabilities, hospitalization, and medical treatments. It categorizes and annotates some 1,000 fiction and nonfiction books for children and youth about health and illness, ability and disability, function and dysfunction of the human body.

With advances in modern technology, more and more children with chronic serious illness and disabilities are living to adulthood. The number who need medical, educational, and social service help for chronic illness and assistance in adapting to or overcoming disability is increasing. Because of new laws and regulations on education of the handicapped, children who have physical or emotional challenges are being accepted into public education where they were formerly excluded. Preschool and public school teachers now have children in their classes with cystic fibrosis or hemophilia, for example, who would have died from their illnesses not many years ago, and children who are blind or deaf, whose families and school systems expect them to learn along with nondisabled children. Youngsters who have leukemia, some forms of which are now considered a chronic rather than a fatal illness, are expected to return to school after treatment produces a remission.

Hospitalized children and those who receive care at clinics and doctors' offices regularly because of chronic illness or permanent disability are now being taught about their conditions and being psychologically prepared before hospitalization or surgery. Such children must have treatment regularly. They experience and fantasize about the noise, size, and action of huge machinery, the toxic effects of chemotherapy, the disfigurement of surgical procedures that save but change lives. When children understand the wide range of nondisabled functioning, deviations from that range can be understood as disabilities, challenges to strive toward more comfortable living. There are, therefore, many books included in this guide on the ability of the body to see, hear, smell, taste, think, breathe, excrete, feel, and function. And there are many books on impairments, disabilities, conditions, diseases, and hospitalization and treatments.

Inevitably, children who look different or who move, speak, or act in a different manner experience teasing, insensitive treatment, and isolation from some other young people and adults. Even when they are functioning as well as possible and adapting to regular school, one remaining painful aspect is often the lack of understanding from other children and adults. Sensitizing ablebodied people to disabilities can help them appreciate the struggles of the disabled to achieve the same functioning that the nondisabled have acquired more easily. The books listed in this guide can help to convey the experience of disability to ablebodied siblings, classmates, and friends as part of the effort to teach them acceptance of others.

Adults should exercise caution when children read books about disability, illness, and death. Young children especially may fear that these same things will happen to them, and they may need to be reassured of their own good health and the protection of adults. Also, some adults may use the themes of accident or acquired disability to frighten or warn children that, if they are not careful in crossing streets or if they do not eat or exercise well, they could contract the diseases or become disabled like the children in the stories. This method of teaching is not effective because children are apt to become fearful of any behavior, uncertain about what to avoid, and helpless in the face of unknown impending disasters. It is much better to reassure children that they have some control over their lives and that their lives can be enhanced by taking good care of their bodies, whatever their health or condition.

Disabled children can be healthy children. One can be in good health wearing a prosthetic arm, using a wheelchair for mobility, or amplifying hearing with an aid. This guide offers books that describe the health of all children and the illness or disability of some.

Acknowledgments

A grant from the National Institute of Mental Health to survey the policies and practices of acute care hospitals in the United States in preparing children for hospitalization and treatment enabled the author to note the gap in information about children's books on health care. Although there are many books available, many health and mental health professionals, hospital teachers, and child developmental specialists in health centers seemed unaware of the range and nature of such titles. Those who did know about them found it difficult to locate books on specific subjects, finding subject headings in current use too general for them to use effectively. When they turned to teachers and children's librarians for help, the resources available were not specific enough. This reference, then, is an effort to respond to the need for more detailed subject headings on health, illness, and disability, and to call attention to the array of stories and factual books for children and youth of all ages. The author appreciates the advice of staff who pointed out the need and who reviewed the subject headings for usability and clarity, and the help of parents and patients who provided their favorite titles.

Librarians have been essential in this compilation, particularly those in the Los Angeles Public Library Children's Services, especially Priscilla Moxom; in the Santa Monica (California) Public Library system, especially Carol Aronoff, Ph.D., the city librarian, and her staff; in the Metropolitan Cooperative Library System that made it possible to find books in 26 independent city and district libraries; and librarians, faculty, and the computer system at the University of Southern California School of Library and Information Management. Research assistants who effectively handled many details include Julie Norman, Virginia Lewis, Karen A. Kushman, and Nancy Kempner. Particular appreciation is expressed to Roy S. Azarnoff, Ph.D., who gave both professional assistance and personal encouragement.

Children's books can convey complex information and sensitive feelings clearly, concisely, and with compassion. Books are not meant to replace human conversation and contact, but they can be a significant aid to young people who want to know more about themselves.

Pat Azarnoff
Santa Monica, California, 1983

Guide to Use

Book Selection

Health, Illness, and Disability: A Guide to Books for Children and Young Adults contains annotated titles, a detailed subject guide and index, a title index, and a list of publishers and ordering addresses. Fact and fiction books from 1960 through mid-1983 were selected that accurately depict or describe the able or disabled human body, especially the psychosocial aspects of care. Stories of "here and now" are emphasized over fables and stories of long ago.

The stories are predominantly of people rather than animals. Some therapists and teachers prefer animal stories for telling children about disability because the books effectively assist young people in coping with stress by distancing the subject or providing a vicarious experience. Others prefer realistic stories about people because children wonder about what seems magical, mysterious, and strange-looking (surgeons in masks and caps, for example, or X-ray machines that move close to the body), and realistic stories can help to balance the fantasies generated by lack of knowledge. Books about animals are differentiated in the subject index.

Only books in print as of mid-1983 are included. Sources used to determine in-print status include book publishers' catalogs and correspondence, *Children's Books in Print, 1982–1983* (New York: Bowker, 1982), and searches by the Baker & Taylor Company. In addition, a certain number of books were again checked with their publishers to verify in-print status just prior to publication.

Sources of Entries

Titles included in this guide were obtained from a variety of sources: publishers' catalogs and correspondence, *Subject Guide to Children's Books in Print, 1982–1983* (New York: Bowker, 1982), catalog cards of the Baker & Taylor Company, and suggestions made by children's librarians, medical and nursing staff, hospital play specialists, teachers, parents of chronically ill children, and medically experienced children and adolescents. Several published and unpublished bibliographies were checked that offered lists of children's books categorized as "nonsexist," for "exceptional children," for the "special child," and "multicultural." Publications that contain some books for children about hospitalization or disabilities are:

Altschuler, Ann. *Books That Help Children Deal with a Hospital Experience*. Washington, D.C.: U.S. Department of Health, Education, and Welfare, 1974.

Baskin, Barbara H., and Karen H. Harris. *Notes from a Different Drummer*. New York: Bowker, 1977.

Bernstein, Joanne. *Books to Help Children Cope with Separation and Loss*. 2nd ed. New York: Bowker, 1983.

Dreyer, Sharon Spredemann. *Bookfinder*. Circle Pines, MN: American Guidance Service, 1977.

Fassler, Joan. *Helping Children Cope*. New York: The Free Press, 1978.

Gillis, Ruth J. *Children's Books for Times of Stress*. Bloomington: Indiana University Press, 1978.

Rees, Alan M., and Blanche A. Young. *The Consumer Health Information Source Book*. New York: Bowker, 1981.

In addition, bibliographies of the following organizations in English-speaking countries were checked:

The American Library Association, 50 East Huron Street, Chicago, IL 60611

The Association for the Care of Children's Health, 3615 Wisconsin Avenue N.W., Washington, D.C. 20016

Pediatric Projects Inc., PO Box 1880, Santa Monica, CA 90406

The Association for the Welfare of Children in Hospital, 78-80 Phillip Street, Parramatta, New South Wales 2150, Australia

Canadian Institute of Child Health, 803-410 Laurier Avenue West, Ottawa, Ontario K1R 7T3, Canada

National Association for the Welfare of Children in Hospital, 7 Exton Street, London SE1 8UE, England

Bibliographic Guide

After reviewing and selecting the books, annotations were written by adapting the publishers' own descriptions and/or Baker & Taylor catalog cards. For example, the author added the name of the disability or condition if that was not given and told more about the story or text when needed in order to indicate the health or illness context. These descriptive or indicative annotations were reviewed by two readers.

The listing of a book in this guide indicates that it is judged to be accurate, informative, and interesting. Beyond that, evaluations are not included. Many of these selections are specialized books on emotional aspects of disease and handicap. Therefore, no book is "best" or even "better" than another. Any particular book may be appropriate for a particular child on a certain occasion, and might not be appropriate for another on the same occasion. The annotation can be helpful in determining choices.

The bibliographic reference for each book or series includes the author(s) or editor(s), grade level as suggested by the publisher or by *Children's Books in Print, 1982–1983*, illustrator(s) or photographer(s), translator(s), publisher, date of publication, number of pages (or unpaged), price of the hardcover edition, publisher and price of the paperback edition (if appropriate), and an indication of fiction or nonfiction. Publishers' names are abbreviated; in the complete list of publishers and ordering addresses at the back of the book, names are alphabetized by the abbreviation.

References are alphabetized by the first author's last name. Mc is placed as though it were written "Mac" and is interfiled with other names beginning with "Mac." Authors are listed under their full names, even though some of their books may have appeared with initials, a pseudonym, or with a middle initial.

Subject Guide

Clusters or groupings of subjects can be an aid to the user of this book who wishes to identify areas that may be related to a particular theme. A descriptive summary of each of the eight themes—

aids/appliances, body, diagnosis, disability, feelings, roles and relationships, signs and symptoms, and treatment—explains the nature of the grouping. The lists in the guide can help to identify related subject headings and enable the user to more effectively utilize the available resources. The subject guide constitutes an initial thesaurus of terms in the field of psychosocial aspects of young people's health care.

Subject Index

A detailed subject index leads the user to the author in the alphabetical annotated listing, or Bibliographic Guide, that forms the main part of the book. Although the latest editions of standard guides were consulted for descriptors of conditions, disabilities, and impairments, such as *Subject Headings Used in the Dictionary of the Library of Congress; M. E. Sears' List of Subject Headings* (Wilson); and *International Classification of Impairments, Disabilities, and Handicaps: A Manual of Classification Relating to the Consequences of Disease* (Geneva: World Health Organization, 1980), more detailed terms have been added. If a nurse wants to show a child a book about having an intravenous pyelogram, in which a color dye is injected in order to view the kidneys more clearly on X-ray film, the term *X ray* will not be of as much help as *intravenous pyelogram*, which leads to books that have detailed drawings or descriptions. If a librarian wants a book about heart surgery for a child about to undergo the procedure, a book about tonsillectomy will not be of much help. The heading of *surgery, heart* is more helpful than the general term *surgery*.

Headings use the language of health care providers, such as *cardiac catheterization, radiation therapy*, and *laser therapy*, to avoid the vagueness and confusion of less specific headings. The subject index contains popular words, when they exist, in addition to technical terms, to assist the reader in understanding jargon or terminology. Some terms now in common use among the public as well as professionals are preferred, such as *anorexia nervosa*. When the simpler, better-known word is now considered inaccurate, derogatory, or inappropriate, the term is omitted, such as mongolism, replaced by *Down's Syndrome*. Exceptions occur when the book title includes better known and still acceptable terminology, such as *rape* instead of the newer term *sexual assault.* When initials are familiar, perhaps more than the technical term (such as CAT Scan, DNA, IVP), the terms are followed by the initials in parentheses.

Subject headings have been selected to avoid value judgments. Instead of unwed mother, which not only omits unwed fathers but also has a disapproving connotation since it usually refers only to adolescents, the headings *adolescent single mother* and *adolescent single father* are used.

Some books that are otherwise accurate and useful employ terms that are currently on the way to oblivion, such as crippled, deformed, distorted. Such terms do not indicate the diagnosis clearly enough and sometimes seem to connote a personal quality rather than a description of the disability. When the cause or nature of the problem is clear in the stories, the part of the body affected is identified and clarified. Thus, *leg disability* is given instead of lame and *spinal disability* instead of crippled.

A title that is listed under more than one subject heading covers more than one subject in enough detail to note. Since some books cover one subject thoroughly while others cover several subjects, the number of times that a book appears in the subject index varies. This should not be taken as an indication of greater worth, but simply that the book covers more subjects. The same holds true for the varied length of the annotations, since some stories depend primarily on their illustrations while others are lengthy in text.

Bibliographic Guide

ABORIGINAL EDUCATION RESOURCE UNIT. *Hughie's Hospital Adventure*. Gr. ps–3. Illus. Aboriginal Ed, 1977. 28 pp. pap. $3.00. Nonfiction.
Hughie is flown to a big city hospital in Australia to have surgery on his ears. All the routines are new and different for him, but the staff tries to help him feel welcome. Children taken to a hospital from a remote or rural area will recognize his experiences of unfamiliarity, fear, and interesting discoveries in the hospital.

ADAMS, Barbara. *Like It Is: Facts and Feelings About Handicaps from Kids Who Know*. Gr. 5–6. Photog. by James Stanfield. Walker, 1979. 96 pp. $8.85. Nonfiction.
Young people tell about their daily lives and feelings concerning their hearing, speech, or visual impairment; orthopedic, developmental, or learning disabilities; or behavior disorders.

ADLER, Irving, and Ruth ADLER. *Taste, Touch and Smell*. Gr. 3–6. Illus. John Day, 1966. 48 pp. $8.79. Nonfiction.
The authors describe these three senses that work through the nervous system. Heat, cold, pressure, and pain are felt through the skin. Taste and smell are chemical senses.

ADLER, Irving, and Ruth ADLER. *Your Ears*. Gr. 4–5. Illus. by Peggy Adler Walsh. John Day, 1963. 48 pp. $5.79. Nonfiction.
The authors describe human ears and how they hear sounds.

1

ADLER, Irving, and Ruth ADLER. *Your Eyes*. Gr. 4–5. Illus. John Day, 1962. 48 pp. $9.89. Nonfiction.
The authors explain the structure and function of the eye, and suggest that visual illusions can fool this vital organ. Aids and appliances that can help visually impaired or blind children are shown.

AGOSTINELLI, Maria E. *On Wings of Love: The United Nations' Declaration of the Rights of the Child*. Gr. ps–3. Illus. Philomel, 1981. 32 pp. $8.95; pap. Collins, $6.91. Nonfiction.
The United Nations has declared that children have the right to food, health care, affection, freedom from abuse, and protection from danger.

AKINS, W. R. *ESP: Your Psychic Powers and How to Test Them*. Gr. 5–6. Illus. by Terry Fehr. Watts, 1980. 59 pp. $7.90. Nonfiction.
Scientific theories about ESP (extrasensory perception) are explained. The most common forms of ESP are telepathy, clairvoyance, and precognition. Simple tests are described that readers can use to become more aware of their own abilities.

ALBERT, Louise. *But I'm Ready to Go*. Gr. 6–8. Bradbury, 1976. 240 pp. $8.95; pap. Dell, $1.25. Fiction.
Judy, a junior-high-school student who has learning disabilities and minimal brain damage, is transferred to special classes. Her struggle to get along with classmates and family and to understand her own abilities and limitations adds to her adolescent confusions.

ALIKI (Aliki Brandenberg). *My Five Senses*. Gr. 1–2. Illus. by the author. Crowell, 1962. Unp. pap. $2.95. Nonfiction.
The pleasure of each of the five senses is shown in illustrations and a simple story.

ALIKI (Aliki Brandenberg). *My Hands*. Gr. ps–3. Illus. by the author. Har-Row, 1962. Unp. $9.89. Nonfiction.
Simple words and pictures of hands of various people show the many things that hands can do.

ALLEN, Anne. *Sports for the Handicapped.* Gr. 6 and up. Walker, 1981. 80 pp. $9.95. Nonfiction.
Capsule stories, lists, addresses, and general sports information point out the many opportunities for the handicapped in aquatics, camping, climbing, fishing, basketball, gymnastics, skiing, and other sports.

ALLEN, Marjorie N. *One, Two Three–Ah-Choo!* Gr. 1–2. Illus. by Dick Gackenbach. Coward, 1980. 62 pp. $6.99. Fiction.
Allergic to feathers and animal fur, young Wally must give up his puppy. He searches for a pet that will not make him sneeze.

ALLINGTON, Richard L., and Kathleen COWLES. *Feelings.* Gr. 1–3. Illus. by Brian Cody. Raintree, 1980. 32 pp. $13.30. Nonfiction.
A boy goes through his day and feels many different feelings such as pride, anger, loneliness, silliness, and shyness.

ALLINGTON, Richard L., and Kathleen COWLES. *Looking.* Gr. ps–1. Illus. by Bill Bober. Raintree, 1980. 32 pp. $13.30. Nonfiction.
Games develop abilities to look closely at common objects.

ALLINGTON, Richard L. and Kathleen KRULL. *Talking.* Gr. ps–2. Illus. by Rick Thrun. Raintree, 1980. 32 pp. $13.00. Nonfiction.
Listening is as important as talking in having conversations. Communication helps to make friends, gain information, get help, persuade, and express feelings.

ALLINGTON, Richard L., and Kathleen COWLES. *Tasting.* Gr. 1–3. Illus. by Noel Spangler. Raintree, 1980. 32 pp. $13.30. Nonfiction.
Recipes and pictures show different things to taste, including sweet, spicy, cold, wet, and salty.

ALLINGTON, Richard L., and Kathleen COWLES. *Touching.* Gr. 1–3. Illus. by Yoshi Miyake. Raintree, 1980. 32 pp. $13.30. Nonfiction.
The skin differentiates between such sensations as smooth, cold, soft, flat, bumpy, and pointed.

ALLINGTON, Richard L., and Kathleen KRULL. *Thinking.* Gr. ps–2. Illus. by Tom Garcia. Raintree, 1980. 32 pp. $13.30. Nonfiction.
A young child tells what he thinks about in his life.

ALLISON, Linda. *Blood and Guts: A Working Guide to Your Own Insides.* Gr. 3–4. Illus. by the author, assisted by David Katz. Little, 1976. 127 pp. $8.95. Nonfiction.
Stories, experiments, and projects explore the organs and body systems that make human life possible.

ALTHEA (Althea Braithwaite). *A Baby in the Family.* Gr. ps–1. Illus. by Ljiljana Rylands. Dinosaur, 1981. Unp. $1.95. Fiction.
The author describes conception and childbirth, emphasizing family love.

ALTHEA (Althea Braithwaite). *Going into Hospital.* Gr. ps–1. Illus. by the author. Dinosaur, 1981. Unp. pap. $1.95. Fiction.
In simple language, hospitalization is explained, such as the ward, a child's own space, mother sleeping overnight, making friends, eating, playing, having intravenous therapy, a cast, blood drawing, using a urinal, going to surgery, and seeing many doctors.

ALTHEA (Althea Braithwaite). *Going to the Doctor.* Gr. ps–1. Illus. by the author. Dinosaur, 1973. Unp. pap. $1.95. Fiction.
In simple language, details of medical care are given, such as a visit to the doctor's office, a home visit, undressing, the black bag of medical tools, taking medicine, an X ray, injection, and reenacting experiences in play.

ALTHEA (Althea Braithwaite). *Having an Eye Test.* Gr. ps–1. Illus. by the author. Dinosaur, 1978. Unp. pap. $1.95. Fiction.
An eye and vision examination are explained simply, such as having vision testing, eye drops, selecting frames, seeing other children wearing glasses, wearing an eye patch for "lazy" eye, and eye surgery.

ALTHEA (Althea Braithwaite). *Having a Hearing Test.* Gr. ps–1. Illus. by Maureen Galvani. Dinosaur, 1981. Unp. $1.95. Fiction.
Hearing games help children show how well they hear. Physical examinations show problems that may be treated. For example, the doctor may provide a hearing aid.

ALTHEA (Althea Braithwaite). *I Can't Talk Like You.* Gr. ps–2. Illus. by Isabel Pearce. Dinosaur, 1982. Unp. pap. $1.95. Fiction.
A boy who leaves special school to attend public school endures some teasing, but friends and a speech therapist help him when his speech impairment interferes with functioning.

ALTHEA (Althea Braithwaite). *I Have Asthma.* Gr. ps–1. Illus. by Jean Howat. Dinosaur, 1982. Unp. $1.95. Fiction.
A boy who has asthma and gets short of breath learns to use an inhaler, which enables him to take part in activities such as playing football.

ALTHEA (Althea Braithwaite). *I Have Diabetes.* Gr. ps–1. Illus. by Maureen Galvani. Dinosaur, 1983. Unp. pap. $1.95. Fiction.
Planning food intake and timing of meals are important to children with diabetes. The author explains various tests that such children do to check the levels of sugar in their blood.

ALTHEA (Althea Braithwaite). *I Use a Wheelchair.* Gr. ps–1. Illus. by Maureen Galvani. Dinosaur, 1983. Unp. pap. $1.95. Fiction.
A girl in a wheelchair is annoyed at being treated differently, since her mind functions well. She emphasizes her ability rather than her disability.

ALTHEA (Althea Braithwaite). *Visiting the Dentist.* Gr. ps–1. Illus. by the author. Dinosaur, 1974. Unp. pap. $1.95. Fiction.
In simple language, dental care is explained, such as toothbrushing, nutrition, sitting in the dental chair, how the machines feel, a nurse or dental hygienist cleaning teeth, filling a cavity, and a new tooth coming in.

ANCKARSVÄRD, Karin. *Doctor's Boy.* Gr. 4–6. Trans. from the Swedish by Annabelle MacMillan. HarBraceJ, 1965. 156 pp. $5.50. Fiction.
Ten-year-old Jon accompanies his doctor-father on medical visits in rural Sweden at the turn of the century, learning medicine and the art of dealing with people who are ill.

ANCONA, George. *I Feel: A Picture Book of Emotions.* Gr. ps–1. Photog. by the author. Dutton, 1977. Unp. $6.95. Nonfiction.
Black-and-white photographs of children in various situations

portray fifteen emotions and stimulate readers to observe and talk about other feelings.

ANDERS, Rebecca. *A Look at Alcoholism*. Gr. 2–3. Photog. by Maria S. Forrai. Lerner, 1978. Unp. $4.95. Nonfiction.
Alcohol abuse causes problems, but various kinds of help are available.

ANDERS, Rebecca. *A Look at Death*. Gr. 3–6. Photog. by Maria S. Forrai. Lerner, 1978. Unp. $4.95. Nonfiction.
Death is explained in simple and direct words, including the death of old people and those who die suddenly or as expected. A funeral is shown and grief is depicted as an important part of survivor recovery.

ANDERS, Rebecca. *A Look at Drug Abuse*. Gr. 2–3. Photog. by Maria S. Forrai. Lerner, 1978. Unp. $4.95. Nonfiction.
Various drugs can cause addiction, from caffeine to heroin, but there are methods of rehabilitation.

ANDERS, Rebecca. *A Look at Mental Retardation*. Gr. 3–6. Photog. by Maria S. Forrai. Lerner, 1976. Unp. $4.95. Nonfiction.
Mental retardation has many causes. Doctors and teachers are interested in helping retarded youngsters learn, play, and grow. Children can help too, by offering friendship to retarded classmates.

ANDERSON, Kay Wooster. *Don't Forget Me, Mommy!* Gr. 9 and up. Marin, 1982. 118 pp. $7.95. Nonfiction.
The author tells the story of the family's efforts to help their son, who is mentally retarded as a result of Down's syndrome, and their feelings of hope and discouragement.

ANDERSON, Mary Quirk. *Step on a Crack*. Gr. 6–8. Atheneum, 1978. 180 pp. $10.95. Fiction.
Fifteen-year-old Sarah's nightmares grow worse when her aunt visits. With her friend's help, Sarah remembers that as a young child she was abused by her mother. They search public records, which reveal that her "aunt" is actually her mother. Sarah realizes she must seek mental health counseling to understand her experiences and resolve her anger.

ANDERSON, Peggy. *Nurse.* Gr. 10 and up. Berkley, 1978. 309 pp. pap. $2.95. Fiction.
Mary, a head nurse in a general hospital, tells about her work, her relationships with other staff and with patients, and the problems and satisfactions of her responsibilities.

ANDERSON, Penny S. *The Operation.* Gr. 2–3. Illus. by Paul Karch. Childrens, 1979. 32 pp. $7.35. Fiction.
Afraid to be hospitalized, Tangie tells her fears about blood, shots, and being alone. Her mother explains anesthesia and tonsillectomy, and stays with her in the hospital throughout her recovery. A postscript encourages the reader to think and talk about the story and gives further information about the hospital.

ANKER, Carol Teig. *Teaching Exceptional Children: A Special Career.* Gr. 7 and up. Messner, 1978. 224 pp. $8.29. Nonfiction.
In describing the job of teaching exceptional children, the author, a former guidance counselor, details types of disabilities and their characteristics, statistics, causes, and educational needs.

ANNEXTON, May, and Brent SCHILLINGER. *Coping with Skin Care.* Gr. 9–12. Illus. by Nancy Lou Gahan. Rosen, 1981. 115 pp. $7.97. Nonfiction.
Arranged alphabetically by subject, this guide to basic skin care discusses the causes of several common problems adolescents experience with skin, hair, and nails and suggests beneficial preventive measures.

ANON. *Go Ask Alice.* Gr. 9–12. P-H, 1971. 189 pp. $5.95; pap. Avon, $1.95. Nonfiction.
Fifteen-year-old Alice's drug addiction and pushing are difficult for her parents to understand and control. When she overdoses and dies, they find her diary, which is this book.

ANTONACCI, Robert J., and Jene BARR. *Physical Fitness for Young Champions.* Gr. 6–7. Illus. by Frank Mullins. McGraw-Hill, 1975. 144 pp. $8.95. Nonfiction.
One of the twelve chapters in this book on how to test and improve fitness is about sports and games for the physically disabled and mentally retarded. Success stories motivate readers to exercise as much as their disabilities and physicians permit.

ARCHER, Jules. *Epidemic! The Story of the Disease Detectives.* Gr. 5 and up. Photog. HarBraceJ, 1977. 149 pp. $5.95. Nonfiction. Epidemiologists at the Centers for Disease Control and the World Health Organization investigate the causes of infectious diseases. The discovery, outbreak, and treatment of thirty diseases are explained, including hepatitis, botulism, typhoid, histoplasmosis, and an incidence of psychosomatic illness among schoolchildren.

ARCHER, Jules. *Who's Running Your Life? A Look at Young People's Rights.* Gr. 7 and up. Illus. HarBraceJ, 1979. 168 pp. $7.95. Nonfiction. Children have the right to be safe, to have food, shelter, and clothing, medical care, schooling, the care of adults, and protection from harm.

AREHART-TREICHEL, Joan. *Immunity: How Our Bodies Resist Disease.* Gr. 7–8. Illus. Holiday, 1976. 160 pp. $6.95. Nonfiction. The development and importance of immunology are described as well as recent achievements and current and projected research in the field.

AREHART-TREICHEL, Joan. *Trace Elements: How They Help and Harm Us.* Gr. 6 and up. Illus. Holiday, 1974. 164 pp. $4.95. Nonfiction. The author discusses the origins and organic function of trace elements, indicating both their beneficial and harmful effects on the human body.

ARNOLD, Katrin. *Anna Joins In.* Gr. 1–6. Illus. by Renate Seelig. Abingdon, 1983. 28 pp. $9.95. Fiction. Because Anna has cystic fibrosis, she takes medicine with her meals and cannot eat some foods; she coughs but is not contagious. She gets help from a medical clinic. She also joins in activities with families and friends and goes to school.

ARTHUR, Catherine. *My Sister's Silent World.* Gr. 2–3. Illus. by Nathan Talbot. Childrens, 1979. 30 pp. $8.65. Fiction. A young girl describes her eight-year-old sister, who is deaf, her hearing aid, and how she watches the way mouths, faces, and tongues move so she can understand language. When they use sign language together, they have their own special signs. Other children call her sister names or think it would be hard to be her friend, but she likes to play and go to school the same as they do.

ASIMOV, Isaac. *How Did We Find Out About Vitamins?* Gr. 5–8. Illus. by David Wool. Walker, 1974. 64 pp. $4.85. Nonfiction.
Small amounts of vitamins in the diet help people to become healthier and live longer. Without vitamins, people can develop vitamin-deficiency diseases. The well-known author gives a history of the discovery and development of vitamins.

ASIMOV, Isaac. *The Human Body: Its Structure and Operation.* Gr. 10 and up. Illus. by Anthony Ravielli. HM, 1963. 340 pp. $11.95; pap. New Amer Lib, $2.50. Nonfiction.
The author describes in detail the parts of the body and their physiology.

AUSTRIAN, Geoffrey. *The Truth About Drugs.* Gr. 7–8. Illus. Doubleday, 1971. 131 pp. $5.95. Nonfiction.
Case histories are used in this introduction to the use of narcotics and the effects of their abuse.

AYLESWORTH, Thomas G. *ESP.* Gr. 7–8. Illus. by George Mac-Clain. Watts, 1975. 63 pp. $7.90. Nonfiction.
Researchers have studied extrasensory phenomena for some time, including clairvoyance, precognition, telepathy, and psychokinesis. These abilities can be used by people to enhance their lives.

AYLESWORTH, Thomas G. *Understanding Body Talk.* Gr. 7–8. Illus. Watts, 1979. 85 pp. $7.90. Nonfiction.
Familiar examples of children at school, with friends, and at home are presented to show how gestures, poses, and expressions are used to define one's space or territory and reflect cultural patterns of behavior.

AYRAULT, Evelyn West. *Sex, Love, and the Physically Handicapped.* Gr. 10 and up. Continuum, 1981. 150 pp. $11.95. Nonfiction.
Believing that sexual expression is a natural right that belongs to everyone, the author suggests adaptive ways for physically disabled people to express and receive love, and encourages self-esteem.

AZARNOFF, Pat, ed. *The Hospital.* Gr. ps–2. Photog. by Phil Bleisher, Sheldon Sroloff, and Bill Brown. Trans. by María Gutiérrez and Herlinda Lozano. Ped Proj, 1976. Unp. $1.25. Nonfiction.
This story, in both English and Spanish, covers admission, treatment, play and school, and going home from the hospital.

AZARNOFF, Pat, ed. *It's Your Body/Es Tu Cuerpo.* Gr. 7–9. Illus. by Kevin Burton. Trans. by María Gutiérrez and Herlinda Lozano. Ped Proj, 1976. Unp. pap. $1.25. Nonfiction.
In both Spanish and English, the book discusses hospitalization for teenagers. Meals, roommates, activities, and medical events are described with humor and facts. Teens should ask questions and know what is happening to them.

B., Bill. *Compulsive Overeater: The Basic Text for Compulsive Overeaters.* Gr. 10 and up. CompCare, 1981. 287 pp. $10.95. Nonfiction.
The author describes how he applied the Twelve Steps (first developed by Alcoholics Anonymous) to control his food intake and feel better about himself.

BACH, Alice. *Waiting for Johnny Miracle.* Gr. 7–8. Har-Row, 1980. 240 pp. $9.95. Fiction.
Becky, a high-school student, struggles with cancer and tries to maintain a normal life, with the loving support of her twin and her parents.

BAKER, Lynn S., in collaboration with Charles G. Roland and Gerald S. Gilchrist. *You and Leukemia: A Day at a Time.* Gr. 7–9. Illus. by the author. Saunders, 1978. 205 pp. $7.95. Nonfiction.
Simple explanations of diagnosis, anatomy, and treatment can be helpful in reassuring leukemia patients. The descriptions include chemotherapy, spinal tap, radiation therapy, blood transfusions, bone marrow transplants, and immunotherapy.

BALDWIN, Anne Norris. *A Little Time.* Gr. 4–5. Viking, 1978. 119 pp. $8.95. Fiction.
A ten-year-old girl and her family have ambivalent feelings about her younger brother, who has Down's syndrome. When he is temporarily placed in a foster home because of the mother's hospitalization, the family experiences a respite from his care. They decide, however, that they want him home.

BALESTRINO, Philip. *Fat and Skinny*. Gr. 2–3. Illus. by Pam Makie. Crowell, 1975. 33 pp. $9.89. Nonfiction.
There are metabolic and dietary factors that influence or determine physical size, shape, and weight.

BALESTRINO, Philip. *The Skeleton Inside You*. Gr. k–3. Illus. by Don Bolognese. Crowell, 1971. 33 pp. pap. $3.97. Nonfiction.
A skeleton is made up of 206 bones that give the body its shape and protect its organs. Joints and ligaments let the bones move. A cast is worn on a broken bone until it heals.

BALIS, Andrea. *What Are You Using? A Birth Control Guide for Teen-Agers*. Gr. 10–12. Illus. Dial, 1981. 119 pp. $5.95. Nonfiction.
The author describes types of contraception, their effectiveness, how to use them, and their possible side effects.

BANISH, Roslyn. *I Want to Tell You About My Baby*. Gr. ps–2. Wingbow Pr, 1982. 47 pp. $5.95. Fiction.
A little boy explains his mother's pregnancy and childbirth, how the infant is cared for, and how he feels about his baby brother.

BARNESS, Richard. *Listen to Me!* Gr. 6 and up. Lerner, 1976. 95 pp. $4.95. Fiction.
Years of addiction lead twenty-one-year-old Sally to the final humiliation of prison.

BARNETT, Naomi. *I Know a Dentist*. Gr. 1–2. Illus. by Linda Boehm. Putnam, 1977. Unp. $4.29. Nonfiction.
The dentist has equipment and instruments, and knows how to prevent and treat tooth decay.

BARRETT, Judith. *Cloudy with a Chance of Meatballs*. Gr. ps–3. Illus. by Ron Barrett. Atheneum, 1980. Unp. $9.95; pap. Atheneum, $2.95. Fiction.
Grandpa tells the children about a land called Chewandswallow that had an abundance of food falling from the sky. Too much food, however, was not an advantage.

BATES, Betty. *Love Is Like Peanuts*. Gr. 7–8. Holiday, 1980. 125 pp. $7.95. Fiction.

A fourteen-year-old girl learns patience and thoughtful caring by babysitting with an eight-year-old child who is brain injured. When she falls in love with the child's brother, she has to make decisions about their relationship.

BATES, Betty. *Picking Up the Pieces.* Gr. 7 and up. Holiday, 1982. 157 pp. $8.95. Fiction.
Nell helps her friend, Dexter, to deal with disability after a car accident.

BAUER, Marion Dane. *Tangled Butterfly.* Gr. 6 and up. HM, 1980. 162 pp. $7.95. Fiction.
Even after seventeen-year-old Michelle attempts suicide, her family still refuses to recognize her problems and take responsibility for getting help for her. A teacher helps her regain self-esteem and get the help she needs.

BAZNIK, Donna. *Becky's Story.* Gr. ps–2. Illus. by Jayne Sestak. ACCH, 1981. 31 pp. pap. $3.00. Fiction.
When Dan is hurt in an accident and hospitalized, his younger sister, Becky, is confused, angry, and jealous. Becky fears she caused the accident and that it might happen to her, too. Her parents reassure her but are involved at the hospital. When she is allowed to visit, the hospital seems strange. Finally Dan comes home and Becky feels better.

BEAME, Rona. *Emergency!* Gr. 4–5. Photog. by the author. Messner, 1977. 64 pp. $6.97. Fiction.
Stories about patients, ambulance aides, nurses, doctors, and police provide insight into the ways a large city cares for its sick and injured.

BECKMAN, Delores. *My Own Private Sky.* Gr. 4–6. Dutton, 1980. 154 pp. $10.25. Fiction.
Eleven-year-old Arthur and his mother move to California because of his allergies. He also has an overbite, is short, and is frightened of swimming and diving. His babysitter shares her fears with him when she is seriously injured in a car accident. They help each other gain confidence.

BECKMAN, Gunnel. *Admission to the Feast.* Gr. 7 and up. Trans. from the Swedish by Joan Tate. Dell, 1973. 139 pp. pap. $.75. Fiction.
A nineteen-year-old searches for answers to life's meaning when she discovers she is about to die from leukemia.

BECKMAN, Gunnel. *Mia Alone.* Gr. 7–8. Trans. from the Swedish by Joan Tate. Viking, 1974. 124 pp. $5.95; pap. Dell, $1.50. Fiction.
Mia is a Swedish high-school student whose parents and school counselor are understanding, but she realizes she must decide for herself if her pregnancy will be ended in an abortion, and how she will deal with her relationships.

BELL, David. *A Time to Be Born.* Gr. 7 and up. Morrow, 1975. 192 pp. $5.95. Nonfiction.
A pediatrician describes the intensive-care nursery of a hospital and how the staff works to make it possible for a child to live.

BEMELMANS, Ludwig. *Madeline.* Gr. k–3. Illus. by the author. Penguin, 1977. Unp. pap. $3.50. Fiction.
After Madeline goes to the hospital for an appendectomy, receiving toys and showing her scar, the other little girls in Sister Clavell's care want to have the operation too.

BENNETT, Hal Zina. *Cold Comfort.* Gr. 10 and up. Potter, 1979. 155 pp. $8.95. Nonfiction.
The author describes the phases of upper respiratory infections and suggests various medical and self-treatments for colds and influenza.

BENNETT, Hal Zina. *The Doctor Within.* Gr. 9 and up. Crown, 1982. 147 pp. $11.50; pap. New Amer Lib, $2.50. Nonfiction.
Natural defenses against disease, such as antibodies and the lymph systems, help the body to heal. The author gives advice on helping the systems by exercise, nutrition, and attitude.

BENNETT, Merilyn Brottman, and Sylvia SANDERS. *How We Talk: The Story of Speech.* Gr. 3–9. Illus. by William R. Johnson. Lerner, 1966. 39 pp. $3.95. Nonfiction.

Speech ability and impairment are described and the anatomy of the voice is detailed.

BENZIGER, Barbara. *Controlling Your Weight*. Gr. 6–7. Illus. by Roland Rodegast. Pocket Bks., 1973. 64 pp. $1.25. Nonfiction.
Good eating habits and exercise are needed to control weight. Crash diets and diet pills should be avoided. The author describes exercises and recipes for low-calorie foods to help young people solve weight-control problems.

BERENSTAIN, Stan, and Jan BERENSTAIN. *The Berenstain Bears Go to the Doctor*. Gr. ps–2. Illus. by the authors. Random House, 1981. Unp. pap. $1.50. Fiction.
Dr. Gert Grizzly gives the Berenstain cubs a regular checkup and booster shots. When Papa Berenstain sneezes, she discovers that he has a cold and needs medicine and rest.

BERENSTAIN, Stan, and Jan BERENSTAIN. *The Berenstain Bears Visit the Dentist*. Gr. ps–2. Illus. by the authors. Random House, 1981. Unp. pap. $1.50. Fiction.
The dentist shows the Bears many instruments, repairs Brother's cavity, and removes Sister's loose tooth.

BERGER, Gilda. *Addiction: Its Causes, Problems and Treatments*. Gr. 6 and up. Watts, 1982. 118 pp. $9.90. Nonfiction.
The author describes physical and psychological causes of addiction, and treatments for the dependence on drugs, alcohol, smoking, caffeine, and various foods.

BERGER, Gilda. *Mental Illness*. Gr. 9 and up. Illus. Watts, 1981. 144 pp. $8.90. Nonfiction.
Mental illnesses include depression and psychosis. There is treatment available; some agencies that can help are listed.

BERGER, Gilda. *Physical Disabilities*. Gr. 6–7. Illus. Watts, 1979. 119 pp. $7.45. Nonfiction.
Readers can learn about eighteen disabilities and multiple handicaps, the problems they cause, and the therapies available for treating them. Young people are encouraged to develop positive attitudes toward the disabled.

BERGER, Gilda. *Speech and Language Disorders.* Gr. 7 and up. Illus. Watts, 1981. 87 pp. $7.45. Nonfiction.
Acquiring language is a learned process. Many speech disorders can be treated.

BERGER, Gilda, and Melvin BERGER. *The Whole World of Hands.* Gr. 2–5. Illus. by True Kelley. HM, 1982. 120 pp. $8.95. Nonfiction.
The authors discuss the structure of the hand, right- and left-handedness, gestures, sign language, fingerprints, and hand wounds.

BERGER, Melvin. *Bionics.* Gr. 7–8. Illus. Watts, 1978. 82 pp. $7.90. Nonfiction.
Bionics is the creation of artificial limbs, organs, and senses, and the recreation of human intelligence with computers and robots.

BERGER, Melvin. *Disease Detectives.* Gr. 4 and up. Illus. Har-Row, 1978. 81 pp. $9.57. Nonfiction.
Bacteriologists, virologists, and toxicologists at the Centers for Disease Control in Georgia investigate epidemics and rare diseases. The narrative traces the exploration of Legionnaires' disease.

BERGER, Melvin. *Enzymes in Action.* Gr. 7–9. Har-Row, 1971. 151 pp. $9.57. Nonfiction.
Enzymes affect the body's chemistry, digestion, and diseases. The author describes enzymes in simple language that incorporates technical terms.

BERGER, Melvin. *Exploring the Mind and Brain.* Gr. 5 and up. Illus. Crowell, 1983. 128 pp. $10.53. Nonfiction.
Scientists are studying learning disabilities, mental disorders, adolescent psychological changes, and the structure of the brain.

BERGER, Melvin. *Medical Center Lab.* Gr. 3 and up. Illus. Har-Row, 1976. 111 pp. $9.89. Nonfiction.
In research labs scientists test new drugs and study the causes and effects of disease. In clinical labs technicians help diagnose and treat patients in the hospital.

BERGER, Melvin. *Sports Medicine.* Gr. 4 and up. Illus. Crowell, 1982. 122 pp. $10.89. Nonfiction.
Sports medicine prevents and treats sports-related injuries and improves performance.

BERGER, Melvin. *Why I Cough, Sneeze, Shiver, Hiccup, and Yawn.* Gr. k–3. Illus. by Holly Keller. Crowell, 1983. 34 pp. $9.57. Nonfiction.
The book describes in simple terms the parts of the nervous system that are involved in involuntary reflexes.

BERGER, Terry. *I Have Feelings.* Gr. 1–2. Photog. by I. Howard Spivak. Human Sci Pr, 1971. Unp. $9.95. Fiction.
A small boy learns to understand his happy and sad feelings. The author presents seventeen feelings, giving a situation and an explanation of each.

BERGER, Terry. *I Have Feelings Too.* Gr. 4–5. Photog. by Michael E. Ach. Human Sci Pr, 1979. Unp. $9.95. Fiction.
When a young girl experiences such emotions as guilt, envy, love, joy, rejection, and worry she learns that others have these feelings as well, and that it is normal for feelings to change.

BERNSTEIN, Joanne E. *Loss and How to Cope with It.* Gr. 6–8. Seabury, 1977. 151 pp. $8.95. Nonfiction.
The death of a loved one affects the survivor's emotional and physical health. Suggestions are given on how to handle the reactions of bereavement.

BERNSTEIN, Joanne E., and Stephen V. GULLO. *When People Die.* Gr. 2–3. Photog. by Rosmarie Hausherr. Dutton, 1977. Unp. $9.95. Nonfiction.
When people die, their bodies stop functioning and they do not hear, feel, speak, or think. When someone close dies, children feel sad and may not want to eat or play. Then, gradually, they act as they did before and enjoy life once more.

BERRY, James R. *Why You Feel Hot, Why You Feel Cold: Your Body's Temperature.* Gr. 2–3. Illus. by William Ogden. Little, 1973. 48 pp. $6.95. Nonfiction.
Simple experiments show the ways in which the body regulates temperature.

BETANCOURT, Jeanne. *Smile! How to Cope with Braces.* Gr. 5 and up. Illus. by Mimi Harrison. Knopf, 1982. 87 pp. pap. $5.95. Nonfiction.
The mechanical aspects of orthodontia are described as well as how it feels, emotionally and physically, to wear braces.

BLANZACO, Andre. *VD: Facts You Should Know.* Gr. 7–12. Illus. Lothrop, 1970. 63 pp. $9.25. Nonfiction.
More than 100,000 people are infected with syphilis each year and a million-and-a-half with gonorrhea, both preventable diseases. The author gives numerous facts and then offers readers a multiple-choice test to check what they have learned.

BLOOM, Freddy. *The Boy Who Couldn't Hear.* Gr. ps–2. Illus. by Michael Charlton. Bodley, 1979. 30 pp. $4.95. Nonfiction.
This story of a day in the life of a child who is deaf conveys the importance of lip reading and the need to understand the problems and emotions of children who are deaf.

BLUE, Rose. *Me and Einstein: Breaking Through the Barrier.* Gr. 3–4. Illus. by Peggy Luks. Human Sci Pr, 1979. Unp. $9.95. Fiction.
Nine-year-old Bobby has dyslexia and does not see letters the way most people do. With counseling and teaching, and the inspiration of knowing that Albert Einstein had dyslexia, he is able to read, meet others who share his problem, and develop feelings of self-worth.

BLUESTONE, Naomi. *"So You Want to Be a Doctor!": The Realities of Pursuing Medicine as a Career.* Gr. 7 and up. Illus. Lothrop, 1981. 241 pp. $12.95. Nonfiction.
This frank narrative of a doctor's work shows the doctor struggling to learn, confronting unpleasant and difficult tasks, and trying to maintain emotional stability.

BLUME, Judy Sussman. *Blubber.* Gr. 4–6. Bradbury, 1974. 160 pp. $8.95; pap. Dell, $1.50. Fiction.
Jill joins most of her fifth-grade classmates in making fun of Linda, who is overweight and called Blubber, until Jill herself becomes the victim of thoughtless teasing.

BLUME, Judy Sussman. *Deenie*. Gr. 6–7. Bradbury, 1973. 159 pp. $8.95; pap. Dell, $1.75. Fiction.
Although Deenie is uncomfortable with people who look "different," she finds, through her own experience of scoliosis treatment, what being disabled means. She wears a body brace for four years to correct the curvature of her spine and has to make many adaptations. The experience helps Deenie mature.

BLUME, Judy Sussman. *Freckle Juice*. Gr. 2–5. Illus. by Sonia O. Lisker. Four Winds, 1971. 40 pp. $5.95. Fiction.
Andrew, who wants freckles, manages to paint on a temporary set, but then is not sure he really wants them.

BLUME, Judy Sussman. *Then Again, Maybe I Won't*. Gr. 5–7. Bradbury, 1971. 176 pp. $8.95; pap. Dell, $1.75. Fiction.
Thirteen-year-old Tony reacts to teenage stresses with psychosomatic stomach pains. With the help of his physician and psychiatrist he recuperates and develops healthier ways of coping.

BODE, Janet. *Rape: Preventing It, Dealing with the Legal, Medical, and Emotional Aftermath*. Gr. 7 and up. Watts, 1979. 103 pp. $6.50. Nonfiction.
Case histories and interviews are used to discuss rape as a social problem. Ideas on prevention and protection are detailed with facts and stories.

BOLIAN, Polly. *Growing Up Slim*. Gr. 7–8. Illus. Am Heritage, 1971. 150 pp. $5.95. Nonfiction.
This teenager's guide to weight loss and control is based on a practical daily program of balanced eating and exercise.

BOOHER, Dianna Daniels. *Rape: What Would You Do If . . ..* Gr. 7 and up. Messner, 1981. 159 pp. $9.80. Nonfiction.
Preventing, fighting or resisting, and getting help after a rape are discussed with stories and facts.

BORNSTEIN, Jerry, and Sandy BORNSTEIN. *What Is Genetics?* Gr. 10–12. Illus. Messner, 1979. 192 pp. $8.29. Nonfiction.
Genetics is the study of chromosomes, the material involved in cell division; cells, the basic structure of life; and DNA, the chemical substance that carries the hereditary code. Heredity and environment determine a person's appearance and characteristics.

BOSTON WOMEN'S HEALTH BOOK COLLECTIVE. *Our Bodies, Ourselves: A Book by and for Women*. Gr. 9–12. Illus. S&S, 1979. 383 pp. $14.95; pap. S&S, $9.95. Nonfiction.
The authors emphasize that women have the right to know about their bodies. They discuss the anatomy and physiology of a woman's body, emotional needs, and self-examination and care.

BOTTNER, Barbara. *Dumb Old Casey Is a Fat Tree*. Gr. 1–4. Illus. Har-Row, 1979. 40 pp. $6.89. Fiction.
Second-grader Casey, who is overweight, learns to feel good about herself by working hard to learn ballet.

BOVE, Linda. *Sesame Street Sign Language Fun*. Gr. 1–2. Illus. Random House, 1980. Unp. $4.95. Nonfiction.
Using Jim Henson's Muppets, American Sign Language is shown in categories such as family and school.

BOWE, Frank. *Comeback: Six Remarkable People Who Triumphed over Disability*. Gr. 7 and up. Har-Row, 1981. 172 pp. $12.50. Nonfiction.
The abilities of real people are emphasized in stories about how they reduced the limitations of blindness, deafness, retardation, paralysis, and multiple handicaps.

BRADBURY, Bianca. *The Girl Who Wanted Out*. Gr. 7–12. Scholastic, 1981. 191 pp. pap. $1.50. Fiction.
Andie must find the courage to face her friends and return to school after a car accident kills her boy friend and leaves her paralyzed and in a wheelchair.

BRADBURY, Bianca. *Those Traver Kids*. Gr. 3–7. Illus. by Marvin Friedman. HM, 1972. 204 pp. $5.95. Fiction.
Four children, ages three to seventeen, are physically and psychologically abused by their stepfather. With courage and the help of friends, they begin to put their lives back together after the man is imprisoned.

BRADLEY, Buff. *Endings: A Book About Death*. Gr. 7–8. Addison-Wesley, 1979. 191 pp. $8.95. Nonfiction.
Several aspects of death, including suicide, euthanasia, grief, and various burial customs, are described to help the young reader understand more about mortality.

BRADY, Mari. *Please Remember Me: A Young Woman's Story of Her Friendship with an Unforgettable Fifteen-Year-Old Boy.* Gr. 7–9. Archway, 1978. 104 pp. pap. $1.75. Nonfiction.
The author met Graham in the recreation therapy program at Memorial Sloan-Kettering Hospital in New York. Graham is rehospitalized seven times for treatment of cancer of the lymph glands and eventually dies. His spirit and courage inspire the author and the child's family and friends.

BRANCATO, Robin. *Winning.* Gr. 5 and up. Knopf, 1977. 211 pp. $7.95; pap. Bantam, $1.95. Fiction.
Paralyzed and on a Stryker frame after an accident in a football game, Gary changes his views about competition, his high-school friendships, and other values. Gary and his tutor, who is recently widowed, help each other through their losses.

BRANDENBERG, Franz. *I Wish I Was Sick, Too!* Gr. 1–2. Illus. by Aliki. Morrow, 1976. Unp. $8.59; pap. Viking, $2.95. Fiction.
When Edward is sick, Elizabeth thinks that he is lucky not to have to go to school or do his chores, but her views change when she becomes ill.

BRANDRETH, Gyles. *This Is Your Body.* Gr. 4–5. Illus. Sterling, 1979. 120 pp. $7.50. Nonfiction.
The author explains the organs, systems, and physiology of the body with many facts and cartoon drawings. Simple experiments and projects are provided to give abundant detail about how the body works.

BRANLEY, Franklyn M. *Oxygen Keeps You Alive.* Gr. k–3. Illus. by Don Madden. Crowell, 1971. Unp. $4.78. Nonfiction.
Oxygen is the most important part of air. Simple words and experiments show how people and animals use oxygen.

BRANSCUM, Robbie. *For Love of Jody.* Gr. 5–6. Illus. by Allen Davis. Lothrop, 1979. 111 pp. $7.92. Fiction.
Having the daily care of her retarded younger sister, whom she thinks her mother favors, makes a twelve-year-old girl feel unloved.

BREINBURG, Petronella. *Doctor Shawn*. Gr. 1–2. Illus. by Errol Lloyd. Crowell, 1974. Unp. $8.95. Fiction.
Shawn, his sisters, and a friend play hospital with banana-slice pills, banana-peel bandages, and their uncooperative, impatient cat.

BRENNER, Barbara. *Bodies*. Gr. ps–1. Photog. by George Ancona. Dutton, 1973. Unp. $8.95. Nonfiction.
Bodies can stand, play in the mud, hold a frog, blow up a balloon, laugh, sleep, sweat, breathe, eliminate, swing, or splash. Bodies are made of cells. An X ray shows the inside of the body. A stethoscope helps a child hear his or her heart.

BRENNER, Barbara. *Faces*. Gr. 2–3. Photog. by George Ancona. Dutton, 1970. Unp. $10.95. Nonfiction.
A picture study of the uniqueness of the human face, this story shows many different faces.

BRIGHTMAN, Alan. *Like Me*. Gr. k–3. Photog. by the author. Little, 1976. Unp. $6.95. Nonfiction.
Some children are slower in learning but are "like me" in their desire to succeed and their need to have friends. The author uses verse and color photographs of real retarded children to highlight the aspects of people that are alike and different.

BRINDZE, Ruth. *Look How Many People Wear Glasses: The Magic of Lenses*. Gr. 5–9. Atheneum, 1975. 101 pp. $7.95. Nonfiction.
The author describes and illustrates the anatomy of vision, a doctor's examination and the making of lenses, and gives suggestions on caring for one's eyes.

BROWN, Barbara B. *Stress and the Art of Biofeedback*. Gr. 10 and up. Illus. Har-Row, 1977. 298 pp. $14.50. Nonfiction.
Concepts and procedures derived from experimental research and clinical practice highlight the use of biofeedback to treat various physiological disorders and to relieve conditions related to stress.

BROWN, Fern. *You're Somebody Special on a Horse*. Gr. 5–6. Illus. by Darrell Wiskur. A Whitman, 1977. 128 pp. $7.50. Fiction.
In a class for the handicapped at the riding academy, a young

woman helps a nervous teenage boy, who is usually in a wheelchair, learn to ride a horse.

BROWN, Marc. *Arthur's Eyes.* Gr. 1–2. Illus. Little, 1979. Unp. $7.95; pap. Avon, $1.95. Fiction.
When his classmates tease him about his new glasses, Arthur the aardvark stops wearing them. Because he does not see as well, he gets into difficulties. Soon he enjoys wearing glasses because he realizes how much better vision they give him.

BROWN, Marcia. *Walk with Your Eyes.* Gr. 3–4. Photog. by the author. Watts, 1979. Unp. $7.90. Nonfiction.
This photographic survey shows how to use the eyes to discover simple beauties and wonders.

BROWN, Roy. *Find Debbie!* Gr. 6 and up. HM, 1976. 160 pp. $7.95. Fiction.
A detective's professional objectivity mixes with his emotions during his search for Debbie, a retarded child who is reported missing but is not particularly missed by her parents or siblings.

BRUUN, Ruth Dowling, and Bertel BRUUN. *The Human Body.* Gr. 5 and up. Illus. by Patricia J. Wynne. Random House, 1982. 96 pp. $7.99; pap. Random House, $6.95. Nonfiction.
The authors, a psychiatrist and a neurologist, describe eight areas and twelve systems of the body. The detailed illustrations show several angles of the parts described.

BUCKALEW, Jr., M. W. *Learning to Control Stress.* Gr. 7–12. Rosen, 1979. 115 pp. $7.95. Nonfiction.
Teenagers can learn techniques for preventing or reducing stress in their lives, such as learning the source of the stress, and relaxation.

BUNTING, Eve. *The Empty Window.* Gr. 4–9. Illus by Judy Clifford. Warne, 1980. Unp. $7.95. Fiction.
Two brothers catch a wild parrot as a gift for their dying friend but are afraid to see their friend face to face.

BURCH, Robert. *D.J.'s Worst Enemy.* Gr. 4–7. Illus. by Emil Weiss. Viking, 1965. 142 pp. $8.95. Fiction.

D.J.'s speech articulation improves when he realizes that it is time to stop being his own worst enemy and to become a part of his family instead.

BURCH, Robert. *Simon and the Game of Chance.* Gr. 6–8. Illus. by Fermin Rocker. Viking, 1970. 128 pp. $4.13. Fiction.
Thirteen-year-old Simon must deal with the deaths of his baby sister and his future brother-in-law, and then with his mother's hospitalization for depression.

BURGESS-KOHN, Jane. *Straight Talk About Love and Sex for Teenagers.* Gr. 10–12. Beacon, 1979. 219 pp. pap. $5.95. Non-fiction.
Answers are given to high-school students about premarital sex, birth control, venereal diseases, homosexuality, pregnancy, and abortion.

BURNS, Marilyn. *The Book of Think: Or How to Solve a Problem Twice Your Size.* Gr. 5 and up. Illus. by Martha Weston. Little, 1976. 125 pp. $8.95; pap. Little, $5.95. Nonfiction.
Imagination exercises that invite the reader to participate emphasize the use of all the senses and intelligence to become more aware of self, other people, and the environment.

BURNS, Marilyn. *Good for Me! All About Food in 32 Bites.* Gr. 6–7. Illus. by Sandy Clifford. Little, 1978. 127 pp. $8.95. Nonfiction.
Activity suggestions and drawings supplement an exploration of the components of food, its use by the body, and its crucial role in daily life.

BURNS, Sheila L. *Allergies and You.* Gr. 4–5. Illus. Messner, 1980. 63 pp. $7.59. Nonfiction.
There are scientific reasons for allergic reactions to pollens, foods, poisons, and animals. Research helps to alleviate the ill effects of allergies.

BURSTEIN, John. *Slim Goodbody: The Inside Story.* Gr. 3–4. Illus. by Craigwood Phillips. Photog. by J. Paul Kirouac. McGraw-Hill, 1977. Unp. $7.95. Nonfiction.
Photographs of interior views of Slim Goodbody's (John Burstein's)

body are combined with verses relating facts about the functioning of the body and advice on maintaining health.

BURSTEIN, John. *Slim Goodbody: What Can Go Wrong and How to Be Strong.* Gr. 3–4. Illus. by Craigwood Phillips. Photog. by Russell Dian. McGraw-Hill, 1978. 47 pp. $7.95. Nonfiction.
Slim Goodbody (John Burstein) shows a child's-eye view of being ill and answers questions about the body and health, emphasizing the ability of the body to heal itself.

BURTON, Adrianne. *Your New Kidney.* Gr. 5 and up. Illus. by Axelle Fortier and David Factor. UCSF, 1978. 60 pp. pap. Single copy free. Nonfiction.
Written for children who need a kidney transplant, this book details the causes for kidney failure, and the tests, surgery and aftermath of a transplant. Children's fears and hopes are considered.

BUTLER, Beverly Kathleen. *Gift of Gold.* Gr. 7–8. Dodd, 1972. 278 pp. $5.95; pap. Pocket Bks, $1.95. Fiction.
Just before college begins, Cathy becomes blind. She has to contend with strangers and relatives who mean well but believe she cannot manage school and work. With humor and intelligence she counters their remarks or avoids them and looks forward to the possibility of having her vision partially restored.

BUTLER, Beverly Kathleen. *Light a Single Candle.* Gr. 7–9. Dodd, 1962. 242 pp. $7.95. pap. Pocket Bks, $1.75. Fiction.
Adjusting to blindness is difficult but sometimes easier for Cathy than dealing with the reactions of people. A training course to use a guide dog gives her freedom of movement, and she returns to high school.

BUTLER, Dorothy. *Cushla and Her Books.* Gr. 7 and up. Illus. Horn Book, 1980. 128 pp. $13.50. Nonfiction.
A severely disabled child with developmental delay enjoys books from a young age. Her supportive family uses stories to teach and entertain her, helping her increase her abilities.

BUTTERWORTH, W. E. *Under the Influence.* Gr. 7–8. Illus. Four Winds, 1979. 247 pp. $9.95. Fiction.

Alan begins to realize the extent of his friend Keith's problem with alcohol when Keith becomes involved in a brawl at a local club, a fight that gets him thrown off the football team, and a car accident.

BYARS, Betsy. *After the Goat Man.* Gr. 6–7. Illus. by Ronald Himler. Viking, 1974. 126 pp. $7.95; pap. Avon, $1.75. Fiction.
Figgy and his grandfather, called the Goat Man because of pet goats that follow him, live in a house that has to be demolished for a highway. When his grandfather disappears, Figgy asks his friend Harold, who has been preoccupied with how overweight and unhappy he is, to help search for him. Getting to know and understand the Goat Man gives Harold a new perspective on important values.

BYARS, Betsy. *The Summer of the Swans.* Gr. 7–8. Illus. by Ted CoConis. Viking, 1970. 142 pp. $9.95. Fiction.
Fourteen-year-old Sara perceives life differently after the panic of searching for her lost retarded younger brother. The story describes a warm sibling relationship with humor.

CALHOUN, Mary. *Medicine Show: Conning People and Making Them Like It.* Gr. 5–8. Illus. Har-Row, 1976. 135 pp. $9.89. Nonfiction.
This narrative of the traveling shows that sold useless but harmless remedies details ways the public can be fooled by claims of cures.

CALLEN, Larry. *Sorrow's Song.* Gr. 4–6. Illus. by Marvin Friedman. Little, 1979. 150 pp. $7.95. Fiction.
Sorrow, a girl who cannot talk, finds and cares for an injured young whooping crane and risks her life to save the bird from boys who try to catch it for their own profit.

CANADA, Lena. *To Elvis, with Love.* Gr. 7–12. Everest House, 1978. 178 pp. $6.95. Nonfiction.
A girl in a wheelchair in a special school and home wants most of all to be Elvis Presley's friend. She is changed by the compassion and generosity shown to her by the performer.

CARLSON, Dale Bick. *Boys Have Feelings Too: Growing Up Male for Boys.* Gr. 7–8. Illus. by Carol Nicklaus. Atheneum, 1980. 165 pp. $9.95. Nonfiction.
Adolescent boys have the problem of great expectations that creates tension and discourages them from expressing their emotions.

CARLSON, Dale Bick. *Call Me Amanda.* Gr. 4–6. Dutton, 1981. 80 pp. $8.50. Fiction.
Eleven-year-old Amanda finds she is a kleptomaniac but has no memory of stealing things. She strives to understand herself better and discover her identity.

CARLSON, Dale Bick. *Loving Sex for Both Sexes: Straight Talk for Teenagers.* Gr. 9 and up. Watts, 1979. 209 pp. $9.90. Nonfiction.
This nonjudgmental guide explores attitudes toward sex, love, and making choices. The author stresses the need for maturity in making decisions about sexuality.

CARLSON, Dale Bick. *Where's Your Head? Psychology for Teenagers.* Gr. 6–12. Illus. by Carol Nicklaus. Atheneum, 1977. 217 pp. $7.95. Nonfiction.
There are various theories of mental and emotional development. The author discusses the causes and symptoms of mental illnesses, the various therapies, and common mental and emotional problems and disorders.

CASEWIT, Curtis W. *The Stop Smoking Book for Teens.* Gr. 7 and up. Photog. Messner, 1980. 160 pp. $7.79. Nonfiction.
Having quit smoking himself, the author explains to teenagers the various commercial systems designed to help people stop smoking. He discusses why teens smoke, the effects of smoking on the body, and ways to stop.

CASTLE, Sue. *Face Talk, Hand Talk, Body Talk.* Gr. 1–2. Photog. by Frances McLaughlin-Gill. Doubleday, 1977. Unp. $9.95. Nonfiction.
Pictures and simple text show ways in which people use gestures to express anger, surprise, doubt, affection, amusement, and other feelings.

CAVALLARO, Ann. *Blimp.* Gr. 6 and up. Lodestar, 1983. 166 pp. $10.34. Fiction.
Kim loses weight with the help of a psychologist and a supportive family. She helps her boy friend, who has more severe emotional problems, to get help too.

CENTER FOR ATTITUDINAL HEALING. *There Is a Rainbow Behind Every Dark Cloud.* Gr. 3–4. Illus. Celestial, 1978. 96 pp. pap. $6.95. Nonfiction.
Children who have cancer, leukemia, and other serious diseases share their feelings and experiences with the support of a therapy staff.

CHALMERS, Mary. *Come to the Doctor, Harry.* Gr. ps–1. Illus. by the author. Har-Row, 1981. 32 pp. $7.64. Fiction.
A little cat named Harry discovers that a visit to the doctor for medical care is nothing to fear.

CHANG Mao-chiu. *The Little Doctor.* Gr. ps–1. Illus. by Yang Wen-hsiu. Hai Feng, n.d. Unp. $1.95. Fiction.
Ping-Ping and her sister play doctor, examining and curing the doll, teddy bear, and rocking horse.

CHARLIP, Remy, and Mary Beth SULLIVAN. *Handtalk: An ABC of Finger Spelling and Sign Language.* Gr. 4–5. Illus. Parents, 1974. Unp. $10.95. Nonfiction.
Some deaf people use finger positions to designate the letters of the alphabet and body gestures to imitate the concepts behind basic vocabulary words.

CHILDRESS, Alice. *A Hero Ain't Nothin' but a Sandwich.* Gr. 6–7. Putnam, 1973. 96 pp. $8.95; pap. Avon, $1.75. Fiction.
A thirteen-year-old boy, on the verge of being addicted to heroin, expresses his thoughts and emotions about ghetto life.

CHRISTOPHER, Matt. *Glue Fingers.* Gr. 3–4. Illus. by Jim Venable. Little, 1975. 37 pp. $6.95. Fiction.
Billy Joe plays football well but is afraid of his teammates' rejection and ridicule because he stutters. His older brothers convince him that ability and intelligence, not how one speaks, are the key to football success. He joins the team and succeeds.

CILIOTTA, Claire, and Carole LIVINGSTON. *Why Am I Going to the Hospital: A Helpful Guide to a New Experience.* Gr. 3–6. Illus. by Dick Wilson. Lyle Stuart, 1981. Unp. $12.00. Fiction.
The people and procedures of a hospital are explained as children in the story are admitted for tests, emergency care, or surgery.

CLAYPOOL, Jane. *Alcohol and You.* Gr. 7–8. Illus. Watts, 1981. 84 pp. $7.90. Nonfiction.
The author defines teenage drinking, explores why teenagers drink, and analyzes the effects of alcohol on the body.

CLEARY, Beverly. *Mitch and Amy.* Gr. 3–7. Illus. by George Porter. Morrow, 1967. 222 pp. $8.95; pap. Dell, $1.75. Fiction.
Nine-year-old twins have learning problems in school, which are eventually resolved. They have conflicts with one another, but help each other when a bully bothers them.

CLEAVER, Vera, and Bill CLEAVER. *Me Too.* Gr. 7–9. Har-Row, 1973. 160 pp. $10.95; pap. New Amer Lib, $1.50. Fiction.
A twelve-year-old girl spends the summer trying to teach her twin sister, who is retarded. Even though she has little success, she matures and appreciates her sister's difficulties.

CLEMENTS, Hanna, and Bruce CLEMENTS. *Coming Home to a Place You've Never Been Before.* Gr. 7 and up. FS&G, 1975. 192 pp. $6.95. Nonfiction.
The authors narrate twenty-four hours in the work of Perception House, a halfway house in Connecticut that assists former drug addicts and pushers, ex-convicts, ex-prostitutes, and other people sixteen years old and up who have had health and mental health problems that got them into criminal activities.

CLIFTON, Lucille. *My Friend Jacob.* Gr. 1–3. Illus. by Thomas DiGrazia. Dutton, 1980. Unp. $7.95. Fiction.
Sam's best friend, Jacob, is older and retarded. They help each other learn.

COBB, Vicki. *How the Doctor Knows You're Fine.* Gr. 2–5. Illus. by Anthony Ravielli. Har-Row, 1973. 48 pp. $4.95. Nonfiction.
It is important for people to know how they feel and give

themselves care, but the doctor uses instruments to determine things happening inside the body that might not be felt by the patient. The instruments and parts of the body are illustrated.

COBB, Vicki. *How to Really Fool Yourself: Illusions for All Your Senses.* Gr. 5 and up. Illus. by Leslie Morrill. Lippincott, 1981. 145 pp. $8.89. Nonfiction.
Many explanations and demonstrations that can be done at home show how and why the senses can be fooled.

COERR, Eleanor B. *Sadako and the Thousand Paper Cranes.* Gr. 3–5. Putnam, 1977. 64 pp. $8.95. Fiction.
In a story based on the life of a real child in Japan, eleven-year-old Sadako is ill with leukemia ten years after the atomic bomb was dropped on her city, Hiroshima. Her friend persuades her that if she can fold a thousand origami paper cranes, she will become healthy. But she dies before she can do that, so her classmates continue folding and all one thousand paper cranes are buried with her.

COHEN, Barbara. *Fat Jack.* Gr. 6 and up. Atheneum, 1980. 192 pp. $9.95. Fiction.
Judy, a quiet, shy girl, becomes friends with Jack, who is unhappy about his overweight. They are encouraged by the school librarian to produce the school play. This work gives them both greater confidence.

COHEN, Daniel. *ESP: The Search Beyond the Senses.* Gr. 7 and up. HarBraceJ, 1973. 187 pp. $6.50; pap. HarBraceJ, $1.75. Nonfiction.
Many people study ways to enhance and use all the senses. The author evaluates research about extrasensory perception, with analyses and case histories.

COHEN, Daniel. *Intelligence: What Is It?* Gr. 5 and up. Illus. Dutton, 1974. 160 pp. $7.95. Nonfiction.
The author details methods of testing animal and human intelligence and describes Piaget's theories about children's cognitive growth.

COHEN, Daniel. *Stress: Understanding the Tension You Feel at Home, at School and Among Your Friends.* Gr. 7 and up. Evans, 1983. 156 pp. $8.95. Nonfiction.
Stress can be caused by reactions to illness, thoughts of suicide, poor relationships, and other experiences. The author suggests to teenage readers ways to identify and cope with stress.

COHEN, Miriam. *See You Tomorrow, Charles.* Gr. ps–3. Illus. by Lillian Hoban. Greenwillow, 1983. Unp. $9.95. Fiction.
The children in first grade are unsure about Charles, their classmate who is blind. Soon they realize he can do most of the same activities as they and some even better.

COLE, Joanna, and Madeleine EDMONDSON. *Twins: The Story of Multiple Births.* Gr. 4–5. Illus. by Salvatore Raciti. Morrow, 1972. 64 pp. $3.56. Nonfiction.
The authors describe the major stages in the prenatal growth of identical and fraternal twins and discuss the role of heredity in their development.

The COLEMAN Family, and Bill DAVIDSON. *Gary Coleman: Medical Miracle.* Gr. 7 and up. Photog. Coward, 1981. 236 pp. $9.95. Nonfiction.
Gary Coleman, a young television and film actor, has a kidney transplant and takes medication to avoid transplant rejection. He and his family tell their life story, with emphasis on his medical and surgical experiences.

COLLINS-AHLGREN, Marianne. *Matthew's Accident.* Gr. k–4. Illus. by Linda C. Tom. Gallaudet, 1975. 32 pp. $5.00. Fiction.
Mother teaches Matthew, who wears a hearing aid, how to cross a street safely. One time he forgets to look at the traffic light before proceeding across. He trips in the rainy street, hurts his hand, and is almost hit by a truck. A police officer helps him and calls his mother. Drawings of hands signing the words or letters help children who are learning Signed English, a tool to supplement the speech of people with hearing impairments.

COLMAN, Hila Crayder. *Accident.* Gr. 7–8. Morrow, 1980. 154 pp. $8.75. Fiction.
After Jenny and Adam are involved in a motorcycle accident,

emotions conflict when she is paralyzed and bitter and he feels guilt.

COLMAN, Hila Crayder. *Diary of a Frantic Kid Sister.* Gr. 4–5. Crown, 1973. 119 pp. $4.95; pap. Pocket Bks, $1.75. Fiction.
Eleven-year-old Sarah writes in her diary feelings of anger and jealousy about her older sister's behavior and attitudes. When their mother has psychiatric help, the girls are also counseled. Sarah begins to understand her own and her sister's feelings.

CONE, Molly. *Paul David Silverman Is a Father.* Gr. 9–12. Photog. by Harold Roth. Dutton, 1983. 64 pp. $9.64. Fiction.
Paul and Cathy are sixteen years old and married, and they have a baby. They struggle to make their marriage work and to cope with caring for their baby.

COOK, Marjorie. *To Walk on Two Feet.* Gr. 6–7. Westminster, 1978. 93 pp. $7.50. Fiction.
A recent double amputee because of a car accident, Carrie musters her courage and realizes that life goes on regardless of other people's curiosity, sympathy, or lack of sympathy.

COOKSON, Catherine. *Go Tell It to Mrs. Golightly.* Gr. 6–7. Lothrop, 1980. 192 pp. $8.40. Fiction.
Eight-year-old Bella, who is blind, has adventures with her understanding grandfather.

COOLIDGE, Olivia. *Come By Here.* Gr. 6–7. Illus. by Milton Johnson. HM, 1970. 239 pp. $9.95. Fiction.
When Minty Lou's parents are killed in an accident, her secure and loving home life is lost. She is sent to the homes of various relatives who are poorer, have less hope than she has been used to, and who abuse her and suppress her positive emotions. She struggles to achieve her hopes of a better life.

COONEY, Nancy Evans. *The Wobbly Tooth.* Gr. k–3. Illus. by Marylin Hafner. Putnam, 1978. Unp. $6.95. Fiction.
When cartwheels on the lawn and chewing a caramel-covered chocolate bar fail to remove a loose tooth, Elizabeth Anne resorts to a neighborhood baseball game.

COOPER, Elizabeth. *Rosie's Hospital Story.* Gr. ps–2. Illus. by Susan Harrison. Silver, 1980. 28 pp. $4.50. Fiction.
Hospitalized because of a broken leg, Rosie makes friends and plays, eats meals, and has treatment.

CORCORAN, Barbara. *Axe-Time, Sword-Time.* Gr. 7–8. Atheneum, 1976. 204 pp. $6.95. Fiction.
Elinor wants to attend college but has difficulty with reading and conceptual learning because of a mild brain injury. She realizes she needs to develop self-confidence before she can improve.

CORCORAN, Barbara. *Child of the Morning.* Gr. k–4. Atheneum, 1982. 132 pp. $9.95. Fiction.
Episodes of briefly losing consciousness concern Susan. After she is tested and diagnosed as having epilepsy, Susan learns to live with her condition and takes medication to control the seizures.

CORCORAN, Barbara. *A Dance to Still Music.* Gr. 6–7. Illus. by Charles Robinson. Atheneum, 1974. 180 pp. $9.95; pap. Atheneum, $1.95. Fiction.
Margaret fears that she will be sent by her disinterested mother and new father to a school for the deaf, so she runs away. Helping an injured fawn, in need of assistance as she is, and developing a friendship with an older woman who takes an interest in her, helps Margaret understand and cope with her deafness and the reality of her family relationships.

CORCORAN, Barbara. *A Row of Tigers.* Gr. 6–7. Illus. by Allan Eitzen. Atheneum, 1969. 165 pp. $4.08. Fiction.
An eleven-year-old girl who is grieving her father's death and a man with a spinal curvature become friends and help each other understand their losses.

COREY, Dorothy. *You Go Away.* Gr. ps–1. Illus. by Lois Axeman. A Whitman, 1976. Unp. $7.75. Fiction.
Parents go away and come back. A small child sees departures and returns and understands that, even when parents are away for a long time, they come back.

CORMIER, Robert. *The Chocolate War.* Gr. 7–9. Pantheon, 1974. 272 pp. $8.95. Fiction.

A high-school student, affected by his mother's recent death, considers the effect of one person on the universe. He decides to resist the bullying and beatings of the school gang and the psychological abuse of one of his teachers.

CORN, Anne L. *Monocular Mac.* Gr. 2–4. Illus. by Diane Dawson. NAVH, 1977. 31 pp. $7.50. Fiction.
Mac's vision impairment is aided by a monocular, a telescopic glass tube that helps him see things more than a few feet away. His family is supportive and understanding.

COSGROVE, Margaret. *Your Muscles—And Ways to Exercise Them.* Gr. 3–6. Illus. by the author. Dodd, 1980. 64 pp. $6.95. Nonfiction.
Understanding one's muscles makes exercise more meaningful and productive. The author describes three kinds of muscles, the teamwork between muscles and bones, and what happens when muscles are not used. Suggestions are given for getting started with gymnastics, calisthenics, aerobics, and yoga.

COVELLI, Pat. *Borrowing Time: Growing Up with Juvenile Diabetes.* Gr. 10 and up. Crowell, 1979. 160 pp. $9.95. Nonfiction.
The author developed diabetes at age ten. Although he learned to give self-care, he resisted it in adolescence. He details the treatments and difficulties of the disease and emphasizes that it is possible to cope with it.

COX-GEDMARK, Jan. *Coping with Physical Disability.* Gr. 10–12. Westminster, 1980. 119 pp. $4.95. Nonfiction.
Chronic illness or disability causes specific problems that must be managed and feelings of anger and guilt that must be resolved. Suggestions are given to help the families of disabled people and the disabled individuals themselves.

CRAIG, Eleanor. *One, Two, Three . . . The Story of Matt, a Feral Child.* Gr. 7 and up. McGraw-Hill, 1978. 294 pp. $10.95; pap. New Amer Lib, $2.50. Nonfiction.
The author, a social worker, describes her work with a boy whose diagnosis is difficult to determine, perhaps brain damage, retarda-

tion, autism, or schizophrenia. She is helpful to him in his development and partial recovery.

CRANE, Caroline. *A Girl Like Tracy.* Gr. 7–9. McKay, 1966. 186 pp. $4.25. Fiction.
Kathy helps care for her nineteen-year-old sister, Tracy, who is retarded, but is overwhelmed when their mother is hospitalized. When Kathy realizes that one day she will have full responsibility for Tracy, she runs away. She returns before long and persuades their mother to bring Tracy to a workshop where Tracy learns social and job skills.

CRAWFORD, Charles P. *Three-Legged Race.* Gr. 6–7. Har-Row, 1974. 145 pp. $9.89. Fiction.
During a one-month friendship, two boys and a girl who are hospitalized get caught up in a world of their own and can sometimes forget their hospital surroundings.

CULIN, Charlotte. *Cages of Glass, Flowers of Time.* Gr. 7 and up. Bradbury, 1979. 197 pp. $9.95; pap. Dell, $2.75. Fiction.
Physically and emotionally battered by her parents, a self-absorbed father and an alcoholic mother, fourteen-year-old Claire Burden considers suicide until two new friends help her believe in a loving world.

CUNNINGHAM, Glenn, with George X. SAND. *Never Quit.* Gr. 6 and up. Illus. Chosen Bks, 1981. 143 pp. $7.95. Nonfiction.
Glenn is burned in a school fire that kills his brother. His story details his long-term treatments and psychological adaptations to chronic illness. He becomes an outstanding track performer.

CUNNINGHAM, Julia. *Far in the Day.* Gr. 4–7. Illus. by Don Freeman. Pantheon, 1972. 98 pp. $6.99. Fiction.
A young French boy who does not speak is adopted by members of an English circus. Despite difficulties, he learns to use his talents to become a successful mime.

CUNNINGHAM, Julia. *The Silent Voice.* Gr. 5–9. Dutton, 1981. 145 pp. $10.75. Fiction.
Auguste, an orphan who can hear but does not speak, is rescued by Astair. Auguste joins Astair's street dancers and mimes. A mime teacher recognizes his talent and helps him.

CURTIS, Patricia. *Cindy, a Hearing Ear Dog.* Gr. 6 and up. Illus. by David Cupp. Dutton, 1981. 55 pp. $10.25. Nonfiction.
Young dogs are selected from pounds and humane shelters and are trained to help deaf owners. The dogs alert them to sounds they cannot hear and provide companionship.

CURTIS, Patricia. *Greff: The Story of a Guide Dog.* Gr. 5–9. Photog. by Mary Bloom. Lodestar, 1982. 53 pp. $9.95. Nonfiction.
A Labrador retriever is trained at the Guide Dog Foundation and meets the blind owner he will assist.

CURTIS, Robert H. *Questions and Answers About Alcoholism.* Gr. 7–8. Illus. P-H, 1976. 91 pp. $7.95. Nonfiction.
The book answers in detail numerous questions that older children might ask about alcohol.

DACQUINO, V. T. *Kiss the Candy Days Good-Bye.* Gr. 5–9. Delacorte, 1982. 160 pp. $9.95. Fiction.
When Jimmy is diagnosed as having diabetes, his whole life seems changed. He, his family, and his girl friend must make adjustments.

DALY, Kathleen N. *Body Words: A Dictionary of the Human Body, How It Works, and Some of the Things That Affect It.* Gr. 4–6. Illus. by Melanie Gaines. Doubleday, 1980. 176 pp. $10.95. Nonfiction.
Children can learn to describe what they feel and where they feel it from a vocabulary of terms for parts of the body and its functions.

DANZIGER, Paula. *The Pistachio Prescription.* Gr. 7 and up. Delacorte, 1978. 154 pp. $8.95. Fiction.
Thirteen-year-old Cassandra has an asthma attack whenever she hears her parents fight and when they tell her they will divorce. She "cures" herself by eating pistachio nuts. She develops insights into her own and other people's needs through her relationship with a school friend and the resolution of her rivalry with her sister.

DAYEE, Frances S. *Private Zone: A Book Teaching Children Sexual Assault Prevention Tools.* Gr. ps–3. Illus. by Marina Megale Horosko. C Franklin Pr, 1982. Unp. $3.00. Nonfiction.

Doctors and parents might need to touch children's genitals to help them clean or care for them, but children have the right to say at other times or to other people, "Don't touch, that's my private zone." If someone touches children anyway, it's important to "yell and tell," to let parents or other adults know.

DEEGAN, Paul. *A Hospital: Life in a Medical Center.* Gr. 5–9. Photog. by Bruce C. Ross-Larson. Creative Ed, 1971. 78 pp. $5.95. Nonfiction.
Detailed photographs and text describe the many parts of a large public hospital and the work of the staff.

DENGLER, Marianna. *A Pebble in Newcomb's Pond.* Gr. 6 and up. Ace, 1980. 160 pp. pap. $1.95. Fiction.
When a teenage girl's unusual behavior and suicide attempt lead her to acknowledge her emotional problems, she finally agrees to consult a psychiatrist. He diagnoses schizophrenia and includes planned nutrition (orthomolecular treatment) as part of therapy.

DE PAOLA, Tomie. *Oliver Button Is a Sissy.* Gr. ps–3. Illus. by the author. HarBraceJ, 1979. 48 pp. $7.95; pap. HarBraceJ, $2.45. Fiction.
A young boy must deal with the teasing and isolation he experiences when he chooses to read, paint, and dance rather than participate in sports.

DIXON, Paige. *May I Cross Your Golden River?* (Also titled: *A Time to Love, a Time to Mourn*) Gr. 7–8. Atheneum, 1975. 262 pp. $8.95. Scholastic, 1975. 284 pp. pap. $1.50. Fiction.
Eighteen-year-old Jordan is handsome, intelligent, and in love when he becomes ill with Lou Gehrig's disease, amyotrophic lateral sclerosis, a weakening and atrophy of the muscles. He plunges into activities to make the most of the short time left to him.

DIXON, Paige. *Skipper.* Gr. 6–7. Atheneum, 1979. 110 pp. $8.95. Fiction.
Still mourning the death of his brother, Skipper searches for his father, whom he has never known. Instead, he finds a disabled cousin who helps him recover and plan his life.

DIZENZO, Patricia. *Why Me? The Story of Jenny.* Gr. 7 and up. Avon, 1981. 142 pp. pap. $1.25. Fiction.
A fifteen-year-old girl tells about the emotional and physical experience of being raped and the aftermath of telling her parents and being examined by a doctor.

DODSON, Susan. *The Creep.* Gr. 7–9. Illus. by Ruth Sanderson. Scholastic, 1979. 218 pp. $9.95; pap. Pocket Bks, $1.95. Fiction.
After ten-year-old Annie is attacked by a child molester, her babysitter agrees to act as a police decoy, despite her fears and shyness, in order to lure the man who has been accosting children.

DOLAN, Jr., Edward F. *Child Abuse.* Gr. 7–8. Watts, 1980. 115 pp. $7.90. Nonfiction.
Physical and emotional abuse, neglect, incest, and child pornography are discussed. Laws are described that are designed to protect children.

DONAHUE, Parnell. *Sports Doc: Medical Advice, Diet, Fitness Tips, and Other Essential Hints for Young Athletes.* Gr. 7 and up. Illus. by Mimi Harrison. Knopf, 1979. 192 pp. $7.99; pap. Knopf, $4.95. Nonfiction.
This anecdotal handbook advises on protecting and caring for the body in sports activities, helping readers to help themselves.

DONAHUE, Parnell, and Helen CAPELLARO. *Germs Make Me Sick: A Health Handbook for Kids.* Gr. 5–6. Illus. by Kelly Oechsli. Knopf, 1975. 96 pp. $5.99; pap. Knopf, $2.95. Nonfiction.
Germs in the body's systems can cause diseases and uncomfortable conditions. The process of infection and contagion is described and ideas given on ways to stay well or get well.

DOSS, Helen Grigsby. *Your Skin Holds You In.* Gr. 4–5. Illus. by Christine Bondante. Messner, 1978. 64 pp. $6.97. Nonfiction.
The structure and functions of skin are described. Advice is given on skin protection and on treating bites, stings, burns, bruises, warts, moles, and blemishes.

DOSS, Helen Grigsby, and Richard L. WELLS. *All the Better to Bite With.* Gr. 4–5. Illus. by Charles Clement. Messner, 1976. 64 pp. $7.29. Nonfiction.
Proper tooth care is essential. The structure and functions of teeth, the importance of good nutrition, brushing, and flossing, and dental check-ups are shown.

DRAGONWAGON, Crescent (Ellen Parsons). *Wind Rose.* Gr. ps–3. Illus. by Ronald Himler. Har-Row, 1976. 31 pp. $4.79. Fiction.
A mother poetically tells her daughter of her conception, the pregnancy and birth, and the feelings her parents had while waiting for her to be born.

DUNBAR, Robert E. *Heredity.* Gr. 4 and up. Illus. Watts, 1978. 64 pp. $7.90. Nonfiction.
The research of Darwin and Mendel led to an understanding of cell structure, DNA, mutation, the effects of heredity and environment, and genetic engineering. The reader is encouraged to discover genetic principles through simple experiments with plants and through observations.

DUNBAR, Robert E. *Mental Retardation.* Gr. 7–9. Watts, 1978. 63 pp. $6.45. Nonfiction.
The author discusses the causes and symptoms of mental retardation, and education and employment programs that are available, and asserts that children and adults who have mental retardation have rights.

DUNCAN, Theodore G. *The Diabetes Fact Book.* Gr. 10 and up. Scribner, 1982. 146 pp. $11.95. Nonfiction.
The author, a physician, gives numerous facts about the diagnosis and treatment of diabetes. He emphasizes personal responsibility for diet, exercise, urine testing, and personal care.

DUNN, Graeme. *Benjamin Goes to the Dentist: An Introduction to the Dentist for Children and Parents.* Gr. 1–3. Illus. by Kerri-Ann Foster. Golden Pr (Sydney), 1980. 30 pp. $5.00. Fiction.
Benjamin takes good care of his teeth, including going for a dental visit. The dentist explains the machines and tools, then she cleans and examines Benjamin's teeth. His sister, Joanne, has to

have two baby teeth removed to make room for the new teeth, so oral surgery is explained and she has an injection. At home they play "dentist." Notes for parents encourage honest explanations, early visits, and proper home care of children's teeth.

DUNNAHOO, Terry. *Who Cares About Espie Sanchez?* Gr. 4–7. Dutton, 1975. 152 pp. $7.95. Fiction.
Fifteen-year-old Espie learns police-assistant work and lives in a foster home to escape her mother's neglect and sexual molestation by her mother's boy friend. When Espie's younger brother overdoses on drugs, despite her efforts to persuade him to withdraw from pills, she reports the supplier and helps in the arrest.

DVORINE, William. *A Dermatologist's Guide to Home Skin Treatment: An Up-To-Date Guide That Explains the Best Available Treatment for Every Common Skin Problem, from Acne to Warts.* Gr. 9–12. Scribner, 1983. 282 pp. $11.74. Nonfiction.
The author advises on diet, over-the-counter preparations, and prescribed medications for acne, herpes, sunburn, and other skin problems.

DYER, Thomas A. *A Way of His Own.* Gr. 6–7. HM, 1981. 154 pp. $7.95. Fiction.
A Native American boy who has a disabled leg is abandoned by his family in the wilderness to die. He survives the unknown as well as his own fears. With the help of a girl he meets, he reunites with his family.

EAGAN, Andrea B. *Why Am I So Miserable If These Are the Best Years of My Life?: A Survival Guide for the Young Woman.* Gr. 8 and up. Har-Row, 1976. 220 pp. $9.57; pap. Avon, $2.25. Nonfiction.
Besides describing the anatomy and physiology of the female body, the author encourages teenage women to learn more about their bodies and their emotions in order to have more control of their own lives.

EAGLES, Douglas A. *Your Weight.* Gr. 4 and up. Illus. Watts, 1982. 63 pp. $7.90. Nonfiction.
The author explains how and why people gain and lose weight;

the advantages, disadvantages, and role of body fat; and how to reach and maintain an appropriate weight.

EDELSTEIN, Barbara. *The Woman Doctor's Diet for Teen-Age Girls*. Gr. 7–8. P-H, 1980. 290 pp. $8.95; pap. Ballantine, $2.50. Nonfiction.
Adolescent girls often have concerns about weight and health. This diet includes discussion of psychological needs and what to eat when going out, and offers many diet plans. Boys, who have similar concerns, would also find some of it helpful.

EDWARDS, Gabrielle. *Coping with Venereal Disease*. Gr. 7–12. Rosen, 1983. 117 pp. $7.97. Nonfiction.
The author describes the causes and prevention of syphilis, gonorrhea, herpes, and AIDS (acquired immune deficiency syndrome) among sexually active young people.

EISENBERG, Michael. *Ulcers*. Gr. 10 and up. Random House, 1978. 238 pp. $8.95. Nonfiction.
The author, a gastroenterologist and surgeon, explains types of ulcers and treatment by surgery, drugs, and diet.

ELGIN, Kathleen, and John F. OSTERRITTER. *Twenty-Eight Days*. Gr. 5–6. Illus. by Kathleen Elgin. McKay, 1973. 64 pp. $6.95. Nonfiction.
The authors describe the meaning of and myths about menstruation and explain the menstrual cycle.

ELGIN, Kathleen, and John F. OSTERRITTER. *The Ups and Downs of Drugs*. Gr. 4–5. Illus. by Kathleen Elgin. Knopf, 1972. 63 pp. $4.99. Nonfiction.
The authors give information on drug use, the nature and effects of various drugs, and a glossary of drug terms.

ELKIND, David. *All Grown Up and No Place to Go*. Gr. 10 and up. Addison-Wesley, 1983. 224 pp. $12.95. Nonfiction.
Many teenagers understand technology better than they understand themselves and others. The author suggests ways to help adolescents become more emotionally mature.

ELKIND, David. *The Hurried Child: Growing Up Too Fast Too Soon.* Gr. 10 and up. Addison-Wesley, 1982. 224 pp. $11.95; pap. Addison-Wesley, $6.95. Nonfiction.
Children have many pressures to act maturely while still young. The author, a child psychologist, offers suggestions for reducing the stress this causes.

ELLIOTT, Ingrid Glatz. *Hospital Roadmap: A Book to Help Explain the Hospital Experience to Young Children.* Gr. ps–3. Illus. Resources, 1982. 36 pp. pap. $6.95. Fiction.
The various places and people children see in the medical center are viewed by following a child's examination, hospitalization, treatment, and discharge. The parents are close by and helpful and the child, although expressing some apprehension, is proud to have mastered the experience. A yellow arrow on the poster that is included with the book leads the reader through drawings of the medical center.

ENGLEBARDT, Leland S. *You Have a Right: A Guide for Minors.* Gr. 6 and up. Lothrop, 1979. 128 pp. $9.75. Nonfiction.
The chapter on child abuse and neglect describes cases in which children are abused. The author suggests varied ways in which children can obtain help for themselves or for other children who need to get away from abusive adults.

EPSTEIN, Sherrie S. *Penny, the Medicine Maker: The Story of Penicillin.* Gr. k–5. Illus. by Mark Springer. Lerner, 1960. Unp. $3.95. Fiction.
Through a cartoon germ named Penny, the story of the discovery of penicillin is told.

ERNST, Kathryn F. *Danny and His Thumb.* Gr. ps–3. Illus. by Tomie de Paola. P-H, 1973. Unp. $3.95; pap. P-H, $1.25. Fiction.
A small boy who enjoys sucking his thumb eventually gives up this habit as he becomes interested in a wide range of activities.

EVANS, Jessica. *Blind Sunday.* Gr. 6–7. Scholastic, 1978. 167 pp. pap. $1.50. Fiction.
Jeff learns to overcome his uneasiness around Jenny, the blind girl

he has started dating, but he worries about the attitudes of his friends.

EYERLY, Jeannette. *Bonnie Jo, Go Home.* Gr. 7–8. Bantam, 1972. 114 pp. pap. $1.50. Fiction.
A pregnant sixteen-year-old from the Midwest travels to New York hoping to arrange an abortion.

EYERLY, Jeannette. *Escape from Nowhere.* Gr. 7–8. Lippincott, 1969. 187 pp. $9.95; pap. Berkley, $1.75. Fiction.
High-school student Carla seeks escape from loneliness and an alcoholic mother by turning to drug use, until she realizes that change comes from within.

EYERLY, Jeannette. *He's My Baby, Now.* Gr. 6 and up. Har-Row, 1977. 156 pp. $10.35. Fiction.
A sixteen-year-old single father has difficulty deciding whether to agree to put up the new baby for adoption. He tries to find ways to keep the baby but must consider the infant's well-being and future as well as his own feelings.

EYERLY, Jeannette. *The Seeing Summer.* Gr. 4–6. Illus. Har-Row, 1981. 128 pp. $9.13. Fiction.
Carey still misses her best friend, who has moved away, when a new family moves into the empty house. The family's ten-year-old daughter, who is blind, compensates well and learns new activities quickly. Carey's initially negative attitudes grow into an understanding of the value of her new friend.

EYERLY, Jeannette. *The World of Ellen March.* Gr. 7–8. Lippincott, 1964. 188 pp. $9.95. Fiction.
Ellen is in a car accident. While hospitalized she begins to realize her parents' divorce was not her fault.

FACKLAM, Margery, and Howard FACKLAM. *The Brain: Magnificent Mind Machine.* Gr. 10–12. Illus. by Paul Facklam. HarBraceJ, 1982. 118 pp. $12.95. Nonfiction.
The brain learns, remembers, dreams, and knows. Brain research described includes laser surgery, repair of brain tissue, biofeedback, hypnosis, and the theory that multiple sclerosis may be caused by a slow-acting virus.

FACKLAM, Margery, and Howard FACKLAM. *From Cell to Clone: The Story of Genetic Engineering*. Gr. 7 and up. Illus. by Paul Facklam. HarBraceJ, 1979. 128 pp. $8.95. Nonfiction.
The authors describe the history and technique of cloning, recombinant DNA, and "test-tube babies." They suggest the practical capabilities of scientists in genetic engineering.

FAGERSTROM, Grethe, and Gunilla HANSSON. *Our New Baby: A Picture Story for Parents and Children*. Gr. k–6. Illus. by Gunilla Hansson. Barron, 1982. 48 pp. $7.95. Fiction.
Parents explain sex and birth to their two children to prepare them for the birth of another baby.

FANSHAWE, Elizabeth. *Rachel*. Gr. k–4. Illus. by Michael Charlton. Bradbury, 1975. Unp. $6.50. Fiction.
Rachel, in a wheelchair, needs some help in regular school but takes part in most events and social activities. She studies, paints, feeds animals, plays games, swims, and plans her future.

FASSLER, Joan. *The Boy with a Problem: Johnny Learns to Share His Troubles*. Gr. ps–3. Illus. by Stuart Kranz. Human Sci Pr, 1971. Unp. $9.95. Fiction.
When the suggestions of his mother, doctor, and teacher do not help Johnny with his problem, he tells his story to an attentive friend.

FASSLER, Joan. *Don't Worry, Dear*. Gr. ps–3. Illus. by Stuart Kranz. Human Sci Pr, 1971. 29 pp. $7.95. Fiction.
Jenny's family is patient, warm, and loving toward her even though she sucks her thumb, wets her bed, and stutters. Her family reassures her that she will outgrow these habits, and she does.

FASSLER, Joan. *Howie Helps Himself*. Gr. 2–3. Illus. by Joe Lasker. A Whitman, 1975. 32 pp. $8.25. Fiction.
Howie wants to make his father proud of him by learning to move his own wheelchair as his classmates do. He feels playful and well some days, clumsy and sad on others, but he continues his struggle to achieve this victory.

FASSLER, Joan. *One Little Girl*. Gr. 2–3. Illus. by M. Jane Smyth. Human Sci Pr, 1969. Unp. $9.95. Fiction.

Laurie, a retarded child, learns to take pride in the things that she can do well.

FEINGOLD, S. Norman, and Norma R. MILLER. *Your Future: A Guide for the Handicapped Teenager.* Gr. 7–8. Rosen, 1981. 177 pp. $7.97. Nonfiction.
Some career problems are unique to the disabled. Current and future job opportunities are described for disabled individuals who wish to achieve a self-sufficient life.

FERRIS, Caren. *A Hug Just Isn't Enough.* Gr. 10 and up. Illus. Gallaudet, 1980. 106 pp. $10.95. Nonfiction.
Photographs of children who are deaf, and brief interviews with their parents, show the pleasures and problems of living with a deaf child.

FERRIS, Jean. *Amen, Moses Gardenia.* Gr. 6 and up. FS&G, 1983. 176 pp. $10.95. Fiction.
Although Farrell's adolescence seems comfortable and without problems, she feels unhappy. In her need for attention and love she attempts suicide.

FIRST, Julia. *Getting Smarter.* Gr. 5–6. P-H, 1974. 89 pp. $4.95. Fiction.
Twelve-year-old Rona feels unattractive and is dismayed to find that she will need to wear glasses.

FIRST, Julia. *Look Who's Beautiful!* Gr. 6–7. Watts, 1980. 122 pp. $7.90. Fiction.
Coping with allergies, braces, overweight, and a beautiful mother, Cornelia feels unloved and unattractive until she gives up a vacation to care for an elderly friend, and wins her mother's pride and respect.

FLEEGE, Francis. *How to Eat: Chewing, Tooth Care, and Diet.* Gr. 8 and up. Dutton, 1980. 96 pp. $7.95. Nonfiction.
An eating plan with careful chewing, and brushing teeth after meals or sweets, will keep the teeth and body healthy.

FLEISCHER, Leonore. *Ice Castles.* Gr. 7–8. Fawcett, 1978. 220 pp. pap. $1.95. Fiction.

Intent on becoming a champion figure-skater, Alexis continues training even after she is blinded in an accident. Support from a friend is essential in encouraging her.

FLENDER, Harold, as told to. *We Were Hooked: Thirteen Young Ex-Addicts Tell About Their Experiences with Heroin, LSD, Speed, and Other Drugs and How They Kicked the Habit.* Gr. 7–8. Random House, 1972. $4.99. Nonfiction.
Firsthand narratives by former addicts provide insights into their struggles to overcome the use of drugs.

FODOR, R. V. *What to Eat and Why: The Science of Nutrition.* Gr. 4–5. Illus. Morrow, 1979. 96 pp. $5.71. Nonfiction.
Good nutrition includes foods containing the five nutrient groups: carbohydrates, fats, proteins, minerals, and vitamins. Proper eating habits help prevent tooth decay and obesity.

FOX, Ray Errol. *Angela Ambrosia.* Gr. 7–12. Knopf, 1979. 176 pp. $7.95. Fiction.
When teenager Angela is hospitalized for leukemia, she makes friends with other young cancer patients and, after treatment, is able to go home.

FRANCKE, Linda Bird. *The Ambivalence of Abortion.* Gr. 7–12. Random House, 1978. 288 pp. $10.00. Nonfiction.
The author provides case histories and interviews from women who have had abortions and from counselors, exploring the emotional and psychological aspects of abortion.

FRANKEL, Edward. *DNA: The Ladder of Life.* Gr. 7 and up. Illus. by Anne Marie Jauss. McGraw-Hill, 1978. 127 pp. $8.95. Nonfiction.
DNA (deoxyribonucleic acid) is a molecule that determines the nature of life. The author describes the chemistry and effects of DNA, as well as hereditary conditions such as hemophilia, color blindness, sickle cell anemia, phenylketonuria, and possibly cancer.

FRANKS, Hugh. *Will to Live.* Gr. 10 and up. Routledge, 1979. 147 pp. $11.50; pap. Routledge, $2.95. Nonfiction.
Robby developed Duchenne muscular dystrophy at the age of six.

The author describes Robby's relationships at school and with his family and details the difficulties of his condition.

FRANZ, Barbara, and William FRANZ. *Nutritional Survival Manual for the Eighties: A Young People's Guide to "Dietary Goals for the United States."* Gr. 7 and up. Illus. Messner, 1981. 159 pp. $8.79. Nonfiction.
The authors present each goal, such as "Eat less fat," with practical suggestions on how to achieve the goal and detailed information about it.

FREESE, Arthur S. *The Bionic People Are Here.* Gr. 7–8. Illus. McGraw-Hill, 1979. 103 pp. $6.95. Nonfiction.
Implants and transplants are explained in detail, with stories of the doctors who conducted the initial research and performed the experimental surgery.

FRENEY, Rosemary, Lia KAPELIS, and Peter HICKS. *Guess Where I've Been!* Gr. ps–3. Illus. AAWCH, 1981. 24 pp. pap. $5.95. Fiction.
Posie is hospitalized for examination and treatment of her leg pain. Procedures and surgery are explained. Posie is reassured that both the staff and her mother, who sleeps in the hospital overnight, will care for her. When she recovers she plays in the playroom, then leaves the hospital and tells her kindergarten friends about her experiences. Messages to parents about how to help their hospitalized children amplify the story.

FRETZ, Sada. *Going Vegetarian: A Guide for Teen-agers.* Gr. 7 and up. Illus. by Eric Fretz. Lothrop, 1983. 256 pp. $11.00. Nonfiction.
Avoiding an unbalanced diet is possible in vegetarian meal-planning with the recipes and charts provided in this detailed guide.

FREVERT, Patricia Dendtler. *It's Okay to Look at Jamie.* Gr. 4–8. Photog. by David Jonasson and Gordon Dunn. Creative Ed, 1983. 47 pp. $6.95. Nonfiction.
Jamie has spina bifida. An open part of her spinal column had to be closed surgically, so she has no feeling below that part of the spine. Her check-up includes an intravenous pyelogram, in which

a colored fluid is injected so that it shows on X rays of the kidneys. A cast mold is made for her new braces to enable her to walk better. Jamie's school and play experiences and the emotional support of her family, teacher, friends, and the medical staff help her keep a positive attitude about the adaptations she has to make in caring for herself.

FREVERT, Patricia Dendtler. *Patrick: Yes You Can.* Gr. 4–8. Photog. by Sally Di Martini. Creative Ed, 1983. 47 pp. $6.95. Nonfiction.
Patrick was born with glaucoma, in which new eye fluid builds up faster than old fluid can drain, creating pressure inside the eye and affecting vision. Surgery, eyedrops, and help from a special teacher enable Patrick to begin reading. At eight years of age, a sports injury leads to total blindness. Home teachers help him learn mobility and Braille reading and typing, and his parents encourage him. Returning to second grade, his friends and special teachers help him make adaptations.

FREVERT, Patricia Dendtler. *Patty Gets Well.* Gr. 4–8. Photog. by David Jonasson. Creative Ed, 1983. 47 pp. $6.95. Nonfiction.
Patty's three-year recovery from leukemia is detailed in this story of the diagnosis, chemotherapy, side effects, and recuperation. Emotional support from her family, friends, and the medical staff encourage Patty to have a positive attitude that enable her to cope with uncomfortable treatment, inconveniences, and fears.

FRIIS, Babbis. *Kristy's Courage.* Gr. 4–6. Trans. from the Norwegian by Lisa Sømme McKinnon. Illus. by Charles Geer. HarBraceJ, 1965. 159 pp. $5.95. Fiction.
After a car accident, seventeen-year-old Kristy must cope with a speech problem and cosmetic changes. She has almost no one to talk with about her feelings. Her determination and social skills eventually lead her to be accepted by her previously unaccepting friends and classmates.

FRYER, Judith. *How We Hear: The Story of Hearing.* Gr. 3–9. Illus. by George Overlie. Lerner, 1961. 30 pp. $3.95. Nonfiction.
Hearing ability and impairment are described, with suggestions for healthy care of the ears.

GALBRAITH, Kathryn Osebold. *Spots Are Special.* Gr. 1–2. Illus. by Diane Dawson. Atheneum, 1976. 32 pp. $5.95. Fiction.
When Sandy's chicken pox keeps her at home, she uses her imagination to play special games just for people with spots—pretend giraffes, leopards, frogs, dalmatians. Only when her brother also catches the disease is he allowed to play; he has to agree that spots are special.

GARDEN, Nancy. *Annie on My Mind.* Gr. 6 and up. Illus. FS&G, 1982. 234 pp. $10.95. Fiction.
Two young women who are in love with each other show how they feel in this story of their romance.

GARDNER, Richard A. *MBD: The Family Book About Minimal Brain Dysfunction.* Gr. 4 and up. Illus. by Alfred Lowenheim. Aronson, 1973. 185 pp. $12.50. Nonfiction.
The nature of brain dysfunction is explained to both parents and children in special sections designed for each.

GARDNER-LOULAN, JoAnn, Bonnie LOPEZ, and Marcia QUACKENBUSH. *Period.* Gr. 4 and up. Illus. by Marcia Quackenbush. Glide, 1979. 89 pp. $7.95. Nonfiction.
The authors give information and suggestions for understanding and coping with menstruation. They describe a pelvic examination in detail.

GARRIGUE, Sheila. *Between Friends.* Gr. 6–7. Bradbury, 1978. 160 pp. $8.95. Fiction.
Jill befriends a retarded schoolmate. At first Jill is hesitant and loses other friends because of this choice. Even her family discourages her. Jill learns more about retardation and shows her family and peers a valuable lesson in loyalty.

GAY, Kathlyn. *Body Talk.* Gr. 3–8. Illus. Scribner, 1974. 108 pp. $8.95. Nonfiction.
Examples and illustrations of gestures and actions explain the nonverbal language of the body.

GAY, Kathlyn, Martin GAY, and Marla GAY. *Get Hooked on Vegetables.* Gr. 6–7. Messner, 1978. 157 pp. $7.29. Nonfiction.
The authors describe different types of vegetarian eating for good

nutrition, as well as the situations vegetarians must contend with.

GELINAS, Paul J. *Coping with Anger.* Gr. 7–12. Rosen, 1979. 120 pp. $7.97. Nonfiction.
In the struggle to survive, there are many frustrations. Some people react to these with anger. The author suggests ways to identify and cope with angry feelings.

GELINAS, Paul J. *Coping with Weight Problems.* Gr. 7–12. Rosen, 1983. 132 pp. $7.97. Nonfiction.
The author is a psychotherapist who specializes in problems of adolescence. He discusses the psychological basis of weight problems and what young people can do to maintain weight control.

GELINAS, Paul J. *Coping with Your Emotions.* Gr. 6–7. Rosen, 1979. 120 pp. $7.97. Nonfiction.
The author offers practical guidance in understanding and dealing with feelings in order to help young people achieve emotional stability and maturity.

GELMAN, Rita Golden, and Susan Kovacs BUXBAUM. *Ouch! All About Cuts and Other Hurts.* Gr. 3–4. Illus. by Jan Pyk. HarbraceJ, 1977. 63 pp. $6.95. Nonfiction.
Descriptions of common mishaps and injuries and of the body's reactions to them are arranged alphabetically for easy reference.

GERSON, Corinne. *Passing Through.* Gr. 7–12. Dial, 1978. 193 pp. $7.95. Fiction.
When her older brother commits suicide, fifteen-year-old Liz is bereaved. From her new friend Sam, who has cerebral palsy, she learns to accept and live with difficulties. This helps her reconcile her loss and some of her differences with her parents.

GIBBONS, Thomas B. *How Doctors Diagnose You and How You Can Help.* Gr. 10 and up. Saunders, 1980. 196 pp. $11.95. Nonfiction.
The author, a physician, describes how a doctor diagnoses from information the patient gives, a physical examination, and tests.

GILBERT, Nan. *The Unchosen.* Gr. 7 and up. Har-Row, 1963. 214 pp. $9.89; pap. Har-Row, $.95. Fiction.

Seventeen-year-old Ellen finally decides to overcome her shyness and weight problem by changing her expectations, reaching out to friends, and dieting.

GILBERT, Sara D. *Fat Free: Common Sense for Young Weight Worriers.* Gr. 6 and up. Macmillan, 1975. 114 pp. $8.95. Nonfiction.
Various weight-reduction methods are reviewed, including diet pills, diuretics, and quick-weight-loss diets. Positive ideas for planning and eating a balanced menu include measuring quantities, keeping records, and setting reasonable goals.

GILBERT, Sara D. *Feeling Good: A Book About You and Your Body.* Gr. 7–8. Four Winds, 1978. 181 pp. $7.95. Nonfiction.
Physical, emotional, and mental changes occur during adolescence, but there are ways to care for one's body and cope with problems or conditions that might occur.

GILBERT, Sara D. *What Happens in Therapy?* Gr. 6 and up. Lothrop, 1982. 144 pp. $8.63; pap. Lothrop, $6.00. Nonfiction.
Various kinds of psychotherapy can be helpful for different problems. The author offers advice about when therapy should be sought.

GILSON, Jamie. *Do Bananas Chew Gum?* Gr. 6 and up. Archway, 1980. 146 pp. pap. $1.95. Fiction.
Sam can memorize and do math well, but he has learning disabilities in reading and writing. Braces on his teeth and the usual preteen concerns add to his problems. With the help of a teacher-specialist, he learns to emphasize listening to information rather than reading it, and gains confidence in the abilities he does have.

GIRION, Barbara. *The Boy with the Special Face.* Gr. 2–3. Illus. by Heidi Palmer. Abingdon, 1978. Unp. $5.95. Fiction.
Perry is sure that his freckles, unruly hair, and odd-shaped nose will keep him from being selected to be in a television commercial.

GIRION, Barbara. *A Handful of Stars.* Gr. 7 and up. Scribner, 1981. 176 pp. $10.95. Fiction.

Julie's high-school years are going well until diagnostic exams, including electroencephalograms and CAT scans, show that her blank-outs are epileptic seizures. Balancing the medications, as the neurologist tries to get the seizures under control, is difficult. She finds that some friends, classmates, and teachers are understanding and others are not, but her family is supportive.

GLASSER, Ronald J. *The Body Is the Hero.* Gr. 10–12. Random House, 1976. 248 pp. $8.95; pap. Bantam, $2.50. Nonfiction.
An account of the human body's immune system and its occasional breakdown is interwoven with tales of important medical discoveries about the system.

GLAZZARD, Margaret H. *Meet Camille and Danille, They're Special Persons: Hearing Impaired.* 53 pp. *Meet Danny, He's a Special Person: Multiply Handicapped.* 47 pp. *Meet Lance, He's a Special Person: Trainable Mentally Retarded.* 43 pp. *Meet Scott, He's a Special Person: Learning Disabled.* 46 pp. Gr. 1–3. Photog. by Hank Young. H & H Ent, 1978. $9.50 each. Nonfiction.
This series introduces real disabled children to their classmates and friends. While showing the normal play activities all children enjoy, the special educational methods are also detailed, and the emotions of children who feel different are described. A story record is included with each book.

ANON. *Go Ask Alice.* Gr. 9–12. P-H, 1971. 189 pp. $5.95; pap. Avon. $1.95. Nonfiction.
Fifteen-year-old Alice's drug addiction and pushing are difficult for her parents to understand and control. When she overdoses and dies, they find her diary, which is this book.

GOLD, Phyllis. *Please Don't Say Hello.* Gr. 5–6. Photog. by Carl Baker. Human Sci Pr, 1975. 45 pp. $9.95. Fiction.
Eddie and his family move into a new neighborhood. The questions of the neighbor children enable Eddie's mother to tell them about his social and learning problems. With special education and the children's support, Eddie matures somewhat. Since the story does not specify, Eddie could have learning disabilities and/or autism.

GOLDSMITH, Ilse. *Anatomy for Children.* Gr. 5–8. Illus. by William Krause. Sterling, 1964. 93 pp. $4.89. Nonfiction.
Each system of the body is explained and diagrammed, including digestion, respiration, circulation, reproduction, glands, skeleton, and sense organs.

GOLLAY, Elinor, and Alwina BENNETT. *The College Guide for Students with Disabilities: A Detailed Directory of Higher Education Services, Programs, and Facilities Accessible to Handicapped Students in the United States.* Gr. 10–12. Westview, 1976. 545 pp. $35.00. Nonfiction.
Information is provided on policies such as accessibility and services available at colleges and universities, listed by state.

GOODBODY, Slim (John Burstein). *The Force Inside You.* Gr. 4–8. Photog. by Bruce Curtis. Illus. by Nurit Karlin. Coward, 1983. 64 pp. $9.95; pap. Coward, $4.95. Nonfiction.
Balance exercises, self-healing, and body awareness help develop the body's physical abilities and skills—the force.

GOODBODY, Slim (John Burstein). *The Healthy Habits Handbook.* Gr. 4–8. Photog. by Bruce Curtis. Illus. by Nurit Karlin. Coward, 1983. 64 pp. $9.95; pap. Coward, $4.95. Nonfiction.
Children can build healthy bodies with attention to such habits as posture, sleep, and nutrition.

GOODE, Ruth. *Hands Up!* Gr. 2–6. Illus. by Tony Kramer. Macmillan, 1983. 64 pp. $8.95. Nonfiction.
The author explains how hands work, right- and left-handedness, motor development, hand-eye-brain coordination, and the myth of double-jointedness.

GOODMAN, Joseph I., and W. Watts BIGGER. *Diabetes Without Fear.* Gr. 7 and up. Avon, 1979. 198 pp. pap. $2.95. Nonfiction.
Many diabetics have misunderstandings or misinformation that lead to fears. With correct information and care, people with diabetes can live active lives.

GOODSELL, Jane. *Katie's Magic Glasses.* Gr. k–3. Illus. by Barbara Cooney. HM, 1978. 43 pp. $5.95; pap. HM, $2.25. Fiction.
When five-year-old Katie is fitted for glasses, she can see what used to be a blur. In rhyme the examination is detailed.

GORE, Harriet Margolis. *What to Do When There's No One but You.* Gr. 4–5. Illus. by David Lindroth. P-H, 1974. 48 pp. $4.95. Nonfiction.
A collection of vignettes relays basic first-aid procedures and accident prevention information.

GRABER, Richard. *A Little Breathing Room.* Gr. 5–7. Har-Row, 1978. 121 pp. $6.79. Fiction.
Thirteen-year-old Ray is close to his younger brother and helps when his brother becomes ill and later when his leg is broken and in a cast. Ray eventually learns to resist their father's verbal and physical abuse. Their mother arranges for Ray to visit grandparents for "a little breathing room."

GREEN, Hannah. *I Never Promised You a Rose Garden.* Gr. 9 and up. HR&W, 1964. 288 pp. $6.95. Fiction.
Through a long, complex therapy, a young woman begins to realize the source of her problems.

GREENBANK, Anthony. *A Handbook for Emergencies: Coming Out Alive.* Gr. 7 and up. Illus. by Jerry Malone and Mel Klapholz. Doubleday, 1976. 192 pp. $8.95; pap. Doubleday, $4.95. Nonfiction.
Dealing with emergencies at home and while camping or boating requires calmness, survival supplies, and information.

GREENBERG, Harvey R. *Hanging In: What You Should Know About Psychotherapy.* Gr. 7 and up. Four Winds, 1982. 256 pp. $12.95. Nonfiction.
The author, a psychotherapist, explains the process of therapy, why it is needed, how it works, how to select types of therapy, and how to recognize when it is not helping.

GREENBERG, Jan. *No Dragons to Slay.* Gr. 6 and up. FS&G, 1983. 152 pp. $10.95. Fiction.
Seventeen-year-old Thomas finds he needs the help of others when he develops cancer. But his parents are too anxious and his friends too frightened to be helpful. He finds a new, older friend who helps him realize the vulnerability of other people as well as his own.

GREENBERG, Jan. *The Pig-Out Blues.* Gr. 7 and up. FS&G, 1982. 150 pp. $9.95. Fiction.
Jodie wants the lead in the school play, but she is overweight, so she tries a crash diet. After she faints she gives up and goes on an eating binge. Jodie is helped by a friend who is not ashamed of her own overweight, by the owner of a health food store, who gives her a job, and by her mother.

GREENE, Carla. *Doctors and Nurses: What Do They Do?* Gr. k–3. Illus. by Leonard Kessler. Har-Row, 1963. Unp. $8.89. Nonfiction.
The ways in which doctors and nurses care for children is shown in drawings and simple language.

GREENE, Constance C. *Beat the Turtle Drum.* Gr. 5–6. Illus. by Donna Diamond. Viking, 1976. 119 pp. $8.95; pap. Dell, $1.95. Fiction.
Sustained by her parents and friends, Kate recalls and grieves for her younger sister, who was killed in an accident.

GREENE, Constance C. *The Ears of Louis.* Gr. 5–6. Illus. by Nola Langner. Viking, 1974. 90 pp. $9.95; pap. Dell, $.95. Fiction.
A small boy, who is constantly being teased about his large ears, proves his worth to his classmates by playing football well.

GREENE, Constance C. *The Unmaking of Rabbit.* Gr. 6–7. Viking, 1972. 125 pp. $9.95; pap. Dell, $.95. Fiction.
Smaller than the other boys and with ears that stick out, eleven-year-old Paul is teased by his classmates. His parents are divorced, and he lives with his grandmother. Although he hopes to be able to live with his parents someday, he realizes, when there is a prospect that his mother will invite him to stay with her and her new husband, that his grandmother needs him more.

GREENE, Laura. *I Am Somebody.* Gr. 1–2. Illus. by Gerald Cross. Childrens, 1980. 30 pp. $7.95. Fiction.
Two boys who do not feel talented on their baseball teams discuss what makes them feel important. They decide that being themselves is what really matters.

GREENE, Shep. *The Boy Who Drank Too Much*. Gr. 6–7. Viking, 1979. 149 pp. $8.95; pap. Dell, $1.50. Fiction.
Lonely and isolated because he is more mature than most of his high-school classmates and hockey teammates, Buff relies heavily upon alcohol until a crisis makes him realize that he is free to live his own life.

GREENFIELD, Eloise. *Darlene*. Gr. k–2. Illus. by George Gord. Methuen, 1980. Unp. $8.95. Fiction.
Darlene, who uses a wheelchair, visits her cousin, but soon wants to go home. Her relatives play games with her until her mother arrives, by which time she is having so much fun she does not want to go home.

GREENFIELD, Eloise, and Alesia REVIS. *Alesia*. Gr. 5 and up. Photog. by Sandra Turner Bond. Philomel, 1981. 59 pp. $9.95. Nonfiction.
Alesia's diary tells about a car accident that disabled her when she was nine years old. It describes her efforts over the years to adapt physically and emotionally, especially during adolescence.

GREENWALD, Arthur, and Barry HEAD. *Going to the Hospital*. Gr. ps–1. Illus. by William Panos. Family Comm, 1977. Unp. pap. $1.95. Fiction.
Children's friend from television, Mister Rogers, reassures them about hospital care, including the staff, time for play, procedures that may be uncomfortable, and going home to rest and tell friends about being hospitalized.

GREENWALD, Arthur, and Barry HEAD. *Having an Operation*. Gr. ps–1. Illus. by Ruth Brunner-Strosser. Family Comm, 1977. Unp. pap. $1.95. Fiction.
Children's television friend, Mister Rogers, tells about preoperative medication, how the operating room looks, recovery, and going home. He suggests children might want to playact about the time in the hospital.

GREENWALD, Arthur, and Barry HEAD. *Wearing a Cast*. Gr. ps–1. Illus. by George Gaadt. Family Comm, 1977. Unp. pap. $1.95. Fiction.

Mister Rogers, of the television show, describes a strong, hard bandage called a cast. He explains about X rays, putting the cast on, activities children can do while wearing casts, and how the cast is removed.

GREENWALD, Sheila. *The Secret in Miranda's Closet.* Gr. 4–7. Illus. by the author. HM, 1977. 138 pp. $6.95. Fiction.
Having an antique doll helps a young girl find individuality and self-assurance when her mother disapproves of traditional sex roles.

GRIESE, Arnold A. *At the Mouth of the Luckiest River.* Gr. 3–4. Illus. by Glo Coalson. Crowell, 1973. 64 pp. $8.79. Fiction.
Tatlek is an Alaskan Indian who has a weak, turned foot. This disability is well regarded by his tribe and is a challenge to Tatlek. He finds many ways to compensate for the disability and to accept it as part of himself.

GROLLMAN, Earl A. *Talking About Death: A Dialogue Between Parent and Child.* Gr. 4–5. Illus. by Gisela Heau. Beacon, 1976. 98 pp. $9.95; pap. Beacon, $4.50. Nonfiction.
This read-along picture book explains death to young children and has an extensive guide for parents, including a list of pertinent organizations, books, tapes, films, and a bibliography.

GROSS, Ruth Belov. *A Book About Your Skeleton.* Gr. k–4. Illus. by Deborah Robison. Hastings, 1979. 32 pp. $7.95. Nonfiction.
Bones protect the body, manufacture blood cells, and support movement of the body.

GRUENBERG, Sidonie M. *The Wonderful Story of How You Were Born.* Gr. 3–5. Illus. by Symeon Shimin. Doubleday, 1970. Unp. $7.95. Fiction.
This detailed story describes conception, pregnancy, breast-feeding, and family love.

GUEST, Judith. *Ordinary People.* Gr. 10–12. Viking, 1976. 263 pp. $11. 95; pap. Ballantine, $2.75. Fiction.
After his brother dies in a boating accident, seventeen-year-old Conrad attempts suicide. After eight months in a hospital he returns to his parents' home and tries to build a new life.

HAAR, Jaap ter. *The World of Ben Lighthart.* Gr. 6–7. Trans. from the Dutch by Martha Hearns. Delacorte, 1979. 123 pp. $5.95; pap. Dell, $1.25. Fiction.
When he becomes blind in an accident, Ben struggles against anger and fear and begins to accept his condition and the adaptations he has to make.

HAINES, Gail Kay. *Brain Power: Understanding Human Intelligence.* Gr. 7–8. Illus. Watts, 1979. 117 pp. $5.45. Nonfiction.
The author describes the learning process, right- and left-brain differences, creativity, and the measurement of intelligence.

HAINES, Gail Kay. *Cancer.* Gr. 4 and up. Watts, 1980. 64 pp. $7.90. Nonfiction.
Cancer is an overgrowth of cells, which can be treated with medicine, radiation, surgery, and the body's own defenses. Vignettes provide explanations of various cancers and research.

HAINES, Gail Kay. *Natural and Synthetic Poisons.* Gr. 4–6. Illus. by Giulio Maestro. Morrow, 1978. 96 pp. $7.44. Nonfiction.
Poison from animals, plants, bacteria, and minerals creates chemical changes that affect the nerves, the circulation, the liver, or other body systems.

HAISLET, Barbara. *Why Are Some People Left-Handed?* Gr. 3–4. Illus. by Sandra Higashi. Creative Ed, 1981. 31 pp. $5.95. Nonfiction.
The author dispels superstitions about left-handedness, names many famous people who are left-handed, and discusses research about the reasons and mechanism of left-handedness.

HALACY, Daniel B., Jr. *X-Rays and Gamma Rays.* Gr. 7–8. Illus. Holiday, 1969. 159 pp. $4.95. Nonfiction.
The author discusses the electromagnetic spectrum, penetrating radiation, and the biological effects of X rays.

HALL, Candace Catlin. *Shelley's Day: The Day of a Legally Blind Child.* Gr. k–6. Illus. by the author. Andrew Mountain Pr, 1980. 24 pp. pap. $2.95. Nonfiction.
Seven-year-old Shelley, who has vision impairment, does first-grade work at school with the help of a special teacher and

selected materials such as a magnifier light and large-print books. At home she plays games, watches television with special glasses, and does her share of housework.

HALL, Elizabeth. *From Pigeons to People: A Look at Behavior Shaping.* Gr. 5 and up. Illus. HM, 1975. 130 pp. $6.95. Nonfiction.
The author describes B. F. Skinner's work in behavior modification, giving many examples of operant conditioning that show how individuals can change habits such as overeating or misbehavior.

HALL, Elizabeth. *Possible Impossibilities: A Look at Parapsychology.* Gr. 5 and up. HM, 1977. 169 pp. $6.95. Nonfiction.
Events that seem to defy the laws of physics and seem beyond the normal ability of people's senses are the subject matter of parapsychology. The phenomena described include precognition, extrasensory perception, psychokinesis, and others.

HALL, Lynn. *Half the Battle.* Gr. 7 and up. Scribner, 1982. 151 pp. $10.95. Fiction.
Eighteen-year-old Blair, who is blind, is dependent on his younger brother, Loren, and resents it. Loren is jealous of the attention his blind brother receives. During an endurance ride on horseback, the brothers have a chance to work out some of their conflicts.

HALL, Lynn. *Sticks and Stones.* Gr. 6–7. Follett, 1972. 220 pp. $5.95; pap. Dell, $1.50. Fiction.
Gossip about Tom and Ward's close friendship results in Tom's backing out of the state music competition. When Tom is hospitalized after a car accident he remembers the importance of relationships and the need to be true to one's own sexuality.

HAMILTON, Eleanor. *Sex, with Love: A Guide for Young People.* Gr. 7–10. Beacon, 1978. 179 pp. $11.06; pap. Beacon, $5.50. Nonfiction.
The author emphasizes the link between sexuality and caring and the importance of responsible behavior. She describes male and female physiology and safe yet fulfilling means of early sexual expression, adult lovemaking, and contraception.

HAMILTON, Virginia. *The Planet of Junior Brown.* Gr. 7–8. Illus. Macmillan, 1971. 210 pp. $9.95. Fiction.
Junior Brown contends with isolation and a neurotic, sometimes psychotic, mother who discourages his musical and artistic talents. Obese, depressed, and unable to go to school, he is helped by a friend who aids runaways.

HAMILTON-PATERSON, James. *House in the Waves.* Gr. 8 and up. S G Phillips, 1970. 157 pp. $9.95. Fiction.
Having spent most of his life in foster homes and psychiatric institutions, a fourteen-year-old boy withdraws into himself until he finds a cryptic message on the beach. That takes him back to another time, where he helps a prisoner (as he has been a prisoner of his own mind) escape and thereby begins his own recovery.

HAMMOND, Janice Marie. *When My Dad Died: A Child's View of Death.* Gr. 1–3. Illus. by the author. Cranbrook, 1981. 31 pp. pap. $3.95. Nonfiction.
Children may experience various normal feelings after the death of their fathers. The author advises adults who want to help children at this difficult time.

HAMMOND, Janice Marie. *When My Mommy Died: A Child's View of Death.* Gr. 1–3. Illus. by the author. Cranbrook, 1980. 31 pp. pap. $3.95. Nonfiction.
Children may have many different feelings about the death of their mothers. Adults can help children grieve.

HAMMOND, Winifred G. *The Riddle of Teeth.* Gr. 3–5. Illus. Coward, 1971. 60 pp. $4.99. Nonfiction.
Easy projects are suggested through which the reader can observe and discover the nature, functions, and care of teeth.

HAMMOND, Winifred G. *The Story of Your Eye.* Gr. 5–6. Illus. by Heidi Palmer. Coward, 1975. 63 pp. $6.99. Nonfiction.
The characteristics and workings of the parts of the human eye and the physiological aspects of sight are described. Projects are suggested to aid understanding.

HANCKEL, Frances, and John CUNNINGHAM. *A Way of Love, a Way of Life: A Young Person's Introduction to What It Means to*

Be Gay. Gr. 9–12. Illus. by Alix Olson and Larry Stein. Lothrop, 1979. 188 pp. $7.95. Nonfiction.
Being gay or lesbian is an attitude as well as a way of loving. Acceptance of self and others is the basis for responsible relationships, sexuality, and health.

HANLON, Emily. *It's Too Late for Sorry.* Gr. 7–8. Bradbury, 1978. 224 pp. $8.95; pap. Dell, $1.75. Fiction.
Ken feels jealous and left out when he and Rachel help a retarded teenage neighbor, Harold. Ken's angry words confuse Harold, who gets lost and hurt while running away. Ken's rethinking of his attitude leads to more maturity and understanding.

HANLON, Emily. *The Swing.* Gr. 5–6. Dutton, 1979. 209 pp. $8.95; pap. Dell, $1.95. Fiction.
Eleven-year-old Beth, who is deaf, uses a swing in a field as a place to get away from the pressures of communicating. Thirteen-year-old Danny uses the swing to remember his dead father and to get away from the pressures of his stepfather. Although a lie Danny tells results in the death of the mountain bears that Beth treasures, the children eventually grow to understand each other's needs and become friends.

HANN, Jacquie. *Up Day, Down Day.* Gr. k–3. Illus. by the author. Scholastic, 1978. Unp. $6.95. Fiction.
One small boy catches a shoe, a tin can, and a cold during a Sunday spent fishing with a friend.

HARMIN, Merrill. *Better Than Aspirin: How to Get Rid of Emotions That Give You a Pain in the Neck.* Gr. 7–8. Illus. Argus, 1976. 95 pp. pap. $2.50. Nonfiction.
Simple exercises and projects aid in gaining knowledge of personal feelings, needs, and goals, clarifying values, and relieving destructive tensions.

HARRIES, Joan. *They Triumphed over Their Handicaps.* Gr. 7 and up. Watts, 1981. 88 pp. $8.50. Nonfiction.
Even if disabled people cannot achieve all their goals, they can try to decrease their limitations. Stories of real people who have deafness, blindness, amputation, or drug abuse problems demon-

strate a variety of ways to overcome some of the handicapping aspects of disability.

HARRIS, Audrey. *Why Did He Die?* Gr. k–5. Illus. by Susan Sallade Dalke. Lerner, 1965. Unp. $3.95. Fiction.
In verse and metaphor, a mother explains death to her young son.

HARRIS, Robie H., and Elizabeth LEVY. *Before You Were Three: How You Began to Walk, Talk, Explore and Have Feelings.* Gr. 1 and up. Photog. by Henry Gordillo. Delacorte, 1981. 160 pp. $7.95. Nonfiction.
This illustrated narrative of children's first three years of life details stages of growth in learning and feeling.

HASKINS, James. *Teen-Age Alcoholism.* Gr. 9–12. Hawthorn, 1976. 156 pp. $7.95. Nonfiction.
Teenage alcoholism has causes, immediate and long-term effects, and possible remedies. Guidelines are provided for recognizing, understanding, and dealing with the problem.

HASKINS, James, and J. M. STIFLE. *The Quiet Revolution: The Struggle for the Rights of Disabled Americans.* Gr. 7 and up. Illus. Har-Row, 1979. 147 pp. $9.89. Nonfiction.
Many people are working for the rights of disabled people through social and health agencies, telethons, mass communication, sit-ins, and legal action.

HASKINS, James, with Pat CONNOLLY. *The Child Abuse Help Book.* Gr. 6 and up. Addison-Wesley, 1982. 115 pp. $9.95. Nonfiction.
Children can learn some ways to help themselves when faced with abuse, neglect, sexual abuse, exploitation, or incest.

HASS, Aaron. *Teenage Sexuality: A Survey of Teenage Sexual Behavior.* Gr. 10 and up. Macmillan, 1979. 202 pp. $10.95. Nonfiction.
In a survey by the author, teenagers discuss their sexual attitudes, preferences, expectations, and activities.

HAUTZIG, Deborah. *Hey Dollface.* Gr. 7 and up. Morrow, 1978. 151 pp. $9.75; pap. Bantam, $1.75. Fiction.

Two fifteen-year-old girls are attracted to each other and confused about their sexuality.

HAUTZIG, Deborah. *Second Star to the Right.* Gr. 7–8. Greenwillow, 1981. 160 pp. $7.95. Fiction.
When fourteen-year-old Leslie loses control of her dieting, she is hospitalized for treatment of anorexia nervosa.

HAWKER, Frances, and Lee WITHALL. *Donna Finds Another Way.* Gr. 3–6. Photog. by Queensland Department of Education and Bruce Campbell. Jacaranda, 1979. 28 pp. $5.95. Nonfiction.
Donna has cerebral palsy and goes to special school. She plays, learns academics, and manages her body with aids and devices. Bliss symbols are shown and the various therapies and appliances are described.

HAWKER, Frances, and Lee WITHALL. *With a Little Help from My Friends.* Gr. 3–6. Photog. by Melinda Hutton. Jacaranda, 1979. 28 pp. $5.95. Nonfiction.
Peter has spina bifida and an ostomy and uses leg braces, walking crutches, and a small "car" to get around. In answering his classmates' questions, he and his mother convey information to the reader. With help and emotional support from his friends, Peter takes part in activities, travel, and fun. When Peter is hospitalized his friends visit and find he has school in the hospital, has to take medicine, has X ray films made of his broken bone, and enjoys television.

HAYDEN, Robert C. *Seven Black American Scientists.* Gr. 5 and up. Addison-Wesley, 1970. 176 pp. $6.95. Nonfiction.
In telling the lives of seven scientists who are black, the author describes their discoveries and medical advances in such areas as blood transfusion, heart care, and nutrition. The scientists included are Charles R. Drew, Daniel Hale Williams, Benjamin Banneker, Charles Henry Turner, Ernest E. Just, Matthew A. Henson, and George Washington Carver.

HAYDEN, Robert C., and Jacqueline HARRIS. *Nine Black American Doctors.* Gr. 5 and up. Addison-Wesley, 1976. 144 pp. $6.95. Nonfiction.

The authors describe the medical and surgical skills of black doctors whose work has advanced the practice of medicine.

HAYMAN, LeRoy. *Triumph! Conquering Your Physical Disability.* Gr. 9 and up. Messner, 1982. 159 pp. $9.29. Nonfiction.
Examples of real disabled persons, including the author, illustrate that as long as one keeps control of thinking and feelings, disabilities remain only physical.

HAYNES, Henry Louis. *Squarehead and Me.* Gr. 4–5. Illus. by Len Epstein. Westminster, 1980. 143 pp. $8.95. Fiction.
After David befriends Robert, who has dyslexia, the pair bicycle from Washington, D.C., to the countryside, where David comes to realize that Robert is intelligent.

HAZEN, Barbara Shook. *To Be Me.* Gr. 1–2. Illus. by Frances Hook. Childs World, 1975. Unp. $7.95. Fiction.
Various children describe and illustrate the personal traits that make each of them unique.

HEIDE, Florence Parry. *Secret Dreamer, Secret Dreams.* Gr. 5 and up. Har-Row, 1978. 95 pp. $9.57. Fiction.
Thirteen-year-old Caroline is unable to communicate; she neither speaks nor fully understands others' conversations. Her special-education teacher writes this story, interpreting Caroline's feelings — striving but frustrated, cared for by her family yet not a part of them.

HELFMAN, Elizabeth S. *Blissymbolics: Speaking Without Speech.* Gr. 6 and up. Illus. Elsevier/Nelson, 1981. 152 pp. $10.95. Nonfiction.
A system of symbol boards created by Charles Bliss is used to teach children who cannot communicate in other ways because of disabilities such as paralysis or cerebral palsy.

HENRIOD, Lorraine. *Special Olympics and Paralympics.* Gr. 4 and up. Illus. Watts, 1979. 66 pp. $7.90. Nonfiction.
The Special Olympics is for children and adults who are retarded. The Paralympics is for people who are physically disabled. Both sports events demonstrate the desire to belong and achieve.

HERMES, Patricia. *Nobody's Fault?* Gr. k–6. HarBraceJ, 1983. 107 pp. $8.95; pap. Dell, $1.75. Fiction.
Emily is angry at her older brother, who sometimes teases her, so she tries to get even. When he dies in a home accident, she feels responsible. With psychiatric help she begins to understand that his death was nobody's fault.

HERMES, Patricia. *What If They Knew?* Gr. 6–7. HarBraceJ, 1980. 121 pp. $6.95; pap. Dell, $1.50. Fiction.
Transferring to a new school, eleven-year-old Jeremy fears that her new friends will discover her carefully guarded secret, that she has epilepsy.

HERZIG, Alison C., and Jane L. MALI. *Oh, Boy! Babies!* Gr. 5 and up. Photog. by Katrina Thomas. Little, 1980. 106 pp. $9.95; pap. Little, $6.95. Nonfiction.
Fifth- and sixth-grade boys take a course about baby care in which they play with and care for real babies. Numerous photographs and vignettes highlight the experiences they have.

HEUSER, Edith. *This Is How My Body Works.* Gr. 1–5. Illus. by Dieter Mettelsiefen. Barron, 1982. 80 pp. $3.95. Nonfiction.
A physician tells about digestion, respiration, circulation, reproduction, and the five senses in this story of the human body.

HINTON, S. E. *That Was Then, This Is Now.* Gr. 7 and up. Viking, 1971. 159 pp. $9.95. Fiction.
Mark and Bryon, both sixteen years old, are among many young people who live in poor neighborhoods, take part in beatings, and witness injuries to their families and friends. They are at a point in their lives when they need to decide whether they will continue being petty thieves and bullies or strive to be something better.

HIRSCH, Karen. *Becky.* Gr. k–3. Illus. by Jo Esco. Carolrhoda, 1981. Unp. $6.50. Fiction.
A girl who is deaf lives with a hearing family while she attends school. They learn to adapt to her special needs, such as the use of sign language.

HIRSCH, Karen. *My Sister.* Gr. 2–3. Illus. by Nancy Inderieden. Carolrhoda, 1977. Unp. $4.95. Fiction.
A young boy loves and understands his older sister, who is retarded. Sometimes he feels sad for her and embarrassed and sometimes he gets angry at the special attention she receives from their parents.

HIRSCH, Linda. *The Sick Story.* Gr. 3–4. Illus. by John Waliner. Hastings, 1977. Unp. $5.95. Fiction.
A common cold gives Miranda an excuse for staying home from school and for issuing dramatic commands to her parents as they try to care for her.

HLIBOK, Bruce. *Silent Dancer.* Gr. 3–6. Photog. by Liz Glasgow. Messner, 1981. 64 pp. $8.29; pap. Wanderer, $4.95. Nonfiction.
The author's sister, who is deaf, dreams of becoming a ballerina. She works in a special class at the Joffrey Ballet School, showing how deaf children can learn to dance.

HOFF, Syd. *The Littlest Leaguer.* Gr. 1–3. Illus. by the author. Dutton, 1976. 48 pp. $5.95; pap. S&S, $2.50. Fiction.
Harold is the shortest member of his Little League baseball team. With the coach's encouragement and his own determination, Harold is able to help win a game because of his height.

HOGAN, Paula, and Kirk HOGAN. *The Hospital Scares Me.* Gr. 1–3. Illus. Raintree, 1980. 32 pp. $9.98. Fiction.
While being treated for a broken ankle, Dan grows less afraid of the hospital, receiving emotional support and explanations of everything that happens to him.

HOLLAND, Isabelle. *Alan and the Animal Kingdom.* Gr. 5–8. Har-Row, 1977. 190 pp. $10.95; pap. Dell, $1.95. Fiction.
Nine-year-old Alan, who stutters when he is upset, lives in various relatives' homes. He distrusts people, relating better to animals. Alan accepts friendship only from a few people, who help Alan mature and gain more control of his life.

HOLLAND, Isabelle. *Dinah and the Fat Green Kingdom.* Gr. 5 and up. Har-Row, 1978. 189 pp. $10.95; pap. Dell, $1.75. Fiction.

Tired of being nagged and teased about her overweight, twelve-year-old Dinah imagines a kingdom where the fattest people are the most beautiful. In real life she finds new friends and an unattractive puppy to care for, and begins to take charge of her life again.

HOLLAND, Isabelle. *Heads You Win, Tails I Lose.* Gr. 7–8. Lippincott, 1973. 159 pp. $9.95; pap. Dell, $1.50. Fiction.
Fifteen-year-old Melissa's parents and teacher urge her to lose weight and her classmates tease and insult her about her obesity. With her parents' continual fighting and eventual separation, Melissa takes an overdose of diet pills. Her physician, a friend, and, finally, her father help her to get some perspective.

HOLLAND, Isabelle. *The Man Without a Face.* Gr. 6–7. Lippincott, 1972. 159 pp. $9.95; pap. Bantam, $1.50. pap. Dell, $1.75. Fiction.
Charles's tutor is a lonely man who has facial scars from burns. Charles, having problems with his family, goes to his tutor for sympathy. Their relationship leads to a loving encounter. Charles must resolve his feelings about homosexuality, although his tutor assures him the incident was not significant. Through the discipline of academics, and the trust and caring of his friend and teacher, Charles learns to deal with the problems of his life.

HOLMES, Burnham. *Early Morning Rounds: A Portrait of a Hospital.* Gr. 7 and up. Photog. by Janet Beller. Four Winds, 1981. 79 pp. $9.95. Nonfiction.
This narrative gives realistic details of medical, surgical, and emergency care along with photographs of real doctors, patients, and procedures.

HOLMES, Burnham. *The First Seeing Eye Dog.* Gr. 7 and up. Illus. by Judith Clark. Silver, 1978. 46 pp. $8.07. Nonfiction.
Morris Frank and his dog, Buddy, pioneered changes needed for blind people who travel, especially in training dogs to guide the blind.

HOLZENTHALER, Jean. *My Feet Do.* Gr. ps–1. Dutton, 1977. 31 pp. $5.95. Nonfiction.
Feet can splash, run, dance, wear shoes or boots, and rest.

HOROS, Carol V. *Rape.* Gr. 10 and up. Illus. Dell, 1981. 176 pp. pap. $2.50. Nonfiction.
Rape has both legal and psychological aspects. The author discusses practical ways to prevent rape.

HOWARD, Marion. *Did I Have a Good Time?: Teenage Drinking.* Gr. 9 and up. Continuum, 1981. 161 pp. $10.95. Nonfiction.
Young people now begin drinking alcohol at an average age of thirteen years. Currently 3.3 million adolescents have alcohol abuse problems. Three young people tell their stories from their first contact with alcohol to the point at which it caused life changes. The comments of professionals are interspersed with the narrative.

HOWE, James. *The Hospital Book.* Gr. 3–4. Photog. by Mal Warshaw. Crown, 1981. 94 pp. $10.95. Nonfiction.
The jobs of hospital staff, including that of child life specialist, are described as well as the equipment used and the purpose for tests. Full-page photographs of real children, staff, procedures, and places in the hospital illustrate the detailed information. In particular, some tests not usually found in children's books are covered, such as the CAT scanner, electrocardiograph, and operating room equipment. The playroom is also shown. The feelings children have are important and are shown as a part of procedures.

HOWE, James. *A Night Without Stars.* Gr. 4–7. Atheneum, 1983. 178 pp. $10.34. Fiction.
In a conversation in the hospital, a boy who had had many operations for burns reassures young Maria about having heart surgery. In turn she helps him feel accepted once again.

HUGHES, Monica. *Hunter in the Dark.* Gr. 5–9. Atheneum, 1983. 131 pp. $9.64. Fiction.
Throughout a year of hospital care, chemotherapy, and other treatments for leukemia, Mike dreams of going hunting again. When he is able to do so he comes to terms with life and death, realizing that life must be lived fully.

HULL, Eleanor. *Alice with Golden Hair.* Gr. 7 and up. Atheneum, 1981. 186 pp. $9.95. Fiction.

At age eighteen, Alice emerges from an institution for the retarded to assume a job in a nursing home and to become part of a world she has never experienced.

HUNT, Irene. *The Lottery Rose.* Gr. 7–12. Scribner, 1976. 185 pp. $6.95; pap. Ace, $1.95. Fiction.
A seven-year-old boy, abused at home, comes to live in a boys' home and gradually learns trust, love, and friendship.

HUNT, Irene. *William.* Gr. 5–6. Scribner, 1977. 188 pp. $7.95; pap. Grosset & Dunlap, $1.95. Fiction.
One of William's sisters is blind from cataracts but has corrective surgery. When their mother dies they are cared for by a single adolescent mother who has no parents.

HUNT, Morton. *Gay: What You Should Know About Homosexuality.* Gr. 7 and up. FS&G, 1977. 210 pp. $7.95. Nonfiction.
Drawing from studies of homosexuality in American society and other cultures, the author explicitly describes forms of homosexual behavior, physical practices, variations of relationships, and the changing consciousness of the public toward gay people.

HUNT, Morton. *The Young Person's Guide to Love.* Gr. 7 and up. FS&G, 1975. 192 pp. $6.95. Nonfiction.
There are many ways to love, at different ages and intensities and for varying lengths of time. The author describes variations of physical love and the influence of ethnic origin, social class, religion, race, education, and experience.

HUNTER, Edith Fisher. *Sue Ellen.* Gr. 5–6. Illus. by Bea Holmes. HM, 1969. 170 pp. $7.95. Fiction.
Eight-year-old Sue Ellen's impoverished family is unable to provide for her needs or stimulate her learning. Her life is changed when she attends a special education class and, for the first time, has individualized teaching, adequate food, rest, and care.

HUTCHINS, Pat. *Happy Birthday, Sam.* Gr. ps–2. Illus. Greenwillow, 1978. Unp. $9.75. Fiction.
A young boy finds that, even on his birthday, he still cannot reach the light switch, doorknob, hangers, or faucets. When his grand-

father sends a small chair as a birthday gift, the boy learns he can stand on it and do things by himself.

HYDE, Margaret Oldroyd. *Cry Softly! The Story of Child Abuse.* Gr. 9–12. Westminster, 1980. 96 pp. $10.95. Nonfiction.
Child abuse is often the result of a larger emotional or psychological problem. The author suggests how to report abuse and help the abused child who feels lonely, guilty, or afraid.

HYDE, Margaret Oldroyd. *Fears and Phobias.* Gr. 6–7. McGraw-Hill, 1977. 117 pp. $10.95. Nonfiction.
Detailed descriptions of the factors and circumstances associated with common fears and phobias incorporate real-life stories and suggestions for controlling irrational fears and aversions.

HYDE, Margaret Oldroyd. *Hotline.* Gr. 9–12. McGraw-Hill, 1976. 192 pp. $6.95. Nonfiction.
A hotline is a telephone service for distressed people, especially adolescents, to talk anonymously about their problems with a trained listener. The author includes a directory of hotlines and a list of centers where runaways can get help.

HYDE, Margaret Oldroyd. *Know About Alcohol.* Gr. 4–5. Illus. by Bill Morrison. McGraw-Hill, 1978. 80 pp. $6.95. Nonfiction.
Facts about the positive and negative sides of drinking are presented. There is a difference between use and abuse. There are ways to deal with alcohol in social situations.

HYDE, Margaret Oldroyd, ed. *Mind Drugs.* Gr. 7–8. McGraw-Hill, 1974. 190 pp. $7.95. Nonfiction.
Heroin, marijuana, LSD, drug abuse, and dependency are described by various experts, whose backgrounds are given. Suggestions are offered about where to get help. A glossary of slang, generic, and chemical names for drugs is included.

HYDE, Margaret Oldroyd. *The New Genetics.* Gr. 7–8. Illus. Watts, 1974. 134 pp. $7.45. Nonfiction.
Genetic research on cystic fibrosis, sickle cell anemia, phenylketonuria, hemophilia, and cancer have made some advances, and genetic counseling has helped many couples.

HYDE, Margaret Oldroyd. *VD: The Silent Epidemic.* Gr. 6 and up. McGraw-Hill, 1981. 63 pp. $4.33. Nonfiction.
The author describes symptoms of various types of venereal diseases, their slang names, and treatment. Venereal diseases can be spread in many ways; suggestions are given for avoiding them or for getting help if symptoms appear.

HYDE, Margaret Oldroyd, and Elizabeth Held FORSYTH. *Suicide: The Hidden Epidemic.* Gr. 7 and up. Watts, 1978. 117 pp. $7.90. Nonfiction.
Statistics on adolescent suicide and information on prevention supplement an exploration of the history, patterns, causes, and effects of and misconceptions about suicide.

HYMAN, Jane. *Deafness.* Gr. 4–8. Illus. Watts, 1980. 64 pp. $6.45. Nonfiction.
The causes of deafness and the diagnostic process are described. Hearing impaired children can use hearing aids, lip reading, learned speech, sign language, and finger spelling.

IPSWITCH, Elaine. *Scott Was Here.* Gr. 6 and up. Illus. Delacorte, 1979. 210 pp. $8.95; pap. Dell, $2.25. Nonfiction.
The story of the courage of a ten-year-old boy who dies of Hodgkin's disease is told through his writings and drawings and his family's recollections.

IRELAND, Karin. *Kitty O'Neill: Daredevil Woman.* Gr. 4–5. Illus. Harvey, 1980. 76 pp. $6.59. Nonfiction.
Kitty O'Neill, although deaf, excels as a stunt woman and holds both the women's land-speed record and the all-time free-fall record.

IVERSON, Genie. *I Want to Be Big.* Gr. ps–1. Illus. by David McPhail. Dutton, 1979. Unp. $7.50. Fiction.
A little girl wants to be big enough to reach elevator buttons, eat supper at a friend's house, and outgrow a scratchy dress — but not so big that she outgrows her favorite bathrobe and night light and has to take care of herself all the time.

JACOBSEN, Karen. *Health.* Gr. k–4. Photog. by Tony Freeman. Childrens, 1981. 48 pp. $9.85. Nonfiction.

The body needs food, exercise, sleep, and proper clothing to remain healthy.

JESSEL, Camilla. *Going to the Doctor.* Gr. ps–1. Illus. Methuen, 1981. Unp. $3.95. Fiction.
When Clare has a sore throat and headache, the doctor examines her and gives her medicine to help her get well.

JETER, Katherine F. *These Special Children: The Ostomy Book for Parents of Children with Colostomies, Ileostomies and Urostomies.* Gr. 9 and up. Illus. by John R. Jeter, Jr. Bull, 1982. 192 pp. $13.95. Nonfiction.
Although written for parents, this detailed book can be understood by many adolescents. An ostomy is a technique that creates an artificial opening in the abdomen for excretion into a removable sac. Children give many suggestions, such as those fourth-graders provide on how to cope with being different.

JOHNSON, Corinne Benson, and Eric W. JOHNSON. *Love and Sex and Growing Up.* Gr. 6 and up. Illus. Lippincott, 1977. 126 pp. $8.95. Nonfiction.
The authors give the facts of human development and reproduction, with encouragement to develop a responsible attitude.

JOHNSON, Eric W. *Love and Sex in Plain Language.* Gr. 7–12. Illus. by Russ Hoover. Har-Row, 1977. 128 pp. $9.95. Nonfiction.
In straightforward style, the author discusses anatomy, intercourse, pregnancy, birth, and family planning. He also includes the social aspects of sexuality, such as peer pressure and personal choices.

JOHNSON, Eric W. *Sex: Telling It Straight.* Gr. 7–8. Illus. Lippincott, 1979. 112 pp. $8.95. Nonfiction.
The healthy and positive aspects of sex are discussed; it is emphasized that sexuality requires personal responsibility.

JOHNSON, Eric W. *VD: Venereal Disease and What You Should Do About It.* Gr. 6–7. Illus. Lippincott, 1978. 126 pp. $6.98. Nonfiction.
The author overviews venereal diseases, their symptoms and treatment, and describes a visit to a public health clinic.

JONES, Hettie. *How to Eat Your ABC's: A Book About Vitamins.* Gr. 3–6. Illus. by Judy Glasser. Four Winds, 1976. 84 pp. $7.95. Nonfiction.
Vitamins and minerals found in foods help keep the body healthy. This book offers recipes and suggests natural, well-balanced menus.

JONES, Marilyn. *Exploring Careers in Special Education.* Gr. 7–12. Rosen, 1981. 120 pp. $7.97. Nonfiction.
Special education teachers and administrators help children who are physically disabled or learning disabled to acquire knowledge and skills. The author describes the education needed and the type of work that is done.

JONES, Penelope. *Holding Together.* Gr. 3–5. Bradbury, 1982. 176 pp. $8.95. Fiction.
Nine-year-old Vickie finds comfort from her sister and father, after her mother dies, by "holding together" with them as a family.

JONES, Rebecca C. *Angie and Me.* Gr. 6–7. Macmillan, 1981. 113 pp. $7.95. Fiction.
Jenna spends the summer in the hospital being treated for juvenile rheumatoid arthritis. Her terminally ill roommate, Angie, helps her understand how to cope with the pain of swollen, tender knees, with the demands of illness, and with the limitations of what one can do. When Angie dies, Jenna must deal with that loss as well.

JORDAN, Hope D. *Haunted Summer.* Gr. 5 and up. Lothrop, 1967. 158 pp. $8.50; pap. Archway, $1.95. Fiction.
Seventeen-year-old Marilla unintentionally drives her car into a boy on a bicycle, then helps him to a hospital and disappears. While the newspaper and the townspeople talk of the mysterious hit-and-run driver, she tries to cope with overwhelming guilt. Eventually she confesses, finds that the boy has recovered, and realizes her mistake in not facing her responsibility sooner.

JOSEPHS, Rebecca. *Early Disorder.* Gr. 7–8. FS&G, 1980. 185 pp. $10.95; pap. Fawcett, $1.95. Fiction.
Willa's adolescence is difficult. In an accomplished, close family,

she feels unattractive and worthless. Her dieting results in anorexia nervosa and a struggle that she and her family make to resolve the causes of the illness.

KALB, Jonah, and David VISCOTT. *What Every Kid Should Know.* Gr. 5–6. Illus. HM, 1976. 127 pp. $5.95. Nonfiction.
An educator and a psychiatrist discuss problems of growing up. They give suggestions on coping with emotions and developing a sense of self-esteem, inner strength, and belief in one's ability to get along with others.

KALINA, Sigmund. *Your Blood and Its Cargo.* Gr. 2–5. Illus. by Arabelle Wheatley. Lothrop, 1974. 48 pp. $6.48. Nonfiction.
The book describes and illustrates the composition of blood, its circulation, and its function in sustaining life.

KALINA, Sigmund. *Your Nerves and Their Messages.* Illus. by Arabelle Wheatley. Lothrop, 1973. Gr. 2–5. 48 pp. $6.48. Nonfiction.
Nerve fibers relay messages to and from the spinal cord. The nervous system is illustrated and explained.

KAMIEN, Janet. *What If You Couldn't . . .? A Book About Special Needs.* Gr. 5–6. Illus. by Signe Hanson. Scribner, 1979. 83 pp. $9.95. Nonfiction.
Experiments enable children to feel what it is like to live with physical, emotional, and mental disabilities. People have varying ways of dealing with their hearing impairment, blindness, retardation, or paralysis.

KAPLAN, Helen Singer. *Making Sense of Sex: The New Facts About Sex and Love for Young People.* Gr. 9 and up. S&S, 1979. 154 pp. $10.95. Nonfiction.
Giving detailed facts and reassurance about teenage sexuality, the author emphasizes mutual caring relationships.

KATA, Elizabeth. *A Patch of Blue.* Gr. 7 and up. Popular Lib, 1965. 142 pp. pap. $2.25. Fiction.
A young blind woman momentarily escapes a difficult home life when a young man befriends her in the park.

KAUFMAN, Barry Neil. *Son-Rise.* Gr. 10 and up. Har-Row, 1976. 154 pp. $8.95; pap. Warner, $2.25. Nonfiction.
After grieving over their son's autism, a couple decides to make a great effort to help him develop as much as possible.

KAVALER, Lucy. *Cold Against Disease: The Wonders of Cold.* Gr. 7–9. Illus. by Andrew Antal. John Day, 1971. 158 pp. $10.95. Nonfiction.
Cold is used by physicians and researchers for storage, surgery, pain reduction, and healing.

KAY, Eleanor. *The Clinic.* Gr. 3–4. Illus. Watts, 1971. 54 pp. $5.90. Nonfiction.
Chris goes to the clinic for a checkup and learns about its functions and staff. There are clinics in hospitals, health centers, industry, mobile units, and in the armed forces; the World Health Organization sponsors clinics in other countries.

KELLEY, Alberta. *Lenses, Spectacles, Eyeglasses and Contacts: The Story of Vision Aids.* Gr. 7–8. Illus. Nelson, 1978. 98 pp. $7.95. Nonfiction.
The scientific and social history of corrected vision is presented. Eye or vision defects, such as myopia, hyperopia, astigmatism, strabismus, and Daltonism, are described, as are corrective methods and aids and the work of ophthalmologists, optometrists, and opticians.

KELLEY, Sally. *Trouble with Explosives.* Gr. 5–6. Bradbury, 1976. 117 pp. $7.95. Fiction.
Explosive sounds, such as P and B, are difficult for Polly, and she stutters. With the help of a psychiatrist, her family, and friends, she almost eliminates her stutter and learns to be assertive.

KELLY, Gary F. *Learning About Sex: The Contemporary Guide for Young Adults.* Gr. 7 and up. Illus. Barron, 1977. 188 pp. pap. $3.50. Nonfiction.
The author discusses the physical, emotional, and social aspects of sexuality, its pleasures, problems, and responsibilities.

KENT, Deborah. *Belonging.* Gr. 5 and up. Dial, 1978. 200 pp. $7.95; pap. Ace, $1.95. Fiction.

Meg, who is blind, insists on attending public high school rather than a special school. She makes some friends and helps with the school magazine. Eventually she sorts out the group of people whose company she prefers.

KERR, M. E. *Dinky Hocker Shoots Smack.* Gr. 6–7. Har-Row, 1972. 198 pp. $9.95; pap. Dell, $1.50. Fiction.
Dinky fails in her attempt to lose weight, despite encouragement from a new friend who is also obese. On the night her mother is to be honored for charity work at a banquet, Dinky paints the title of this story on a wall. This act mobilizes her parents' attention, and they recognize the need to help her.

KERR, M. E. *I've Love You When You're More Like Me.* Gr. 9 and up. Har-Row, 1977. 183 pp. $9.89. Fiction.
Teenager Sabra wants to be an actress but has to deal with emotional problems and ulcers. Her friends, including one who is gay, help her explore her individuality.

KESSLER, Ethel, and Leonard KESSLER. *Two, Four, Six, Eight: A Book About Legs.* Gr. ps–3. Illus. by Leonard Kessler. Dodd, 1980. 46 pp. $7.95. Nonfiction.
The authors compare animal and human legs and locomotion.

KETTELKAMP, Larry. *Dreams.* Gr. 5–9. Illus. Morrow, 1968. 96 pp. $7.63. Nonfiction.
The way people sleep and dream has been researched for years. Dreaming is important for mental health. The author explains the stages of sleep and discusses the study by parapsychologists of dreams that seem to predict the future.

KETTELKAMP, Larry. *The Healing Arts.* Gr. 6–7. Illus. Morrow, 1978. 128 pp. $7.44. Nonfiction.
The philosophies and practices of methods of healing are surveyed, including the manipulative, medicinal, mental, natural, spiritual, and surgical.

KETTELKAMP, Larry. *Hypnosis: The Wakeful Sleep.* Gr. 5–9. Illus. by the author. Morrow, 1975. 96 pp. $7.95. Nonfiction.
Hypnosis is a state of altered consciousness. It can be used as an anesthetic in some surgery, obstetrics, and dentistry, and as therapy for personality disturbances.

KETTELKAMP, Larry. *Lasers: The Miracle Light*. Gr. 4–7. Illus. Morrow, 1979. 128 pp. $7.44. Nonfiction.
This book offers nontechnical explanations about lasers and their important applications in medicine and other fields.

KETTELKAMP, Larry. *A Partnership of Mind and Body: Biofeedback*. Gr. 7–8. Illus. Morrow, 1976. 96 pp. $7.63. Nonfiction.
People can control unconscious body functions through an effort of will that makes those functions, such as blood pressure and brain waves, perceptible to the senses.

KETTELKAMP, Larry. *Sixth Sense*. Gr. 5–9. Illus. by the author. Morrow, 1970. 95 pp. $7.63. Nonfiction.
Psychic experiences include extrasensory perception, telepathy, and clairvoyance. The author describes investigations conducted to test the validity of such experiences and to see how they can help people understand and use more of their own abilities.

KEYES, Fenton. *Your Future in a Paramedic Career*. Gr. 7–12. Illus. Rosen, 1979. 132 pp. $7.97. Nonfiction.
In emergencies paramedics examine the patient, coordinate information and treatment by phone with a physician at a medical center, and bring the patient to an emergency room when necessary. The training and work of paramedics is described.

KEYES, Fenton. *Your Future in Social Work*. Gr. 7–12. Illus. Rosen, 1978. 160 pp. $7.97. Nonfiction.
In describing the education and responsibilities of a social worker, the author presents such workers as a personal resource in times of emotional need.

KIDD, Ronald. *That's What Friends Are For*. Gr. 7–9. Nelson, 1978. 127 pp. $6.96. Fiction.
For Gary and Scott a summer filled with friendship comes to an end when Gary learns that he is dying of leukemia. Feelings of fear, guilt, and sadness are explored in a story that also has humor.

KIEV, Ari. *The Courage to Live*. Gr. 10 and up. Crowell, 1979. 148 pp. $7.95. Nonfiction.

Depressed people can be helped to recognize and understand the motivation behind their self-destructive acts. The author suggests ways to help depressed people.

KINGMAN, Lee. *Head over Wheels.* Gr. 5 and up. HM, 1978. 186 pp. $8.95. Fiction.
Seventeen-year-old twin brothers are injured in a car accident; one of them becomes a quadriplegic. Each family member is affected. The story emphasizes courage, hope, and a maturing process, as well as humor.

KINGMAN, Lee. *The Peter Pan Bag.* Gr. 7–8. HM, 1970. 219 pp. $5.95; pap. Dell, $1.50. Fiction.
When seventeen-year-old Wendy runs away from home, she becomes involved with a group of people who take drugs. She admires them for being individuals and doing what they prefer. After she experiments with drugs and loses a friend who becomes emotionally ill and is hospitalized, and another friend who accidentally dies, Wendy decides to go back to her family.

KIPNIS, Lynne, and Susan ADLER. *You Can't Catch Diabetes from a Friend.* Gr. 4–5. Photog. by Richard Benkof. Triad Pub FL, 1979. 63 pp. $9.95. Nonfiction.
The lives of four young children who have diabetes give insights into the effects of this disease on children, their families, and their friends.

KLAGSBRUN, Francine. *Too Young to Die: Youth and Suicide.* HM, 1976. 201 pp. $6.95; pap. Pocket Bks, $2.50. Nonfiction.
Through research, case histories, and conversations with suicidal young people and their friends, the author explores the motives underlying suicide among youths. She suggests ways to recognize symptoms of depression.

KLEIMAN, Gary, and Sandford DODY. *No Time to Lose.* Gr. 7 and up. Morrow, 1983. 284 pp. $13.95. Nonfiction.
The first author became diabetic at six years of age and blind at eighteen, later developing kidney problems. With humor, courage, and determination, he pursued as normal a life as possible and is currently a counselor in a university diabetic unit.

KLEIN, Aaron E. *Medical Tests and You*. Gr. 9–12. Illus. by Carol Basen. Grosset & Dunlap, 1977. 124 pp. pap. $4.95. Nonfiction.
Diagnostic tests are described and illustrated with photographs and drawings. The reason for each test is explained, the pain or discomfort anticipated, and risks and side effects noted. Procedures include X rays and passages of tubes and catheters.

KLEIN, Aaron E. *You and Your Body: A Book of Experiments to Perform on Yourself*. Gr. 4–5. Illus. by John Lane. Doubleday, 1977. 95 pp. $7.95. Nonfiction.
A series of simple experiments introduce the basic systems of the body and how they function.

KLEIN, Gerda Weissmann. *The Blue Rose*. Gr. 3–7. Photog. by Norma Holt. Lawrence Hill, 1974. 64 pp. $8.95; pap. Lawrence Hill, $3.95. Nonfiction.
With lyrical symbolism a mother writes of the special qualities of her daughter, who is retarded.

KLEIN, Norma. *Confessions of an Only Child*. Gr. 4–5. Illus. by Richard Cuffari. Pantheon, 1974. 93 pp. $5.95; pap. Dell, $1.25. Fiction.
Antonia enjoys being an only child but accepts a new baby in the family after her infant brother dies.

KNIGHT, David C. *Silent Sound: The World of Ultrasonics*. Gr. 7–8. Illus. Morrow, 1980. 93 pp. $6.95. Nonfiction.
Ultrasound is sound at an extremely high frequency. Among its uses are eye surgery, the safe detection of kidney stones and tumors, measurement of a fetus, diagnosis of the extent of burns, cleaning of instruments and teeth, and therapy in which ultrasonic vibrations create internal heat.

KNIGHT, David C. *Viruses: Life's Smallest Enemies*. Gr. 4–5. Diagrams by Christine Kettner. Morrow, 1981. 127 pp. $7.95. Nonfiction.
Viruses are a major cause of human disease. They damage healthy cells and cause such illnesses as cancer, polio, and the common cold.

KNIGHT, David C. *Your Body's Defenses.* Gr. 5–6. Illus. McGraw-Hill, 1975. 95 pp. $8.95. Nonfiction.
The body has protective and defensive response systems and immunity processes, including skin and mucous membranes, antigens, antibodies, and postrecovery defenses. There are ways to reinforce their effectiveness.

KOTTLER, Dorothy, and Eleanor WILLIS. *I Really Like Myself.* Gr. ps–1. Illus. by J. William Myers. Aurora, 1974. Unp. $2.95. Nonfiction.
Young people share the ways they have learned to develop self-esteem in order to cope with problems of growing up.

KREMENTZ, Jill. *How It Feels When a Parent Dies.* Gr. 3 and up. Photog. by the author. Knopf, 1981. 111 pp. $9.95. Nonfiction.
Eighteen children from seven to sixteen years of age talk of their experiences and emotions when their parents died. The photographs and stories tell of hearing the news of the death, funerals, grieving, physical effects, and feelings of confusion, anguish, guilt, sadness, and anger.

KRISHEF, Robert K. *Our Remarkable Feet.* Gr. 4–5. Illus. by Harold K. Lamson. Lerner, 1968. 46 pp. $3.95. Nonfiction.
The structure and uses of the foot are shown.

KROLL, Steven. *That Makes Me Mad!* Gr. k–3. Illus. by Hilary Knight. Pantheon, 1976. 36 pp. $5.99. Fiction.
Cartoon drawings, statements, and vignettes show situations that make a child angry.

KROPP, Paul. *Wilted.* Gr. 6–12. Coward, 1980. 111 pp. $7.95; pap. Dell, $1.75. Fiction.
In addition to adolescent concerns and family problems, fourteen-year-old Danny has to begin wearing glasses.

LAIKEN, Deidre S., and Alan J. SCHNEIDER. *Listen to Me, I'm Angry.* Gr. 7–8. Illus. by Bernice Myers. Lothrop, 1980. 125 pp. $7.44. Nonfiction.
All people experience negative feelings on occasion. In reassuring terms the reader is told how to recognize, accept, and constructively express feelings of anger.

LANCE, James W. *Headache: Understanding, Alleviation.* Gr. 6 and up. Illus. Scribner, 1975. 232 pp. $8.95; pap. Scribner, $3.45. Nonfiction.
The author explains the causes and symptoms of various kinds of headaches, including migraine. He details proven and likely preventive and remedial procedures and medications.

LANDAU, Elaine. *Death: Everyone's Heritage.* Gr. 7–8. Messner, 1976. 127 pp. $7.29. Nonfiction.
Various aspects of death are discussed, such as euthanasia, suicide, caring for the terminally ill, and cremation.

LANDAU, Elaine. *Why Are They Starving Themselves?: Understanding Anorexia Nervosa and Bulimia.* Gr. 9 and up. Messner, 1983. 160 pp. $9.29. Nonfiction.
People who have had either anorexia nervosa or bulimia, two of the major eating problems, tell their personal stories, emphasizing physical and emotional aspects. Centers and programs are listed that specialize in treatment.

LANE, Donald. *Asthma: The Facts.* Gr. 10 and up. Oxford, 1979. 163 pp. $11.95. Nonfiction.
The causes, symptoms, and specific treatments of asthma are known, but patients do even better with knowledge about themselves and by helping themselves.

LANGONE, John. *Death Is a Noun: A View of the End of Life.* Gr. 7–8. Little, 1972. 228 pp. $7.95. Nonfiction.
A medical journalist discusses abortion, suicide, and euthanasia in this examination of the moral and legal aspects of death.

LANGONE, John. *Goodby to Bedlam: Understanding Mental Illness and Retardation.* Gr. 10–12. Little, 1974. 168 pp. $5.95. Nonfiction.
Social attitudes toward mental illness and retardation have changed. The causes of, and therapy for, neuroses, character disorders, schizophrenia, retardation, psychosomatic disorders, and brain dysfunctions are described.

LANGONE, John. *Like, Love, Lust: A View of Sex and Sexuality.* Gr. 7–12. Avon, 1981. 143 pp. pap. $2.25. Nonfiction.

A candid treatment of sex and love examines such subjects as sex education, homosexuality, romantic love, platonic relationships, pornography, and jealousy.

LAPP, Carolyn. *Dentist's Tools.* Gr. 2–3. Illus. by George Overlie. Lerner, 1973. 30 pp. $3.95. Nonfiction.
Drawings and information explain thirty-two items dentists use to care for teeth, including the explorer, scaler, aspirator, burs, and amalgam carrier.

LARRANAGA, Robert D. *Sniffles.* Gr. 2–3. Illus. by Patricia S. Seitz. Carolrhoda, 1973. Unp. $5.95. Fiction.
An unusual toy dog remains on the department-store shelf until a little boy who is allergic to stuffed animals comes along.

LARSEN, Hanne. *Don't Forget Tom.* Gr. k–4. Illus. Trans. from the Danish by Peggy Blakely. Crowell, 1978. Unp. $9.89. Fiction.
Six-year-old Tom, who is brain injured, gets sad and angry when he cannot care for himself or do what other children do. His family and home teacher help him do handicrafts, cook, and play music. He learns self-care and takes his medication.

LASKER, Joe. *He's My Brother.* Gr. 4–5. Illus. by the author. A Whitman, 1974. 38 pp. $8.25. Fiction.
A warm, close family copes with the learning disability of its youngest child, Jamie. He feels inadequate but loved. Although not retarded Jamie has difficulty making judgments in social situations, learning basic school subjects, and taking tests.

LASKER, Joe. *Nick Joins In.* Gr. 2–3. Illus. by the author. A Whitman, 1980. 32 pp. $8.25. Fiction.
Going from home instruction to public school, Nick is afraid as he enters a regular classroom in his wheelchair for the first time. His parents and teachers help him adjust to the activity and space. His classmates, although curious at first, include him in classroom activities and games. He helps other children, too.

LEE, Essie E. *Alcohol: Proof of What?* Gr. 7–8. Illus. Messner, 1976. 191 pp. $8.79. Nonfiction.
True stories of young people who cope with alcoholism in a parent, relative, or themselves describe the effects of alcohol abuse on the body and on family relationships.

LEE, H. Alton. *Seven Feet Four and Growing.* Gr. 7–9. Westminster, 1978. 95 pp. $7.50. Fiction.
Fifteen-year-old Bill must adjust to remarks people make about his height and to his need for oversize clothes, bed, and space. He meets a tall girl, who encourages him to become more confident.

LEE, Mary Price. *A Future in Pediatrics: Medical and Non-Medical Careers in Child Health Care.* Gr. 9 and up. Illus. Messner, 1982. 159 pp. $9.29. Nonfiction.
The child health specialties include pediatric medicine, nursing, social work, psychiatry, medical technology, physical therapy, and nutrition.

LEE, Mildred Scudder. *The Skating Rink.* Gr. 7–8. Seabury, 1969. 126 pp. $7.95. Fiction.
Sixteen-year-old Tuck has stuttered since he saw his mother drown when he was three years old. He is unhappy and unsettled until he is encouraged by a man who teaches him exhibition skating. Tuck becomes successful, has more control of his body, feels better about himself, and begins to understand his lonely sister and his stepmother better.

LEE, Robert C. *It's a Mile from Here to Glory.* Gr. 7–8. Little, 1972. 150 pp. $7.95. Fiction.
Sixteen-year-old Early is short and does not get along with his peers, but he runs well. Injuries from a motorcycle accident, and hospitalization, prevent him from further competition. Early's physical therapist and coach help him rehabilitate his body and spirit so he is able to enter the state track meet. He learns to feel better about himself and his friends.

LEE, Virginia. *The Magic Moth.* Gr. 3–4. Illus. by Richard Cuffari. HM, 1972. 63 pp. $7.95. Fiction.
While ten-year-old Maryanne is dying of heart disease, a white moth comes out of a cocoon that she has treasured. Her family sees it coming to life as her spirit is being released. They begin to understand the positive effect her life has had on them.

LEGGETT, Linda Rodgers, and Linda Gambee ANDREWS. *The Rose-Colored Glasses: Melanie Adjusts to Poor Vision.* Gr. 2–4.

Illus. by Laura Hartman. Human Sci Pr, 1979. 31 pp. $7.95. Fiction.
After a car accident leaves her with a visual impairment, a young girl tries to adjust to wearing rose-tinted bifocal glasses and, with the teacher's help, tells her classmates what it is like to have low vision.

LERNER, Marguerite Rush. *Color and People: The Story of Pigmentation.* Gr. k–6. Illus. Lerner, 1971. Unp. $5.95. Nonfiction.
Skin pigmentation performs similar functions for humans and animals. The author discusses the scientific and medical aspects of skin color in simple terms.

LERNER, Marguerite Rush. *Lefty: The Story of Left-Handedness.* Gr. 1–4. Illus. by Rov Andre. Lerner, 1960. 32 pp. $3.95. Nonfiction.
Although most people are right-handed, those who are left-handed find ways to adapt. The author overviews the causes, characteristics, and studies of left-handedness.

LERNER, Marguerite Rush. *Twins: The Story of Twins.* Gr. k–6. Illus. by Lawrence Spiegel. Lerner, 1961. Unp. $4.95. Nonfiction.
The author explains how twins are formed and the difference between identical and fraternal twins.

LESH, Terry. *Meditation for Young People.* Gr. 6 and up. Lothrop, 1977. 128 pp. $5.95. Nonfiction.
The author describes in detail various forms of meditation, including biofeedback and stress-reducing relaxation.

LeSHAN, Eda J. *Learning to Say Good-By: When a Parent Dies.* Gr. 3 and up. Illus. by Paul Giovanopoulos. Macmillan, 1976. $5.95; pap. Avon, $3.95. Nonfiction.
After a parent dies children need love, attention, and explanations from an adult who understands their feelings of loss and their fears and fantasies.

LeSHAN, Eda J. *What Makes Me Feel This Way? Growing Up with Human Emotions.* Gr. 4–7. Illus. by Lisl Weil. Macmillan, 1972. 128 pp. $8.95; pap. Macmillan, $1.95. Nonfiction.

Feelings are important and need to be understood so that people can feel all right about themselves. Examples are given to explain the influence of feelings on everyday experiences.

LeSIEG, Theo. *The Eye Book*. Gr. 1–2. Illus. by Roy McKie. Random House, 1968. Unp. $4.99. Nonfiction.
Rhymes and pictures tell young children what eyes can see.

LEVINE, Edna S. *Lisa and Her Soundless World*. Gr. 2–3. Illus. by Gloria Kamen. Human Sci Pr, 1974. Unp. $9.95. Fiction.
The children will not play with eight-year-old Lisa because she does not talk. After a physician diagnoses hearing loss, her parents buy a hearing aid for her and enroll her in a special school to learn sign language and lip reading as well as academics. Now she can hear some sounds and begins to learn to say words. Although it is unusual that Lisa's deafness is discovered so late, the story's details help the reader understand deafness well.

LEVINSON, Nancy. *World of Her Own*. Gr. 7–8. Harvey, 1981. 128 pp. $6.59. Fiction.
Annie's family moves her from a private school for the deaf to the local high school's mainstreaming program. Although Annie is overwhelmed at first by uncaring, thoughtless teachers and classmates, eventually she accommodates to her new school and friends. She especially enjoys a friendship with another deaf classmate who reads lips as she does.

LEVOY, Myron. *Alan and Naomi*. Gr. 6 and up. Har-Row, 1977. 192 pp. $9.89. Fiction.
Twelve-year-old Alan tries to be friends with Naomi, a Jewish refugee whose father was killed by Nazi police. When she witnesses Alan beaten by anti-Semitic bullies, she withdraws emotionally and is hospitalized for mental health care.

LIEBERMAN, E. James, and Ellen PECK. *Sex and Birth Control: A Guide for the Young*. Gr. 9 and up. Har-Row, 1981. 277 pp. $11.95. Nonfiction.
An overview is given of birth control, abortion, venereal diseases, pregnancy, marriage, and parenthood. Social, moral, and psychological points of view about being sexually active are discussed.

LIETZ, Gerald S. *Bacteria.* Gr. 2–5. Illus. by Stephen Peck. Garrard, 1964. 65 pp. $4.98. Nonfiction.
Bacteria are one-celled plants or microorganisms. Bacteria serve many useful purposes. Germs are harmful bacteria causing infection and disease.

LIFTON, Betty Jean, and Thomas C. FOX. *Children of Vietnam.* Gr. 6–7. Photog. by Thomas C. Fox. Atheneum, 1972. 111 pp. $4.95. Nonfiction.
Two journalists report the medical and psychological effects on children of the war in Vietnam, with details on burns, loss of limbs, and deaths occurring after bombings and raids.

LIMBURG, Peter. *Story of Your Heart.* Gr. 3–7. Illus. by Ellen Going Jacobs. Coward, 1979. 94 pp. $6.99. Nonfiction.
This book details a heart operation and explains the anatomy and physiology of the heart. It discusses congenital heart defects and other heart problems and gives suggestions for keeping the heart healthy.

LINDSAY, Rae. *The Left-Handed Book.* Gr. 4 and up. Illus. Watts, 1980. 63 pp. $7.90. Nonfiction.
The author dismisses the superstitions about left-handed people and notes famous left-handers who excelled.

LINDSAY, Rae. *Sleep and Dreams.* Gr. 4 and up. Illus. by Leigh Grant. Watts, 1978. 63 pp. $7.90. Nonfiction.
The author describes the sleep habits of humans and animals, including sleepwalking, sleeptalking, snoring and insomnia.

LIPKE, Jean Coryllel. *Conception and Contraception.* Gr. 5–11. Illus. by Robert Fontaine. Lerner, 1971. 54 pp. $4.95. Nonfiction.
The author includes the responsibilities of conception in this detailed description of reproduction and contraceptive methods.

LIPKE, Jean Coryllel. *Heredity.* Gr. 5–7. Illus. by Patricia Bateman. Lerner, 1971. 61 pp. $3.95. Nonfiction.
Drawings and diagrams help explain inherited illnesses, blood types, the effects of drugs on a fetus, and the benefits and drawbacks of genetic engineering.

LIPKE, Jean Coryllel. *Puberty and Adolescence.* Gr. 5–12. Illus. by Patricia Bateman. Lerner, 1971. 43 pp. $4.95. Nonfiction.
The author describes the physical and emotional characteristics of adolescence, such as menstruation, night emissions, and fluctuations in mood. She also advises on personal care, such as shaving and the use of deodorants.

LIPSON, Tony, and the staff of the Royal Alexandra Hospital for Children. *Benjamin Goes to Hospital: An Introduction to Hospital for Children and Parents.* Gr. 1–3. Illus. by Bruce Treloar. Golden Pr (Sydney), 1979. 30 pp. $5.00. Fiction.
Mother explains to Benjamin why he has to be hospitalized for a tonsillectomy. He meets other children there and plays. Mother has to leave, but Daddy visits after work. Benjamin has an X ray, and a sample of his blood is drawn. The anesthetist and nurse explain about surgery. After Benjamin recovers he goes home and considers the experience exciting. Notes for parents urge them to understand and accept children's fears about being in the hospital and to prepare them for it.

LIPSYTE, Robert. *One Fat Summer.* Gr. 7 and up. Har-Row, 1977. 152 pp. $8.79; pap. Bantam, $1.75. Fiction.
Bobby, who weighs two hundred pounds, goes out in the summer only when it is cool enough to cover himself with clothes. He is persuaded by his friend to take a job looking after a doctor's estate, and he begins to think of himself differently.

LISKER, Sonia O. *Lost.* Gr. ps–3. Illus. by the author. HarBraceJ, 1975. 48 pp. $6.75. Fiction.
The pictures in this book convey the fears of a child who is separated from his parents while visiting the zoo. He helps himself feel better by comforting a younger child who is also lost.

LITCHFIELD, Ada Bassett. *A Button in Her Ear.* Gr. 2–4. Illus. by Eleanor Mill. A Whitman, 1976. 32 pp. $8.25. Fiction.
Angela's hearing loss is diagnosed by her physician and an audiologist. She learns to use a hearing aid and explains its advantages to her classmates.

LITCHFIELD, Ada Bassett. *A Cane in Her Hand.* Gr. 4–5. Illus. by Eleanor Mill. A Whitman, 1977. Unp. $8.25. Fiction.

Valerie learns fuller use of her senses and the advantages of a cane when her low vision gets worse. A special teacher and materials for children who are visually impaired help her manage schoolwork. She deals with her feelings of fear, anger, and then pride at mastering cane travel.

LITCHFIELD, Ada Bassett. *Captain Hook, That's Me.* Gr. 2–6. Illus. by Sonia O. Lisker. Walker, 1982. 32 pp. $8.95. Fiction.
Eight-year-old Judy, who can run and skate and do lots of things well, is afraid the children in her new school will feel sorry for her because she has a steel hook instead of a left hand.

LITTLE, Jean. *From Anna.* Gr. 4–6. Illus. by Joan Sandlin. Har-Row, 1973. 208 pp. pap. $2.95. Fiction.
Not until nine-year-old Anna and her family flee Nazi Germany and settle in Canada do they find that her inability to read is the result of vision impairment. Anna develops confidence with the help of glasses, a special-class teacher who encourages her growing ability to read and teaches her classmates to be more accepting, and her father's belief in her.

LITTLE, Jean. *Listen for the Singing.* Gr. 6–7. Dutton, 1977. 215 pp. $9.95. Fiction.
Anna's vision impairment makes high school difficult. Coping with it, and with her family's problems in a new country, matures her, and she is able to help her family as well.

LITTLE, Jean. *Mine for Keeps.* Gr. 4–6. Illus. by Lewis Parker. Little, 1962. 186 pp. $9.95. Fiction.
Sally moves from a residential school for the handicapped to her family's home. Now she has to explain cerebral palsy and her crutches to new friends, cope with schoolwork in a regular school, and get used to caring more for herself.

LITTLE, Jean. *Take Wing.* Gr. 7–8. Illus. by Jerry Lazare. Little, 1968. 176 pp. $7.95. Fiction.
Laurel has to care for her younger brother, who is retarded. She has no friends or time for herself. Their parents are at first unwilling to acknowledge the boy's disability or Laurel's need for friendships, but they are convinced by an aunt. Laurel's parents try to place the boy in a special class, although school personnel are not

helpful at first. Laurel begins to make friends and develop her own life.

LIVINGSTON, Carole. *I'll Never Be Fat Again!* Gr. 6 and up. Lyle Stuart, 1980. 287 pp. $12.00; pap. Ballantine, $2.50. Nonfiction.
Able to lose weight and keep it off despite her love of eating, the author tells what she has learned about weight and figure control after an adolescence and young adulthood spent on pills, medicines, physicians, and psychiatrists.

LOEBL, Suzanne. *Conception, Contraception: A New Look.* Gr. 9 and up. Illus. McGraw-Hill, 1974. 144 pp. $6.95. Nonfiction.
Many scientists, especially Margaret Sanger, have studied reproduction and population control. The author includes information on methods of contraception and the work of Dr. Sanger.

LONDON, Kathy, and Frank CAPARULO. *Who Am I? Who Are You?: Coping with Friends, Feelings, and Other Teenage Dilemmas.* Gr. 10 and up. Addison-Wesley, 1983. 144 pp. pap. $6.95. Nonfiction.
Using letters from teenagers, the book describes situations and offers suggestions for developing mature relationships and building self-esteem.

LOW, Joseph. *Little Though I Be.* Gr. ps–3. Illus. by the author. McGraw-Hill, 1976. Unp. $5.95. Fiction.
Feeling that his father favors his two brothers, who are tall and strong, a little boy seeks the help of his animal friends to gain his father's recognition of his special trait—his intelligence.

LOWRY, Lois. *A Summer to Die.* Gr. 5–6. Illus. by Jenni Oliver. HM, 1977. 154 pp. $8.95; pap. Bantam, $1.95. Fiction.
Meg has envied her sister's beauty, popularity, and happiness. Now she must face her sister's death from leukemia.

LUBOWE, Irwin I., and Barbara HUSS. *A Teen-Age Guide to Healthy Skin and Hair.* Gr. 7 and up. Illus. Dutton, 1979. 222 pp. $12.50. Nonfiction.
In addition to advice on keeping healthy, Dr. Lubowe discusses acne, allergies, cancer, sexually transmitted diseases, and viruses.

LUND, Doris Herold. *Eric.* Gr. 10–12. Lippincott, 1974. 345 pp. $11.95; pap. Dell, $2.25. Nonfiction.
Eric, an adolescent who has terminal leukemia, strives to participate in school, athletics, and social life as much as possible through treatment and a positive outlook.

McCoy, Kathy. *The Teenage Body Book Guide to Sexuality.* Gr. 9–12. Illus. by Bob Stover. Wallaby, 1983. 128 pp. pap. $7.95. Nonfiction.
The author discusses the sexual feelings of teenagers and answers questions concerning puberty, sexual activity, birth control, sexually transmitted diseases, and pregnancy.

MACCRACKEN, Mary. *Lovey: A Very Special Child.* Gr. 9–12. Signet, 1977. 189 pp. pap. $1.95. Fiction.
An eight-year-old child who had been physically and emotionally abused becomes emotionally ill. She is helped by a dedicated teacher in a school for children with severe emotional disturbances.

McGUIRE, Leslie. *Susan Perl's Human Body Book.* Gr. 2–3. Illus. Platt, 1977. Unp. $7.95. Nonfiction.
Pictures of children of different racial and ethnic backgrounds accompany a simple explanation of the functions of the skeleton, skin, muscles, brain, lungs, and heart.

MACK, Nancy. *Tracy.* Gr. 2–3. Photog. by Heinz Kluetmeier. Raintree, 1976. 31 pp. $11.15. Nonfiction.
Tracy, who has cerebral palsy, goes to school with children who have no apparent disabilities and learns to manage well.

McKILLIP, Patricia. *The Night Gift.* Gr. 6–9. Illus. by Kathy McKillip. Atheneum, 1976. 192 pp. $6.95; pap. Atheneum, $1.95. Fiction.
Claudia is self-conscious about her cleft palate, for which she has had several corrective operations. She and her friend Barbara and several others decorate a room for Barbara's brother, Joe, who is returning home after hospitalization for attempted suicide. Doing something for someone else helps Claudia feel better about herself.

MACLACHLAN, Patricia. *The Sick Day.* Gr. 2–3. Illus. by William Pene du Bois. Pantheon, 1979. Unp. $6.95. Fiction.
When Emily catches the flu, her father takes care of her while her mother goes to work. When her father catches the flu, Emily comforts him.

McLAREN, Annabel, ed. *Going to Hospital.* Gr. ps–3. Illus. by Sara Silcock. Macdonald, 1980. 28 pp. $3.00. Fiction.
When Emma is hospitalized for asthma, she is examined, plays in the waiting area playroom, has medicine, uses masks, and meets the other children. Emma's mother stays overnight with her. A therapist gives Emma exercises and teaches her mother how to help Emma with the exercises at home. Games and activities are suggested for the reader.

McLENDON, Gloria H. *My Brother Joey Died.* Gr. 4–6. Photog. by Harvey Kelman. Messner, 1982. 64 pp. $8.29. Fiction.
A child goes through a difficult adjustment to the sudden illness and death of her younger brother.

McNAMARA, Louise Greep, and Ada Bassett LITCHFIELD. *Your Busy Brain.* Gr. 2–3. Illus. by Ruth Hartshorn. Little, 1973. 31 pp. $5.95. Nonfiction.
The structure and functions of the human brain are explained.

McPHAIL, David. *The Bear's Toothache.* Gr. k–3. Illus. by the author. Little, 1972. Unp. $9.95; pap. Penguin, $2.95. Fiction.
A young boy helps a bear take out its aching tooth.

McPHEE, Richard. *Tom and Bear: The Training of a Guide Dog Team.* Gr. 5 and up. Photog. by the author. Crowell, 1981. 149 pp. $9.89. Nonfiction.
In diary format the author gives his observations of a young blind man growing in his ability to work with a Guide Dog.

McQUADE, Walter, and Ann AIKMAN. *Stress: What It Is, What It Can Do to Your Health, How to Fight Back.* Gr. 10 and up. Bantam, 1975. 246 pp. pap. $1.95. Nonfiction.
Chronic stress can lead to cancer, colitis, and hypertension. The authors suggest ways to recognize and diminish stress.

MADDUX, Hilary C. *Menstruation*. Gr. 10 and up. Illus. Tobey, 1975. 210 pp. $5.95; pap. Tobey, $2.95. Nonfiction.
Following a description of female anatomy and physiology, the author suggests a balanced diet, exercise, and medical care for unusual problems. She emphasizes positive attitudes of self-care during menstruation.

MADISON, Arnold. *Drugs and You*. Gr. 5–6. Illus. Messner, 1971. 80 pp. $7.29; pap. Pocket Bks, $1.50. Nonfiction.
The uses and effects of such drugs as alcohol, heroin, caffeine, and LSD are discussed, as well as the problems of addiction, illegal production, and sales.

MADISON, Arnold. *Smoking and You*. Gr. 4 and up. Photog. Messner, 1975. 64 pp. $5.29. Nonfiction.
The author presents the history of smoking and describes how smoking affects the lungs, heart, and other organs.

MADISON, Arnold. *Suicide and Young People*. Gr. 6 and up. Seabury, 1978. 146 pp. $6.95; pap. HM, $3.95. Nonfiction.
Suicide is now the second highest killer of people between ten and twenty-four years of age. Suicidal equivalents are combining alcohol or drugs with driving. Many groups work to help young people cope with relationships and circumstances that could lead to such attempts.

MADISON, Winifred. *Growing Up in a Hurry*. Gr. 6–7. Little, 1973. 168 pp. $6.95; pap. Pocket Bks, $1.75. Fiction.
Sixteen-year-old Karen stutters when she is with her rich, busy, disinterested parents, who, she thinks, prefer her attractive sisters to her. With her boyfriend, however, she feels cared for and does not stutter. When Karen becomes pregnant, her mother finally gets involved and persuades her to have an abortion.

MADSEN, Jane M., with Diane Bockoras. *Please Don't Tease Me*. Gr. 2–3. Illus. by Kathleen T. Brinko. Judson, 1983. 32 pp. $3.50. Fiction.
A young girl is reassured by her mother when classmates tease her about her appearance. She has leukocytoclastic angiitis, which has resulted in arthritis and swellings. The story is designed to encourage empathy toward and understanding of disabled people.

MANES, Stephen. *I'll Live.* Gr. 7–12. Avon, 1982. 157 pp. pap. $2.25. Fiction.
Eighteen-year-old Dylan's father, who is dying of cancer, commits suicide. Dylan considers suicide as well but his attempt fails and he decides to live.

MANN, Peggy. *Twelve Is Too Old.* Gr. 6–7. Doubleday, 1980. 139 pp. $8.95. Fiction.
Eleven-year-old Jody's sister uses drugs. Jody dreads her upcoming twelfth birthday and the problems of adolescence that she anticipates.

MARCUS, June Z. *Susan.* Gr. 1–4. Illus. by Diane Dawson. NAVH, 1979. 37 pp. $7.50. Fiction.
Susan is unwilling to become friends with Maria, who has a vision impairment, until new friends persuade her that Maria can do most activities and is a good friend.

MARCUS, Rebecca B. *Being Blind.* Gr. 5 and up. Illus. Hastings, 1981. 119 pp. $9.95. Nonfiction.
The causes and problems of blindness are discussed as well as the ways blind people cope with their handicap. New methods and programs for rehabilitating and educating the blind are explained.

MARINO, Barbara Pavis. *Eric Needs Stitches.* Gr. 5–8. Photog. by Richard Rudinski. Addison-Wesley, 1979. 30 pp. $7.95. Fiction.
Eric needs reassurance when his dad brings him to the emergency room for stitches. His father is in the room during the procedure and holds his hand. The doctor shows Eric the instruments and explains what he is doing, telling Eric he should be proud of himself for holding still even when it hurts.

MARKS, Jane. *Help: A Guide to Counseling and Therapy Without a Hassle.* Gr. 7–8. Messner, 1976. 190 pp. $7.79; pap. Dell, $1.75. Nonfiction.
Teenagers can get help in choosing and benefiting from professional counseling or therapy. The author explains the advantages and disadvantages of individual and group therapy, ways of dealing with parents, and methods of determining progress.

MARR, John S. *A Breath of Air and a Breath of Smoke.* Gr. 3–7. Illus. by Lynn Sweat. Evans, 1971. 48 pp. $4.95. Nonfiction.

The author explains what happens inside the body every time a breath is taken and how the lungs and other organs are affected when smoke from cigarettes is inhaled.

MARR, John S. *The Food You Eat.* Gr. 3–4. Illus. by Lynn Sweat. Evans, 1973. 47 pp. $4.95. Nonfiction.
The ways in which foods are digested and utilized by the body are discussed.

MARSHALL, Shelly. *Young, Sober and Free.* Gr. 10 and up. Hazelden Fdn, 1978. 137 pp. $4.95. Nonfiction.
Personal stories of people who are recovered alcoholics encourage young readers to avoid alcohol use.

MASSIE, Robert K., and Suzanne MASSIE. *Journey.* Gr. 9–12. Illus. Knopf, 1975. 417 pp. $12.50; pap. Warner Bks, $1.95. Nonfiction.
Parents of an eighteen-year-old boy who has hemophilia document his lifelong struggle to stay alive and the emotional and psychological adjustments he and his parents have to make.

MATHIS, Sharon Bell. *Listen for the Fig Tree.* Gr. 6–7. Viking, 1974. 175 pp. $9.95; pap. Avon, $1.95. Fiction.
A blind teenager copes with the usual adolescent concerns as well as family problems, such as her mother's alcohol abuse. Her character is developed as she finds the strength and determination to deal with life.

MATHIS, Sharon Bell. *Teacup Full of Roses.* Gr. 7–8. Viking, 1972. 125 pp. $8.95; pap. Avon, $1.75. Fiction.
Paul's drug addiction affects the lives of his brothers, Joe and David. Joe joins the Navy after graduation from night school, giving the money he had saved for college to their fifteen-year-old brother, David. Paul finds the money and uses it to buy drugs. David is shot when he follows Joe, who is searching for the drug pusher.

MAY, Julian. *How to Build a Body.* Gr. 4–5. Illus. by Brendan Lynch. Creative Ed, 1970. Unp. $6.95. Nonfiction.
An illustrated guide to child physiology provides information on the structure, composition, and function of the human anatomy.

MAYERSON, Evelyn. *Sanjo.* Gr. 9–10. Lippincott, 1979. 320 pp. $8.95. Fiction.
Sanjo, who has Down's syndrome, is an adult but is cared for as a child by her parents. The lyrical writing describes the various people in her life and events she must deal with, including her sexuality.

MAZER, Harry. *The Dollar Man.* Gr. 7 and up. Delacorte, 1974. 204 pp. $5.95; pap. Dell, $1.50. Fiction.
An overweight fourteen-year-old boy feels he must find his father in order to establish his own identity.

MAZER, Harry. *The War on Villa Street.* Gr. 7 and up. Delacorte, 1978. 182 pp. $7.95. Fiction.
Willis acquires inner strength after enduring many beatings from his father and the scorn of a gang to which he once wanted to belong. He coaches a retarded boy in running for the school's field day and gains self-confidence.

MEDDAUGH, Susan. *Too Short Fred.* Gr. k–3. Illus. by the author. HM, 1978. 39 pp. $5.95. Fiction.
Fred thinks he is too short to dance with girls, until the tallest girl in the class dances with him. He also uses his imagination to contend with a boy who bullies him.

MELTON, David. *A Boy Called Hopeless.* Gr. 7–8. Illus. Independence Pr, 1976. 231 pp. $7.95. Fiction.
Fifteen-year-old Mary Jane describes her family's reactions when they find that her younger brother is brain-injured. They decide to participate in a program of rehabilitation for him.

MEYERS, Robert. *Like Normal People.* Gr. 10–12. New Amer Lib, 1978. 292 pp. $5.50. Nonfiction.
A newspaper reporter describes his brother and sister-in-law, who are retarded, and their attempts to lead a normal life despite public and family pressures.

MIHALY, Mary E. *Getting Your Own Way: A Guide to Growing Up Assertively.* Gr. 7–8. Evans, 1979. 176 pp. $6.96. Nonfiction.
Real-life anxiety situations, quizzes, and exercises illuminate

how to deal with criticism, protect individualism, handle sexual pressures, and relax with oneself and others.

MILES, Betty. *Looking On.* Gr. 5 and up. Knopf, 1978. 187 pp. $6.95; pap. Avon, $1.95. Fiction.
Being overweight adds to Rosalie's teenage awkwardness, insecurity, and daydreaming. She determines to change her appearance and be a more active participant in living, rather than an observer.

MILGRAM, Gail Gleason. *The Teenager and Sex.* Gr. 7–8. Illus. by Joyce Lord. Rosen, 1974. 158 pp. $3.99. Nonfiction.
In order to help adolescents form their own values, the author discusses human sexuality, marriage, and the family.

MILTON, Hilary. *Blind Flight.* Gr. 6–7. Watts, 1980. 138 pp. $7.90. Fiction.
Debbie's blindness increases the capability of her other senses. She needs all her senses when her uncle is unable to fly the plane and she has to land it, with instructions from people on the ground.

MILTON, Hilary. *Emergency! 10-33 on Channel 11!* Gr. 5–6. Watts, 1977. 134 pp. $7.90; pap. Dell, $1.50. Fiction.
A CB unit becomes the only line of communication between the victims of a road accident and the two young rescuers who attempt to locate and help them.

MINSHULL, Evelyn W. *The Steps to My Best Friend's House.* Gr. 6–9. Illus. by Unada. Westminster, 1980. 143 pp. $8.95. Fiction.
Carol's new friend, Trish, appears to have problems with her mother. Although Trish says her mother is emotionally ill because of her husband's death, Carol and her family begin to realize that Trish, herself, has emotional difficulties over the death of her father.

MINTZ, Thomas, and Lorelie Miller MINTZ. *Threshold: Straight Answers to Teenagers' Questions About Sex.* Gr. 5–9. Illus. by Lorelie Miller Mintz. Walker, 1978. 120 pp. $7.95. Nonfiction.
In question-and-answer format, a psychiatrist talks about

physical and emotional changes in teenagers. The emphasis is on coping with changes in feelings.

MITCHELL, Joyce Slayton. *Free to Choose: Decision Making for Young Men.* Gr. 7 and up. Delacorte, 1976. 182 pp. $8.95. Nonfiction.
The author gives information to help young men make their own choices about sexuality, relationships with women, use of drugs and alcohol, spirituality, sports, and education.

MITCHELL, Joyce Slayton. *Other Choices for Becoming a Woman.* Gr. 9–12. Delacorte, 1976. 258 pp. $7.95; pap. Dell, $1.25. Nonfiction.
A wider range of choices in sexuality, drugs, alcohol, and education now confront high-school students. The author emphasizes choices of life-styles that strengthen healthy bodies and minds.

MITCHELL, Joyce Slayton. *See Me More Clearly: Career and Life Planning for Teens with Physical Disabilities.* Gr. 9–12. HarBraceJ, 1980. 284 pp. $8.95. Nonfiction.
Disabled students can get help in making decisions concerning their lives.

MOE, Barbara. *Pickles and Prunes.* Gr. 9–12. McGraw-Hill, 1976. 122 pp. $6.95. Fiction.
Thirteen-year-old Anne becomes friends with a pediatric patient in the hospital where her mother works as a nurse. Her friend Laurie becomes more ill and both girls have to confront Laurie's death.

MOERI, Louise. *The Girl Who Lived on the Ferris Wheel.* Gr. 7–8. Dutton, 1979. 117 pp. $8.95; pap. Avon, $1.75. Fiction.
Clotilde repeatedly attempts to escape, both physically and emotionally, the terrifying situation of child abuse that threatens her at home.

MONCURE, Jane Belk. *About Me.* Gr. ps–2. Illus. by Linda Sommers. Childs World, 1976. 32 pp. $7.95. Fiction.
A small child takes delight in the things she can do with her feet, hands, ears, and eyes.

MONCURE, Jane Belk. *People Who Help People*. Gr. ps–3. Illus. by Helen Enders. Childrens, 1976. Unp. $6.95. Nonfiction.
Many adults, including the doctor, care about children and help look after them.

MONTGOMERY, Elizabeth Rider. *The Mystery of the Boy Next Door*. Gr. 2–3. Illus. by Ethel Gold. Garrard, 1978. 44 pp. $6.18. Fiction.
When a new boy moves to their neighborhood, the other children misunderstand his caution. They finally realize, through a series of clues, that the new boy is deaf. They learn sign language so they can communicate with him.

MONTGOMERY, Elizabeth Rider. *"Seeing" in the Dark*. Gr. 2–3. Illus. by Troy Howell. Garrard, 1979. 44 pp. $6.18. Fiction.
Kay, a blind girl, enters a new school expecting to be unhappy, but makes new friends as the other children learn that she is not so different from them.

MORGENROTH, Barbara. *Demons at My Door*. Gr. 6–7. Atheneum, 1980. 145 pp. $8.95. Fiction.
Aly believes that demons have been haunting her and that her friends are turning against her, but her problems have less to do with demons than with trying to please her father.

MORRISON, Carl V., and Dorothy Nafus MORRISON. *Can I Help How I Feel?* Gr. 5–9. Illus. by James McCrea and Ruth Mc-Crea. Atheneum, 1976. 124 pp. $7.95. Nonfiction.
Feelings of sadness, depression, jealousy, and anger are part of everyone's life at some time. Children can learn to cope with such emotions. Story vignettes illustrate various emotions and offer advice about managing them.

MORRISON, Velma F. *There's Only One You: The Story of Heredity*. Gr. 4–6. Illus. by William Jaber. Messner, 1978. 64 pp. $6.97. Nonfiction.
Genetics is the study of inherited characteristics. Heredity influences appearance, eye color, and conditions such as muscular dystrophy, hemophilia, cystic fibrosis, allergies, some forms of diabetes, and hearing impairments. Some babies are born with

disabilities that could be the result of excess X rays, infectious diseases, and mothers' use of alcohol, tobacco, and other drugs.

MURRAY, Gloria, and Gerald G. JAMPOLSKY, eds. *Straight from the Siblings: Another Look at the Rainbow.* Gr. 3 and up. Illus. Celestial, 1982. 95 pp. $7.95. Nonfiction.
The emotional and physical experiences of siblings' illnesses are described by and for children who have brothers and sisters with life-threatening illnesses. The children's comments are derived from discussion and support groups at the Center for Attitudinal Healing.

MYERS, Irma, and Arthur MYERS. *Why You Feel Down & What You Can Do About It: A Psychotherapist Tells Everything You Want to Know About Teenage Depression.* Gr. 9 and up. Scribner, 1982. 122 pp. $9.95. Nonfiction.
Physical, intellectual, and emotional changes occur during depression. People can help themselves by looking at the demands of relationships with family and friends and by finding therapeutic help.

MYLANDER, Maureen. *The Great American Stomach Book: How Your Digestion Works and What to Do When It Doesn't.* Gr. 10 and up. Ticknor, 1982. 269 pp. $11.95. Nonfiction.
The author details common and unusual conditions of the stomach. Children may experience such illnesses as hepatitis A, constipation or diarrhea, celiac disease, colic, or abdominal pain.

NAVH. *Cathy.* Gr. k–4. Illus. by Diane Dawson. NAVH, 1979. 31 pp. $7.50. Fiction.
After Cathy has cataract surgery, glasses enable her to see better. Her friends and special teacher help her with special aids. She, in turn, helps a new girl in school, who also has a vision impairment, to be more accepting of vision aids and to make friends.

NAVH. *Larry.* Gr. k–4. Illus. by Diane Dawson. NAVH, 1979. 29 pp. $7.50. Fiction.
Larry is an albino, with light skin and hair, sensitivity to bright sun, and vision impairment. In school, Larry sits near the board and has special instruction with other children who use magnifiers, large type, tape cassettes, and Braille. He and his

friends are active in the usual children's games. A boy who teases them is helped to understand by visiting the special class.

NAWCH Research Team. *Andrew Goes for an X-Ray. Andrew Goes to the Outpatients. Andrew Has a Blood Test.* Gr. ps–1. Illus. NAWCH, 1980. Unp. $3.00 each. Fiction.
This series of colorful fold-out books explains the steps in a boy's physical examination. His mother is shown accompanying him, and photos of the staff at work detail the procedures.

NAYLOR, Phyllis Reynolds. *Getting Along in Your Family.* Gr. 4–7. Illus. by Rick Cooley. Abingdon, 1976. 112 pp. $5.50. Nonfiction.
The author presents numerous suggestions to reduce family conflict and to help children cope with problems such as alcoholism.

NEFF, Fred. *Keeping Fit: A Handbook for Physical Conditioning and Better Health.* Gr. 5 and up. Photog. by James E. Reid. Lerner, 1977. 56 pp. $6.95. Nonfiction.
Physical fitness and proper nutrition are important to maintain health. The author explains and illustrates basic and more advanced exercise programs and suggests better nutrition.

NEIMARK, Anne E. *A Deaf Child Listened: Thomas Gallaudet, Pioneer in American Education.* Gr. 7 and up. Lothrop, 1983. 160 pp. $8.00. Nonfiction.
This biography of the first American to open a school for the deaf illuminates the problems of deaf children. Gallaudet helped develop American Sign Language.

NEIMARK, Anne E. *Touch of Light: The Story of Louis Braille.* Gr. 4–6. HarBraceJ, 1970. 186 pp. $6.95. Nonfiction.
Fifteen-year-old Louis Braille develops a six-dot system of writing that is eventually named after him, and grows up to become a leading educator in France in the nineteenth century.

NEUFELD, John. *Lisa, Bright and Dark.* Gr. 7 and up. S G Phillips, 1969. 125 pp. $9.95; pap. New Amer Lib, $1.75. Fiction.
Despite her friends' attempts to help sixteen-year-old Lisa out of her depression by talking to her unbelieving parents and to unhelpful school personnel, Lisa has a near-fatal accident. After

this episode and seeing Lisa's other strange behaviors, her father finally decides to seek therapy for her.

NEWMAN, Alyse. *It's Me, Claudia!* Gr. k–3. Illus. by the author. Watts, 1981. 32 pp. $7.90. Fiction.
Claudia wants to hide her ears because she thinks they stick out, so she wears a large hat. The hat covers her face as well, so no one knows who she is. She has to come out to be recognized.

NEWMAN, Susan. *Ice Cream Isn't Always Good.* Gr. 1–2. Photog. by Barbara Treaster. Proj Two, 1971. Unp. $1.37. Fiction.
Lisa, a young girl, forgets her mother's warning and gets into a man's car when he offers her ice cream. When he will not let her leave his house, she is able to telephone the operator, who sends a police officer to rescue her and arrest the stranger. Lisa realizes, "Ice cream doesn't taste good when a nasty man gives it to you."

NIXON, Joan Lowery. *The Specter.* Gr. 7–8. Delacorte, 1982. 184 pp. $10.95. Fiction.
Seventeen-year-old Dina is distracted from her anger about having Hodgkin's disease when she becomes involved with a hospital roommate's mysterious life.

NOLEN, William A. *Spare Parts for the Human Body.* Gr. 4–7. Illus. Random House, 1971. 114 pp. $4.99. Nonfiction.
Progress in replacing or assisting defective body organs includes metal and plastic devices and transplants from human and animal sources.

NOLEN, William A. *Surgeon Under the Knife.* Gr. 9 and up. Illus. Coward, 1976. 223 pp. $8.95; pap. Dell, $1.95. Nonfiction.
The author is a surgeon who describes his own heart surgery and explains the techniques and procedures available to heart patients.

NOURSE, Alan Edward. *Clear Skin, Healthy Skin.* Gr. 6–7. Illus. by Ric Estrada. Watts, 1976. 61 pp. $7.90. Nonfiction.
A physician offers advice on the home treatment of mild cases of acne, discussing cleaning habits, diet, makeup, and hair care, and outlines the advantages and disadvantages of more serious medical treatments.

NOURSE, Alan Edward. *Fractures, Dislocations and Sprains.* Gr. 5–6. Illus. Watts, 1978. 63 pp. $7.90. Nonfiction.
A physician explains various injuries to which bones, cartilage, joints, tendons, and ligaments are susceptible, describes the treatment of each kind of injury, and explains the healing processes.

NOURSE, Alan Edward. *Hormones.* Gr. 6–7. Illus. Watts, 1979. 87 pp. $7.90. Nonfiction.
The functions of insulin, cortisone, and hormones produced by the thyroid and pituitary glands are explained. Dysfunctions such as cancer and related research are discussed.

NOURSE, Alan Edward. *Menstruation: Just Plain Talk.* Gr. 4 and up. Illus. Watts, 1980. 64 pp. $7.40. Nonfiction.
The menstrual cycle can be understood and managed. Abnormalities include malformations, irregular or missed periods, pain, excessive flow, premenstrual tension, and endometriosis.

NOURSE, Alan Edward. *The Tooth Book.* Gr. 6–7. Illus. McKay, 1977. 79 pp. $6.96. Nonfiction.
Each tooth has a function and unique shape. The dentist and orthodontist work to prevent or correct problems of decay, infection, misalignment, and replacement.

NOURSE, Alan Edward. *Viruses.* Gr. 6–7. Illus. Watts, 1976. 65 pp. $7.90. Nonfiction.
Viruses cause infectious diseases such as bronchitis, pneumonia, hepatitis, chicken pox, mumps, polio, mononucleosis, and the common cold. Some viral diseases can be prevented by vaccines.

NOURSE, Alan Edward. *Vitamins.* Gr. 6–7. Illus. Watts, 1977. 66 pp. $4.33. Nonfiction.
Vitamins, in tablet form or in foods, are nutrients needed in the diet to maintain good health.

NOURSE, Alan Edward. *Your Immune System.* Gr. 4. Watts, 1982. 72 pp. $7.90. Nonfiction.
The body's immune defense system usually functions well. When it does not, the result can be allergies, rejection of a transplant, arthritis, and other disabling diseases or conditions. Researchers are finding new ways to stimulate normal immune responses.

NULL, Gary, and Steve NULL. *Why Your Stomach Hurts: A Handbook of Digestion and Nutrition.* Gr. 4–7. Dodd, 1979. 216 pp. $8.95. Nonfiction.
In encyclopedia format the author explains the functions of the digestive system, factors that affect its ability to digest, absorb, and utilize nutrients, and how to maintain a sense of personal well-being.

NUMEROFF, Laura Joffe. *Phoebe Dexter Has Harriet Peterson's Sniffles.* Gr. 1–2. Illus. Morrow, 1977. Unp. $7.63. Fiction.
Phoebe finds that staying home with a cold is not at all boring if one has an imagination.

O'DELL, Scott. *Kathleen, Please Come Home.* Gr. 7 and up. Houghton, 1978. 196 pp. $7.95; pap. Dell, $2.25. Fiction.
Fifteen-year-old Kathy imitates her friend Sybil, and uses drugs. She falls in love with a young man and becomes pregnant, but he is killed by immigration officers. Slightly injured in a car accident that kills Sybil, Kathy miscarries. When she finally decides to go home, she finds that her mother has sold the house and is searching for her.

ODOR, Ruth S. *What's a Body to Do?* Gr. 2–6. Illus. Childs World, 1980. 112 pp. $7.95. Nonfiction.
Exercise, good food, and rest help keep bodies strong. Cigarettes, alcohol, and other drugs harm children's health.

OETTINGER, Katherine B., with Elizabeth C. MOONEY. *Not My Daughter: Facing Up to Adolescent Pregnancy.* Gr. 10 and up. P-H, 1979. 184 pp. $8.95. Nonfiction.
After discussing sexuality, the authors give guidelines on how to decide whether a pregnant, single adolescent should have an abortion. Addresses of many resource groups are given.

OKIMOTO, Jean Davies. *It's Just Too Much.* Gr. 6–7. Putnam, 1980. 126 pp. $9.95; pap. Pocket Bks, $1.95. Fiction.
Still trying to accept the fact that she does not yet need a bra but she does need braces, twelve-year-old Cynthia also must adjust to her mother's new husband and her father's new girlfriend.

OLSHAN, Neal H. *Depression.* Gr. 7 and up. Watts, 1982. 119 pp. $8.90. Nonfiction.

This study of depression explores the possible physical, genetic, emotional, and sociological causes of depression and discusses various treatments.

OLSHAN, Neal H., and Julie Dreyer WANG. *Fears & Phobias: Fighting Back.* Gr. 7–8. Illus. Watts, 1980. 122 pp. $7.90. Nonfiction.
It is normal to be afraid sometimes, but when people fear harmless things or places or have excessive fears of doctors, dentists, hospitals, or shots, there are ways to help them overcome these phobias. This self-help guide encourages youngsters to overcome debilitating fears through systematic desensitization and isolating and identifying phobias.

OMINSKY, Elaine. *Jon O.: A Special Boy.* Gr. 1–2. Photog. by Dennis Simonetti. P-H, 1977. Unp. $8.95. Nonfiction.
Jon O. has Down's syndrome and takes longer to learn to walk, talk, understand school subjects, and deal with social situations. Except for saying that something had happened to Jon O. "when he was still in his Mommy's stomach," this story of a real boy gives accurate details of Jon's problems and conveys his family's love and regard for him.

ONEAL, Zibby. *The Language of Goldfish.* Gr. 7 and up. Viking, 1980. 179 pp. $8.95. Fiction.
Thirteen-year-old Carrie is confused and anxious about growing up and life changes. After her unusual behavior and a suicide attempt, she is able to work with a psychiatrist to learn to understand and manage her feelings better.

ORGEL, Doris. *Next Door to Xanadu.* Gr. 5–6. Illus. by Dale Payson. Archway, 1971. 148 pp. pap. $.75. Fiction.
The self-esteem of a lonely, overweight ten-year-old gets a boost when a new neighbor becomes her friend.

PACKARD, Mary. *A Visit to the Dentist.* Gr. 1–5. Illus. by Dora Leder. S&S, 1981. 64 pp. pap. $3.95. Fiction.
Cara's family play-acts a dentist's examination, having X rays, and filling a cavity to help her understand her first visit. Activities that accompany the story encourage the reader to learn about dental care.

PARKER, Mark. *Horses, Airplanes, and Frogs.* Gr. k–2. Illus. by Dan Siculan. Childs World, 1977. 32 pp. $6.50. Fiction.
Although blind, Nick enjoys most of the same activities as other children. He asks his mother to describe horses, airplanes, and frogs but understands better when a new friend finds the actual objects for him to touch.

PARKER, Richard. *He Is Your Brother.* Gr. 6–7. Nelson, 1974. 98 pp. $6.96. Fiction.
Mike's reluctant attention to his withdrawn, autistic younger brother, Orry, and his sharing with Orry his interest in trains, result in unanticipated adventure, respect, and growth for both of them.

PARKINSON, Ethelyn M. *Rupert Piper and the Boy Who Could Knit.* Gr. 3–7. Illus. by Jim Padgett. Abingdon, 1979. 160 pp. $6.95. Fiction.
Rupert and his friends find it difficult to accept a boy named Shirley who prefers knitting. The girls of the town do not understand a girl who dresses like a boy and prefers active sports.

PATENT, Dorothy Hinshaw. *Bacteria: How They Affect Other Living Things.* Gr. 7–8. Illus. Holiday, 1980. 128 pp. $9.95. Nonfiction.
The characteristics, functions, and types of bacteria are discussed; how some bacteria maintain health while others cause illness is explained. Research on using bacteria to improve the quality of human life is summarized.

PATENT, Dorothy Hinshaw. *Germs.* Gr. 3–7. Illus. Holiday, 1983. 40 pp. $9.64. Nonfiction.
Bacteria, viruses, and protozoans can cause diseases. The author describes how germs affect the body and how people can be immunized.

PAYNE, Sherry Newirth. *A Contest.* Gr. k–3. Illus. by Jeff Kyle. Carolrhoda, 1982. 40 pp. $5.95. Fiction.
Ten-year-old Mike, who has cerebral palsy, transfers from special school to public school. He manages his wheelchair and works to be accepted by his classmates.

PEACOCK, Carol Antoinette. *Hand-Me-Down Dreams*. Gr. 10–12. Schocken, 1981. 167 pp. pap. $8.95. Nonfiction.
A psychiatric social worker recounts the true stories of four girls who are poor and dependent on their unsupportive mothers. The girls cope with rejection and neglect, drugs and alcohol, and teenage pregnancy. Each has some success in taking charge of her own life.

PEAVY, Linda, and Ursula SMITH. *Food, Nutrition and You*. Gr. 6–9. Scribner, 1982. 197 pp. $12.95. Nonfiction.
Carbohydrates, vitamins, fats, and proteins give the body the ability to grow and develop. Also discussed are mouth care, food additives, sports nutrition, fast foods, increased appetite in adolescence, and anorexia.

PECK, Richard. *Are You in the House Alone?* Gr. 10–12. Viking, 1976. 156 pp. $8.95; pap. Dell, $1.25. Fiction.
When a high-school student is raped by her boy friend, she, her family, and the community are all affected by it.

PENNEY, Peggy L. *Surgery: From Stone Scalpel to Laser Beam*. Gr. 7 and up. Lodestar, 1977. 143 pp. $6.95. Nonfiction.
True stories are told of surgical methods from ancient times to the present. The development of anesthesia and sterilization of equipment used in surgery were important advances.

PERKINS, Al. *The Ear Book*. Gr. ps–2. Illus. by William O'Brian. Random House, 1968. Unp. $4.95. Nonfiction.
Pleasant sounds are described in simple words and colorful, humorous pictures.

PERL, Lila. *Junk Food, Fast Food, Health Food: What America Eats and Why*. Gr. 5 and up. HM, 1980. 192 pp. $10.95; pap. HM, $4.95. Nonfiction.
The impact of technology on the food industry has resulted in fast-food restaurants, large sales of health food, and varied diets. The book lists many food additives.

PERL, Lila. *Me and Fat Glenda*. Gr. 3–6. HM, 1972. 185 pp. $4.95; pap. Pocket Bks, $.75. Fiction.
Sara is shunned by neighbors and friends because of her father's junk sculpture and garbage truck, her friend Glenda because she

is obese. They form a mutually accepting friendship, which gives Glenda the support she needs to begin to lose weight.

PETER, Diana. *Claire and Emma.* Gr. 3–4. Photog. by Jeremy Finlay. John Day, 1977. Unp. $9.89. Nonfiction.
In this real-life story, four-year-old Claire and two-year-old Emma, two sisters who learn daily to cope with problems arising from their deafness, lead happy, active lives.

PETERSEN, Palle. *Sally Can't See.* Gr. 3–4. Illus. John Day, 1974. Unp. $8.79. Nonfiction.
Twelve-year-old Sally swims, rides a horse, does well in school, and is blind. She uses Braille, a white cane, and trained senses to be active and enjoy school. The Braille alphabet is pictured; photographs of Sally involved in many school and play activities demonstrate her capability.

PETERSON, Jeanne Whitehouse. *I Have a Sister, My Sister Is Deaf.* Gr. 1–2. Illus. by Deborah Ray. Har-Row, 1977. Unp. $8.95. Nonfiction.
In loving, lyrical word pictures, a girl describes her younger, deaf sister who reads people's lips and eyes, likes to leap and climb, and enjoys feeling the cat purring but cannot hear the doorbell.

PEVSNER, Stella. *Keep Stompin' Till the Music Stops.* Gr. 4–6. Seabury, 1977. 136 pp. $7.95; pap. Scholastic, $1.95. Fiction.
Richard's dyslexia keeps him from reading or following conversations well. He feels insecure and distrustful. Richard figures out, from family conversations at a reunion, that there is a plan to place his grandfather in a residence in another state. He is pleased to find that he can learn and helps his grandfather.

PFEFFER, Susan Beth. *What Do You Do When Your Mouth Won't Open?* Gr. 6 and up. Illus. by Loran Tomei. Delacorte, 1981. 114 pp. $8.44. Fiction.
Twelve-year-old Reesa is afraid to speak in public. When she must read her winning essay to a large audience, she overcomes her fear with the help of a psychologist and a library book on public speaking.

PHELAN, Terry Wolfe. *The S.S. Valentine.* Gr. 2–6. Illus. by Judy Glasser. Four Winds, 1979. 40 pp. $5.95. Fiction.

Andy figures out how to involve a disabled classmate, Connie, in the class play, by turning Connie's wheelchair into the *S.S. Valentine.*

PHILIPS, Barbara. *Don't Call Me Fatso.* Gr. k–5. Illus. by Helen Cogancherry. Raintree, 1980. 32 pp. $13.30. Fiction.
Overweight Rita gains control over her life as she realizes the advantages of exercise and healthy eating habits. The personal and interpersonal problems experienced by overweight children are shown in this brief story.

PHILLIPS, Carolyn E. *Michelle.* Gr. 3. Regal, 1980. 176 pp. pap. $7.95. Nonfiction.
An eight-year-old girl makes a courageous adjustment to amputation and chemotherapy, trying to live as normal a life as possible.

PHIPSON, Joan. *A Tide Flowing.* Gr. 5–9. Atheneum, 1981. 156 pp. $8.95. Fiction.
A young quadriplegic girl helps a lonely adolescent boy find strength and peace.

PIEPER, Elizabeth. *A School for Tommy.* Gr. 3–4. Illus. by Mina Gow McLean. Childrens Pr, 1979. 30 pp. $8.35. Fiction.
Seven-year-old Tommy goes to public school in a wheelchair. He explains the chair and crutches to his classmates and shows his ability to play. His teacher is cautious about having a disabled child in class. A postscript encourages readers to think and talk about the ways in which people are alike and different and how to be friends with handicapped people.

PINKWATER, Manus. *Fat Elliot and the Gorilla.* Gr. 4–5. Illus. by the author. Four Winds, 1974. 47 pp. $4.34. Fiction.
Elliot dislikes being fat and learns to eat less and exercise more with the help of an imaginary gorilla and a talking scale.

PIZER, Vernon. *Glorious Triumphs: Athletes Who Conquered Adversity.* Gr. 7–9. Dodd, 1980. 209 pp. $6.96. Nonfiction.
Some athletes have achieved sports successes despite a variety of physical disabilities and adverse circumstances. The narrative describes fourteen athletes whose disabilities included amputation, frailty, and cancer.

PIZER, Vernon. *You Don't Say: How People Communicate Without Speech.* Gr. 6 and up. Illus. by Janet McCaffery. Putnam,
1978. 95 pp. $7.95. Nonfiction.
People communicate through facial expressions, gestures, pic-
tographs, and glyphs. Braille uses raised dots to indicate words
that can be felt. Bliss symbols are pictures on a board to which
nonspeaking people can point to indicate their ideas and needs.
Amerind is a signal system for hearing people who cannot talk.
Sign language uses hand gestures for people who are deaf or hearing impaired.

PLACE, Marian T., and Charles G. PRESTON. *Juan's Eighteen-
Wheeler Summer.* Gr. 4 and up. Dodd, 1982. 160 pp. $8.95.
Fiction.
Juan helps his neighbor, Pete, to truck vegetables and fruits
throughout California. When the tractor and trailer flip over and
burn in an accident Juan saves Pete by pulling him out, and
becomes a hero to his family and friends.

PLATT, Kin. *The Boy Who Could Make Himself Disappear.* Gr. 9
and up. Dell, 1968. 247 pp. pap. $1.75. Fiction.
Roger's harsh, perfectionist mother and detached father offer little
help as he struggles to overcome speech problems. Eventually his
isolation and fantasies lead to schizophrenia. The boy's psychiatrist, and an older man who has befriended him, may be able to
help him to recover.

PLAUT, Martin E. *The Doctor's Guide to You and Your Colon: A
Candid, Helpful Guide to Our #1 Hidden Health Complaint.* Gr.
10 and up. Har-Row, 1982. 138 pp. $10.95. Nonfiction.
The author describes ordinary and rare conditions of the intestines, such as diarrhea, constipation, colitis, and cancer. He
suggests many home treatments and recommends avoiding surgery if at all possible.

POLLAND, Barbara Kay. *Feelings: Inside You and Outloud Too.*
Gr. 2–3. Photog. by Craig De Roy. Celestial, 1975. Unp. pap.
$5.95. Nonfiction.
Questions, statements, and photographs about feelings such as
fear, love, and pain encourage readers to recognize and accept

their emotions, express them openly, and deal with them constructively.

POMERANTZ, Charlotte. *The Mango Tooth.* Gr. 2–3. Illus. by Marylin Hafner. Greenwillow, 1977. Unp. $6.95. Fiction.
Posy loses the first of four teeth by biting into a mango, and makes a profit on each one.

POOLE, Victoria. *Thursday's Child.* Gr. 7 and up. Little, 1980. 352 pp. $10.95. Nonfiction.
The Poole family gives emotional support to their teenage son while they search for medical help as he becomes more ill. Eventually he is given a heart transplant at Stanford University Medical Center. Many details are given of hospital life and the impact of the child's illness on the family.

POWERS, Bill. *A Test of Love.* Gr. 7–8. Photog. by Bill Aron. Watts, 1979. 90 pp. $8.40; pap. Dell, $1.25. Fiction.
Faced with an unwanted pregnancy, sixteen-year-old Patsy must decide whether to have the baby or an abortion. She is helped by her trusting, supportive relationships with her mother and friends.

PRINCE, Alison. *The Turkey's Nest.* Gr. 7–8. Morrow, 1980. 223 pp. $8.75. Fiction.
Pregnant and unmarried, yet determined to have her baby, Kate leaves London to live on a farm.

PRINGLE, Laurence. *Lives at Stake: The Science and Politics of Environmental Health.* Gr. 6 and up. Illus. Macmillan, 1980. 144 pp. $9.95. Nonfiction.
The author examines existing data about the air, water, and food people consume. He analyzes the methods used to test the environment and presents the varied factors that affect improvements in environmental health.

PRINGLE, Laurence. *Radiation: Waves and Particles, Benefits and Risks.* Gr. 7–12. Illus. Enslow, 1982. 128 pp. $9.95. Nonfiction.
Radiation can be beneficial in diagnosing and treating illness.

There is a danger of too much radiation, so judgments must be made to balance risks and benefits.

PURSELL, Margaret Sanford. *A Look at Birth.* Gr. 1–3. Photog. by Maria S. Forrai. Lerner, 1977. 36 pp. $4.95. Nonfiction.
Photographs and brief explanations show conception, the stages of pregnancy, and birth.

PURSELL, Margaret Sanford. *A Look at Physical Handicaps.* Gr. 3–6. Photog. by Maria S. Forrai. Lerner, 1976. 34 pp. $3.95. Nonfiction.
Temporary or long-term disabilities have various causes and effects and require the handicapped to learn to live with their special problems.

RABE, Berniece. *The Balancing Girl.* Gr. ps–2. Illus. by Lillian Hoban. Dutton, 1981. Unp. $10.25. Fiction.
Margaret, a first-grader who is very good at balancing objects while in her wheelchair and on crutches, thinks up her best balancing trick for the school carnival.

RABINOWICH, Ellen. *Underneath I'm Different.* Gr. 6–9. Delacorte, 1983. 182 pp. $11.72. Fiction.
Although sixteen-year-old Amy is overweight, she and a young man who sculpts plump figures fall in love. When he is hospitalized for emotional illness, Amy maintains their friendship despite his rejection.

RAMIREZ, Carolyn. *Foot and Feet.* Gr. 2–3. Illus. by Frieda Gates. Harvey, 1973. 47 pp. $5.09. Nonfiction.
Riddles about feet emphasize their importance.

RASKIN, Ellen. *Spectacles.* Gr. k–4. Illus. Atheneum, 1972. Unp. pap. $1.95. Fiction.
The illustrations help explain the strange sights of weird creatures and monsters that Iris sees before her mother decides to bring Iris for a vision examination.

RAYNER, Claire. *The Body Book.* Gr. 3–4. Illus. by Tony King. Barron, 1978. 43 pp. $6.95. Nonfiction.
Children's questions are answered about how their bodies work, how babies are conceived and born, and what happens as people grow old and die.

RAYNER, Claire. *Everything Your Doctor Would Tell You If He Had the Time.* Gr. 10–12. Illus. Putnam, 1980. 224 pp. $14.95; pap. Putnam, $7.95. Nonfiction.
The author answers hundreds of questions about each of the systems of the body and their functions.

REDPATH, Ann. *Jim Boen: A Man of Opposites.* Gr. 4–8. Illus. by Ned Skubic. Creative Ed, 1980. 48 pp. $6.95. Nonfiction.
At nineteen years of age, Jim's neck was broken in a sports accident, leaving him paralyzed. The story tells of his positive attitude about recovery, the discipline of therapeutic exercises, and looking forward to greater improvement while accepting current limitations.

REEVES, John R. T. *Questions and Answers About Acne.* Gr. 7 and up. Illus. by Henry Tassitano. P-H, 1977. 111 pp. $6.95. Nonfiction.
Treatment of acne varies from home care to prescribed medications to office treatments.

REID, Robert. *Marie Curie.* Gr. 4–6. New Amer Lib, 1978. 168 pp. pap. $2.25. Nonfiction.
From this story of the life and work of the discoverer of radium and the X ray process, the reader can learn about scientific methods and the difficulties and pleasures of studying science.

REYNOLDS, Moira Davison. *Aim for a Job in a Medical Laboratory.* Rosen, 1982. 130 pp. $7.97. Nonfiction.
New technology makes laboratory work interesting to science-minded students. The author describes the education and work of laboratory technicians and researchers. The information is also useful to patients who want to know how specimens of their blood, urine, and other body materials are processed and interpreted.

REYNOLDS, Pamela. *Will the Real Monday Please Stand Up.* Gr. 6–7. Lothrop, 1975. 184 pp. $8.95; pap. Pocket Bks, $1.75. Fiction.
Fourteen-year-old Monday, beset by uncertainties, recounts the secrets and problems of her relationship with her parents, her

brother Johnny's involvement with a drug crowd, and her covert romance with a nineteen-year-old soccer star.

RICE, Eve. *Ebbie.* Gr. 1–2. Illus. by the author. Greenwillow, 1975. Unp. $5.95. Fiction.
Eddie's name becomes Ebbie when he loses his two front teeth and cannot pronounce correctly. When his family also calls him Ebbie, he convinces them he wants to be called Eddie.

RICHARDS, Arlene Kramer, and Irene WILLIS. *What to Do If You or Someone You Know Is Under 18 and Pregnant.* Gr. 6 and up. Illus. Lothrop, 1983. 256 pp. $9.55; pap. Lothrop, $7.00. Non-fiction.
The authors describe the practical, medical, economic, and legal aspects of abortion, adoption, parenting, and marriage so that teenage readers can make informed choices.

RICHTER, Alice Numeroff, and Laura Joffe NUMEROFF. *You Can't Put Braces on Spaces.* Gr. 1–2. Illus. by Laura Joffe Numeroff. Greenwillow, 1979. 54 pp. $5.71. Fiction.
His younger brother enviously watches as Neil has braces fitted on his teeth but must wait for his own until his new teeth grow in.

RICHTER, Betts. *Something Special Within.* Gr. ps–5. Illus. by Alice Jacobsen. De Vorss, 1982. 48 pp. pap. $4.00. Nonfiction.
Love and caring are part of feeling good about oneself. The book offers examples.

RICHTER, Elizabeth. *The Teenage Hospital Experience: You Can Handle It!* Gr. 9–12. Photog. by the author. Coward, 1982. 128 pp. $11.95. Nonfiction.
Teenagers who are interviewed about being in the hospital tell about their conditions, treatments, rights, discomforts, and feelings. Then professionals describe admissions, nursing, surgery, anesthesia, and questions teens might be too embarrassed to ask.

RIEDMAN, Sarah Regal. *Allergies.* Gr. 4–5. Illus. Watts, 1978. 63 pp. $7.90. Nonfiction.
The known and suspected causes of allergies are explained, as well as the symptoms, diagnosis, and treatment of common and unusual allergies.

RIEDMAN, Sarah Regal. *Biological Clocks.* Gr. 5 and up. Illus. by Leslie Morrill. Har-Row, 1982. 128 pp. $10.10. Nonfiction.
Rhythms linked to the motions of the earth and its moon affect plants and insects. Humans have sleep and wake cycles that are affected by changes in schedule and stress.

RIEDMAN, Sarah Regal. *Diabetes.* Gr. 6–8. Watts, 1980. 62 pp. $6.45. Nonfiction.
Diabetes is a chronic condition in which the body does not use glucose as a source of energy. Insulin medication may help, as well as diet and exercise.

RIEDMAN, Sarah Regal. *Food for People.* Gr. 4–7. Illus. by Helen Ludwig. Har-Row, 1976. 190 pp. $9.95. Nonfiction.
The author discusses how much food people eat and need, getting the most nutrition from food, and planning nutritious meals.

RISKIND, Mary. *Apple Is My Sign.* Gr. 5–8. HM, 1981. 146 pp. $8.95. Fiction.
A young boy who is deaf grows up on a small farm and then leaves for school in a large city. His story, told by a hearing woman who grew up with deaf parents, shows a happy, loving family and a strong boy with self-esteem who deals with a hearing world.

ROBERTS, Sarah. *Nobody Cares About Me!* Gr. ps–1. Illus. by Joe Mathieu. Random House, 1982. 40 pp. $4.99. Fiction.
Big Bird, of television's *Sesame Street* (Children's Television Workshop), becomes sick, but it is not as much fun as he had imagined, even though his friends visit.

ROBERTS, Willo Davis. *Don't Hurt Laurie!* Gr. 7–8. Illus. by Ruth Sanderson. Atheneum, 1977. 166 pp. $9.95; pap. Atheneum, $2.95. Fiction.
Laurie, an abused child, is aided by her nine-year-old stepbrother to find the help she needs.

ROBINET, Harriette. *Jay and the Marigold.* Gr. 2–4. Illus. by Trudy Scott. Childrens, 1976. 48 pp. $5.95. Fiction.
Jay has cerebral palsy. He realizes, as he watches a marigold grow, that he too will grow and bloom in his own way.

ROBINSON, Jean. *The Strange but Wonderful Cosmic Awareness of Duffy Moon.* Gr. 4–5. Illus. by Lawrence Di Fiori. HM, 1974. 142 pp. $6.95; pap. Dell, $1.25. Fiction.
Duffy is short for an eleven-year-old, and unhappy about it. To gain success and power he takes a home study course in "cosmic awareness," and relies on it to help him stand up to unfriendly peers. Eventually he discovers he has inner strengths of his own.

ROBINSON, Veronica. *David in Silence.* Gr. 6–7. Illus. by Victor Ambrus. Lippincott, 1965. 126 pp. $8.95. Fiction.
David, who is deaf, makes friends with Michael. Michael's other friends reject David when they misunderstand his communication. Chased away, David runs through a dark tunnel and falls into the water. Michael rescues him and later persuades his friends to let David advise them on the raft they are building. His advice proves useful. When the boys attempt to raft through the tunnel, they turn back, frightened. They express admiration for David's courage in going into the tunnel alone.

ROBISON, Deborah, and Carla PEREZ. *Your Turn, Doctor.* Gr. ps–2. Illus. by Deborah Robison. Dial, 1982. Unp. $7.95. Fiction.
In this humorous story Gloria dreams that she does not want to be prodded, poked, or given shots any more. She and her doctor switch roles and she gives her doctor the same treatment she has received.

ROCKWELL, Anne, and Harlow ROCKWELL. *Sick in Bed.* Gr. ps–2. Illus. Macmillan, 1982. Unp. $7.95. Fiction.
When a little boy has a sore throat and fever, he describes his feelings and experiences such as a throat culture and an injection.

ROCKWELL, Harlow. *My Dentist.* Gr. 1–2. Illus. Greenwillow, 1975. Unp. $8.40. Fiction.
Detailed pictures and a simple story tell about the dentist's chair that goes up and down, the curved mirror, the drill and attachments, and other items the child patient is likely to see in the dentist's office.

ROCKWELL, Harlow. *My Doctor.* Gr. ps–1. Illus. Macmillan, 1973. Unp. $9.95. Fiction.

During a medical check-up a small boy becomes fascinated by the interesting equipment that is shown and explained to him.

RODOWSKY, Colby F. *P.S. Write Soon.* Gr. 6–7. Watts, 1978. 149 pp. $7.90; pap. Dell, $1.50. Fiction.
A young girl cannot accept her paralyzed leg and leg brace. She denies her disability in letters to a pen pal she has never met by recounting activities and adventures she has never had.

RONAYNE, Eileen. *Memoirs of a Tall Girl.* Gr. 7 and up. Scholastic, 1978. 168 pp. pap. $1.75. Fiction.
A seventh-grader, taller than many of her classmates, learns to cope with the problems her height causes, including dealing with a boy who enjoys kissing tall girls.

ROSEN, Lillian. *Just Like Everybody Else.* Gr. 12 and up. Har-BraceJ, 1981. 155 pp. $10.95. Fiction.
A fifteen-year-old girl who loses her hearing after a bus accident feels confused and frightened. A boy who is also deaf helps her understand what it means to be "different," and to cope with the difficulties.

ROSENBERG, Mark L. *Patients: The Experience of Illness.* Gr. 10 and up. HR&W, 1980. 192 pp. $14.95; pap. HR&W, $8.95. Nonfiction.
This photoessay portrays ill people who become "patients" through the process of diagnosis, treatment, and recovery. Interviews with real patients give details of the experience of being ill and hospitalized.

ROSENBERG, Maxine B. *My Friend Leslie: The Story of a Handicapped Child.* Gr. 1–3. Photog. by George Ancona. Lothrop, 1983. 48 pp. $8.59. Nonfiction.
Leslie's best friend recounts Leslie's kindergarten year of successes and struggles, the responses of other children to her several disabilities, and her adapted activities. Leslie is legally blind and has a moderate hearing loss, a cleft palate, muscular weakness, and ptosis, or drooping eyelids.

ROSENBERG, Nancy, and Louis Z. COOPER. *Vaccines and Viruses.* Gr. 7–8. Illus. Grosset & Dunlap, 1971. 159 pp. $7.95. Nonfiction.
Although vaccines have been found against many diseases such as mumps, German measles (rubella), measles, smallpox, malaria, and polio, some cannot as yet be prevented, such as chicken pox, hepatitis, and colds.

ROSS, Pat. *Molly and the Slow Teeth.* Gr. 1–2. Illus. by Jerry Milord. Lothrop, 1980. 43 pp. $6.67. Fiction.
Because second-grader Molly is afraid she will never lose her baby teeth, she tries to fool the tooth fairy.

ROTHENBERG, Mira. *Children with Emerald Eyes: Histories of Extraordinary Boys and Girls.* Gr. 10 and up. Dial, 1977. 294 pp. $10.95. Nonfiction.
The stories of schizophrenic and autistic children show the beauty and the problems of their lives. The psychologist-author emphasizes acceptance of these emotionally ill children.

ROTHMAN, Joel. *This Can Lick a Lollipop: Body Riddles for Kids. Esto Goza Chupando un Caramelo: Las Partes del Cuerpo en Adivinanzas Infantiles.* Gr. 2–3. Photog. by Patricia Ruben. Trans. from the English by Argentina Palacios. Doubleday, 1979. Unp. $6.61. Nonfiction.
Bilingual riddle verses challenge children to demonstrate their skill in naming body parts.

ROUNDS, Glen. *Blind Outlaw.* Gr. 4–5. Illus. by the author. Holiday, 1980. 94 pp. $8.95. Fiction.
A mute boy tames a blind wild horse with patience and an understanding of the horse's fears.

ROY, Howard L. *Bobby Visits the Dentist.* Gr. k–3. Illus. by Ann Silver. Gallaudet, 1975. 48 pp. $5.00. Fiction.
A dental hygienist cleans Bobby's teeth and teaches him how to brush his teeth. Then a dentist checks his teeth. Drawings of hands signing the words or letters help children who are learning Signed English, a tool to supplement the speech of people who have a hearing impairment.

ROY, Howard L. *We're Going to the Doctor.* Gr. k–4. Illus. by Ann Silver. Gallaudet, 1974. 27 pp. $5.00. Fiction.
Mother bear brings her son, Andy, to the doctor for a physical examination, which includes height and weight measurements, vision testing, and audiological testing. The doctor determines that Andy needs a new battery for his hearing aid. Drawings of hands signing the words or letters help children who are learning Signed English, a tool to supplement the speech of people who have a hearing impairment.

ROY, Ron. *Frankie Is Staying Back.* Gr. 2–5. Illus. by Walter Kessel. HM, 1980. 82 pp. $8.95. Fiction.
Frankie will not be promoted to fourth grade. His friend Jonas, who is an excellent student, pretends to read poorly and not be able to complete his homework so that he can stay back with Frankie.

ROZMAN, Deborah A. *Meditation for Children.* Gr. 5 and up. Celestial, 1982. 160 pp. $5.95. Nonfiction.
Quieting their thoughts, feelings, and bodies enables children to find emotional and spiritual resources. Meditation is used with some medical treatments to help children manage discomfort.

RUBY, Lois. *What Do You Do in Quicksand?* Gr. 7–8. Viking, 1979. 199 pp. $9.95; pap. Fawcett, $1.95. Fiction.
Matt is a seventeen-year-old single father who balances high-school classes, an evening job, and the care of his new baby. Help is offered by a sixteen-year-old neighbor, which leads to problems that need to be resolved.

RUDOLPH, Wilma, as told to Bud GREENSPAN. *Wilma: The Story of Wilma Rudolph.* Gr. 5–6. Illus. New Amer Lib, 1977. 172 pp. pap. $2.25. Nonfiction.
An Olympic track champion tells of her frailness and weak leg as a child and the obstacles she overcame to become an athlete.

RUSH, Anne Kent. *Getting Clear: Body Work for Women.* Gr. 10–12. Illus. Random House, 1973. 290 pp. $7.95; pap. Random House, $4.95. Nonfiction.
Various exercises described and illustrated encourage women to achieve physical and mental self-awareness.

RUSSELL, Robert. *To Catch an Angel: Adventures in the World I Cannot See.* Gr. 7 and up. Vanguard, 1962. 317 pp. $12.95. Nonfiction.
A successful teacher, father, and husband, who was blinded at the age of five years, tells of his efforts to overcome limitations.

SACHS, Elizabeth-Ann. *Just Like Always.* Gr. 4–6. Atheneum, 1981. 160 pp. $9.95. Fiction.
Two girls, hospitalized for scoliosis, become best friends despite the differences between them.

SACHS, Marilyn. *A December Tale.* Gr. 5–9. Doubleday, 1976. 87 pp. $7.95. Fiction.
When her father remarries he sends ten-year-old Myra and her six-year-old brother, Henry, to a neighbor's home to live. From there they are sent to a foster home, where Henry is beaten. Myra, inspired by the story of heroic Joan of Arc, figures out how to leave the foster family, bringing Henry to the neighbor's home for safety.

SAMSON, Joan. *Watching the New Baby.* Gr. 4–7. Photog. by Gary Gladstone. Atheneum, 1977. 65 pp. $7.95. Nonfiction.
The photographs and text cover the development of the fetus and the infant's appearance, senses, crying, and loving.

SAMUELS, Gertrude. *Run, Shelley, Run!* Gr. 6–7. Har-Row, 1974. 174 pp. $10.95; pap. New Amer Lib, $1.75. Fiction.
Shelley's father deserts the family. Her mother is alcoholic. As Shelley grows up she is placed in foster homes, from which she runs away. Through the understanding and caring of a neighbor, Shelley begins to find a happier life.

SAVITZ, Harriet May. *The Lionhearted.* Gr. 7–8. John Day, 1975. 149 pp. $8.95. Fiction.
A young girl enters a new high school in a wheelchair. She reaches out for acceptance and friendship with an overweight classmate and a popular senior boy.

SAVITZ, Harriet May. *Run, Don't Walk.* Gr. 4–6. Watts, 1979. 122 pp. $6.90; pap. New Amer Lib, $1.25. Fiction.
After Samantha is told that she cannot enter a marathon because

she is in a wheelchair, she begins to realize why Johnnie, another student in a wheelchair, is determined to fight for what he wants.

SAVITZ, Harriet May. *Wheelchair Champions: A History of Wheelchair Sports.* Gr. 7–9. Crowell, 1978. 117 pp. $7.79. Nonfiction.
Stories are told of athletes who have such disabilities as paraplegia and quadriplegia. They have become sports champions in national games despite their disabilities.

SCARRY, Richard. *Richard Scarry's Nicky Goes to the Doctor.* Gr. k–1. Illus. by the author. Western Pub, 1972. $6.08; pap. Western Pub, $1.95. Fiction.
Nicky, a rabbit, has a physical examination and a booster shot. When he tells his brothers and sisters about it, they want to go to the doctor too.

SCHAEFER, Nicola. *Does She Know She's There?* Gr. 10 and up. Doubleday, 1978. 235 pp. $7.95. Nonfiction.
The mother of a child with brain damage describes the constant care that is needed and relates the effects of the condition on the family.

SCHALEBEN-LEWIS, Joy. *Careers in a Hospital.* Gr. 3–7. Photog. by Heinz Kluetmeier. Raintree, 1976. 48 pp. $13.30. Nonfiction.
The book describes and illustrates the work of the staff in a hospital, including doctors, technologists, nurses, dieticians, anesthetists, cleaners, laundry workers, therapists, administrators, and volunteers.

SCHALEBEN-LEWIS, Joy. *The Dentist and Me.* Gr. 2–3. Illus. by Murray Weiss. Raintree, 1977. 30 pp. $11.15. Fiction.
Adam and Nikki visit their dentists, have their teeth cleaned and checked, and learn to care for their teeth.

SCHLEE, Ann. *Ask Me No Questions.* Gr. 5 and up. HR&W, 1976. 228 pp. $14.50. Fiction.
The mistreatment of children in an English workhouse and the outbreak of cholera there is reported by a young woman who lived nearby at that long-ago time.

SCHNEIDER, Tom. *Everybody's a Winner: A Kid's Guide to New Sports and Fitness.* Gr. 3 and up. Illus. by Richard Wilson and Tom Schneider. Little, 1976. 139 pp. $8.95; pap. Little, $5.95. Nonfiction.
New games are described that do not require competition and winners every time. Some sports are fun to play, and children can learn and benefit from them. The author provides abundant information about exercises, games, and sports; the new modes are explained.

SCHUMAN, Benjamin N. *The Human Eye.* Gr. 5–6. Illus. by Michael K. Meyers. Atheneum, 1968. 78 pp. $3.95. Nonfiction.
The anatomy of the eye and how it functions are discussed.

SCOPPETTONE, Sandra. *Happy Endings Are All Alike.* Gr. 7 and up. Har-Row, 1978. 202 pp. $9.89. Fiction.
Jaret and Peggy are girl friends who resist family concerns to maintain their love for one another. A teenage boy rapes Jaret and threatens to reveal her lesbianism. She prosecutes, which causes anguish for all concerned, and returns to her relationship with Peggy.

SCOPPETTONE, Sandra. *The Late Great Me.* Gr. 7 and up. Bantam, 1977. 249 pp. pap. $2.25. Fiction.
A high-school student recounts the circumstances and stages of her use of alcohol and her own and her mother's reluctance to acknowledge the seriousness of the problem.

SCOPPETTONE, Sandra. *Trying Hard to Hear You.* Gr. 7–8. Har-Row, 1974. 264 pp. $8.95; pap. Bantam, $2.25. Fiction.
Sixteen-year-old Camilla loves Phil but finds out he is homosexual. Friends who discover that Phil and his friend Jeff are gay put pressure on them to end their relationship. To prove he can be straight, Phil goes out on a date. But he gets drunk, has a car accident, and both are killed. Their friends reflect on what has happened and how their attitudes contributed.

SEABROOKE, Brenda. *Home Is Where They Take You In.* Gr. 7–9. Morrow, 1980. 192 pp. $7.95. Fiction.
Twelve-year-old Benicia is neglected by her alcoholic mother and

her mother's boy friend. Neighbors help Benicia to understand her circumstances and to help herself.

SEARIGHT, Mary. *Your Career in Nursing.* Gr. 7 and up. Photog. Messner, 1970. 191 pp. $7.79. Nonfiction.
The education and training of nurses, the various specializations available in nursing, and the opportunities for those interested in a nursing career are discussed.

SEGAL, Lore. *Tell Me a Mitzi.* Gr. ps–3. Illus. by Harriet Pincus. FS&G, 1970. Unp. $12.95. Fiction.
In one of three stories, young Mitzi and her family take care of one another when they all have colds at the same time.

SEIXAS, Judith S. *Alcohol: What It Is, What It Does.* Gr. 4–5. Illus. by Tom Huffman. Greenwillow, 1977. 56 pp. $5.71. Nonfiction.
The author explains the effects of alcohol on the body and mind, including some alcohol found in foods.

SEUSS, Dr. (Theodore Geisel) *The Foot Book.* Gr. ps–1. Illus. by the author. Random House, 1968. Unp. $5.99. Fiction.
Humorous verse accompanies pictures of many different feet.

SGROI, Suzanne M. *VD: A Doctor's Answers.* Gr. 7–8. Illus. Har-BraceJ, 1974. 182 pp. $6.50. Nonfiction.
The author describes the symptoms and treatment of syphilis and gonorrhea and ways to prevent it, and lists centers throughout the United States where medical help is available.

SHAPIRO, Irwin. *The Gift of Magic Sleep: Early Experiments in Anesthesia.* Gr. 2–6. Illus. by Pat Rotondo. Coward, 1979. 64 pp. $5.99. Nonfiction.
Anesthesia, discovered in the 1800s, was developed for use in the medical and dental fields.

SHAPIRO, Patricia Gottlieb. *Caring for the Mentally Ill.* Gr. 7 and up. Watts, 1982. 87 pp. $7.90. Nonfiction.
The author describes early and current methods of therapy and efforts to gain rights for patients with mental illness.

SHERBURNE, Zoa. *Leslie.* Gr. 6–7. Morrow, 1972. 175 pp. $5.95. Fiction.
Leslie becomes involved in a hit-and-run accident when two high-school boys who use drugs drive her home from a party.

SHERBURNE, Zoa. *Why Have the Birds Stopped Singing?* Gr. 7 and up. Morrow, 1974. 189 pp. $7.63. Fiction.
During an epileptic seizure, sixteen-year-old Katie seems to be transported back in time. She is mistaken for her great-great-great-grandmother, who also had epilepsy, at a time when the disease was more misunderstood than it is now.

SHOWERS, Paul. *A Baby Starts to Grow.* Gr. k–3. Illus. by Rosalind Fry. Crowell, 1969. 33 pp. $10.89. Nonfiction.
The story tells simply of the growth of a baby before its birth.

SHOWERS, Paul. *A Drop of Blood.* Gr. 2–3. Illus. by Don Madden. Har-Row, 1967. Unp. $8.79; pap. Har-Row, $2.95. Nonfiction.
Blood carries oxygen and nutrients throughout the body. New blood forms rapidly when any blood is lost.

SHOWERS, Paul. *Find Out by Touching.* Gr. 2–3. Illus. by Robert Galster. Crowell, 1961. Unp. $8.79. Nonfiction.
A simple game helps stimulate a child's sense of touch.

SHOWERS, Paul. *Follow Your Nose.* Gr. 1–2. Illus. by Paul Galdone. Crowell, 1963. Unp. $8.79; pap. Crowell, $2.95. Nonfiction.
Simple text and illustrations explain the sense of smell, its relationship to the sense of taste, and the functions of the nose.

SHOWERS, Paul. *Hear Your Heart.* Gr. 2–3. Illus. by Joseph Low. Crowell, 1968. 35 pp. $3.75; pap. Crowell, $1.25. Nonfiction.
In simple language the author describes the structure, size, and function of the heart.

SHOWERS, Paul. *How Many Teeth?* Gr. 2–3. Illus. by Paul Galdone. Crowell, 1962. Unp. $8.79; pap. Crowell, $1.45. Nonfiction.
Through the experiences of several children, the author tells how

baby teeth grow, fall out, and are replaced by permanent teeth; why teeth are needed; and how to take care of them.

SHOWERS, Paul. *How You Talk.* Gr. k–3. Illus. by Robert Galster. Har-Row, 1967. Unp. $9.89; pap. Har-Row, $1.45. Nonfiction.
Speech is the result of breathing, the use of the mouth and the nose, the larynx, and the lungs. Babies learn speech through practice and encouragement.

SHOWERS, Paul. *Look at Your Eyes.* Gr. 1–2. Illus. by Paul Galdone. Crowell, 1962. Unp. $8.79; pap. Crowell, $3.95. Nonfiction.
A little boy observes his eyes in a mirror and learns about the eyes, eyelids, eyelashes, and tears.

SHOWERS, Paul. *No Measles, No Mumps for Me.* Gr. 2–3. Illus. by Harriett Barton. Crowell, 1980. 33 pp. $9.95. Nonfiction.
Vaccinations can prevent measles, mumps, polio, whooping cough, and other diseases that used to make people very sick.

SHOWERS, Paul. *Sleep Is for Everyone.* Gr. ps–3. Illus. by Wendy Watson. Har-Row, 1974. 33 pp. $9.89. Nonfiction.
Young and growing people need more sleep than adults. Sleep is the time when the brain dreams and the body rests, although the heart still beats and the lungs still breathe.

SHOWERS, Paul. *Use Your Brain.* Gr. 1–2. Illus. by Rosalind Fry. Crowell, 1971. 33 pp. $8.95; pap. Crowell, $2.95. Nonfiction.
When a person takes drugs, such as alcohol, the brain does not work as well.

SHOWERS, Paul. *What Happens to a Hamburger?* Gr. k–3. Illus. by Anne Rockwell. Har-Row, 1970. 33 pp. $9.89; pap. Har-Row, $3.95. Nonfiction.
In simple language the author gives a detailed explanation of the anatomy and physiology of the digestive system.

SHOWERS, Paul. *You Can't Make a Move Without Your Muscles.* Gr. k–3. Illus. by Harriett Barton. Har-Row, 1982. 33 pp. $9.89. Nonfiction.

More than 600 muscles in the human body help us to move. The muscles are described and illustrated.

SHOWERS, Paul. *Your Skin and Mine.* Gr. 3–4. Illus. by Paul Galdone. Crowell, 1965. Unp. $8.79. Nonfiction.
Skin covers people everywhere; it protects, cools, and feels. Skin color, nails, and fingerprints are explained.

SHOWERS, Paul, and Kay Sperry SHOWERS. *Before You Were a Baby.* Gr. k–3. Illus. by Ingrid Fetz. Crowell, 1968. 34 pp. $10.89. Nonfiction.
The story of conception, pregnancy, and birth is presented in simple terms and drawings.

SHREVE, Susan Richards. *Loveletters.* Gr. 6–7. Knopf, 1978. 217 pp. $6.95. Fiction.
As Kate waits to have her baby in a home for single pregnant adolescents, she thinks of her childhood friend Tommy, who has become emotionally ill.

SHUFF, Frances. *Your Future in Occupational Therapy Careers.* Gr. 7–12. Illus. Rosen, 1977. 120 pp. $7.97. Nonfiction.
In describing the education and work of occupational therapists, the author informs young readers about their therapeutic activities and interactions.

SHYER, Marlene F. *Welcome Home, Jellybean.* Gr. 6–8. Scribner, 1978. 160 pp. $9.95; pap. Schol Bk Serv, $1.95. Fiction.
Thirteen-year-old Gerri, who is retarded, begins living at home after living in a residential care setting. She disrupts the family, especially her brother's friendships and schoolwork. Their father leaves home, but her brother grows to understand Gerri's behavior as an effort to belong in the family.

SIEGEL, Dorothy Schainman. *Winners: Eight Special Young People.* Gr. 7–8. Messner, 1978. 189 pp. $8.79. Nonfiction.
Eight young people who have leukemia, hemophilia, blindness, deafness, or other disabilities tell of their determined struggles to lead active, self-reliant lives.

SILVERSTEIN, Alvin, and Virginia B. SILVERSTEIN. *Alcoholism.* Gr. 6–7. Lippincott, 1975. 128 pp. $7.89. Nonfiction.

Alcohol abuse is the result of a craving for alcohol so intense that it can seem to be the most important part of living. Problem drinking can be diagnosed, treated, and cured in various ways for most people.

SILVERSTEIN, Alvin, and Virginia B. SILVERSTEIN. *Allergies.* Gr. 4–5. Illus. Lippincott, 1977. 128 pp. $9.30. Nonfiction.
Basic information is given about allergic reactions, including descriptions of the various types of allergies and summaries of research into causes and treatments.

SILVERSTEIN, Alvin, and Virginia B. SILVERSTEIN. *Cancer.* Gr. 5–6. Illus. by Andrew Antal. John Day, 1977. 102 pp. $8.79. Nonfiction.
The causes and treatments of various kinds of cancer, and the ways in which individuals can help prevent this disease, are described.

SILVERSTEIN, Alvin, and Virginia B. SILVERSTEIN. *Circulatory System: The Rivers Within.* Gr. 6–7. Illus. by George Bakacs. P-H, 1970. 74 pp. $6.95. Nonfiction.
This detailed work discusses the composition of blood cells, the circulation process, healing, and transfusions.

SILVERSTEIN, Alvin, and Virginia B. SILVERSTEIN. *The Code of Life.* Gr. 5–9. Illus. by Kenneth Gosner. Atheneum, 1972. 89 pp. $4.50. Nonfiction.
The human body has its own genetic code, in genes, chromosomes, and DNA, determining the appearance and structure of each person.

SILVERSTEIN, Alvin, and Virginia B. SILVERSTEIN. *The Digestive System: How Living Creatures Use Food.* Gr. 6–7. Illus. by Mel Erikson. P-H, 1970. 74 pp. $8.95. Nonfiction.
From smelling and seeing food to processing it through the body, digestion helps living things get food.

SILVERSTEIN, Alvin, and Virginia B. SILVERSTEIN. *The Endocrine System: Hormones in the Living World.* Gr. 6–7. Illus. by Mel Erikson. P-H, 1971. 68 pp. $6.95. Nonfiction.
Glands that produce secretions called hormones help children grow and keep their bodies running smoothly.

SILVERSTEIN, Alvin, and Virginia B. SILVERSTEIN. *Epilepsy.* Gr. 6–7. Illus. Lippincott, 1975. 64 pp. $9.95. Nonfiction.
The authors explain the nature, symptoms, and treatment of the several kinds of epilepsy, and dispel common misconceptions about epilepsy by describing research into its causes and effects.

SILVERSTEIN, Alvin, and Virginia B. SILVERSTEIN. *The Excretory System: How Living Creatures Get Rid of Wastes.* Gr. 4–5. Illus. by Lee J. Ames. P-H, 1972. 74 pp. $6.95. Nonfiction.
The ways in which wastes are excreted, with the complementary role of the lungs, skin, urinary system, and digestive systems, are described. Malfunctions include bedwetting, diarrhea, and constipation. Some of the remedies are artificial kidneys, dialysis machines, and certain medications.

SILVERSTEIN, Alvin, and Virginia B. SILVERSTEIN. *Futurelife: The Biotechnology Revolution.* Gr. 7 and up. Illus. by Marjorie Thier; photog. P-H, 1982. 105 pp. $9.95. Nonfiction.
Bionic limbs and artificial organs currently help disabled people. The authors believe the future will bring regeneration of amputated limbs, genetic engineering, and new diagnostic machines.

SILVERSTEIN, Alvin, and Virginia B. SILVERSTEIN. *The Genetics Explosion.* Gr. 7–8. Illus. Four Winds, 1980. 154 pp. $9.95. Nonfiction.
An analysis is offered of genetic engineering, its potential benefits, and the risks of cloning and recombinant DNA research.

SILVERSTEIN, Alvin, and Virginia B. SILVERSTEIN. *Heartbeats: Your Body, Your Heart.* Gr. 3–5. Illus. by Stella Ormai. Lippincott, 1983. 60 pp. $9.89. Nonfiction.
The authors describe the anatomy of the heart, transplants, artificial valves, and how to keep the heart healthy.

SILVERSTEIN, Alvin, and Virginia B. SILVERSTEIN. *Itch, Sniffle and Sneeze: All About Asthma, Hay Fever and Other Allergies.* Gr. 3–4. Illus. by Roy Doty. Four Winds, 1978. Unp. $7.95. Nonfiction.
About one in five people is allergic to something. The authors explain how to find out what one is allergic to and what to do about it. Included are asthma, hay fever, and dust and pollen allergies.

SILVERSTEIN, Alvin, and Virginia B. SILVERSTEIN. *The Respiratory System: How Living Creatures Breathe.* Gr. 5–6. Illus. by George Backacs. P-H, 1969. 60 pp. $4.50. Nonfiction.
The respiratory system is the mechanism for breathing. Humans and animals have different ways of getting oxygen to the cells of their bodies.

SILVERSTEIN, Alvin, and Virginia B. SILVERSTEIN. *Runaway Sugar: All About Diabetes.* Gr. 3–5. Illus. by Harriett Barton. Lippincott, 1981. 34 pp. $9.50. Nonfiction.
The causes of diabetes are not as well known as the symptoms and treatment. The book explains normal and diabetic digestion.

SILVERSTEIN, Alvin, and Virginia B. SILVERSTEIN. *The Skeletal System: Frameworks for Life.* Gr. 3–7. Illus. by Lee J. Ames. P-H, 1972. 74 pp. $5.95. Nonfiction.
The human skeleton works together with the muscles and other systems of the body. The skeletal system of human beings is similar to and different from that of animals, birds, and insects.

SILVERSTEIN, Alvin, and Virginia B. SILVERSTEIN. *The Skin: Coverings and Linings of Living Things.* Gr. 4–5. Illus. by Lee J. Ames. P-H, 1972. 90 pp. $4.95. Nonfiction.
The skin covers and lines humans, animals, and plants. The skin can be allergic and can have rashes and other problems, but there are many treatments available.

SILVERSTEIN, Alvin, and Virginia B. SILVERSTEIN. *Sleep and Dreams.* Gr. 7–8. Illus. Lippincott, 1974. 159 pp. $9.25. Nonfiction.
The book traces scientific discoveries about sleep and sleep patterns and the nature of dreams.

SILVERSTEIN, Alvin, and Virginia B. SILVERSTEIN. *So You're Getting Braces: A Guide to Orthodontics.* Gr. 5–6. Photog. by the authors. Har-Row, 1978. 128 pp. pap. $3.95. Nonfiction.
The process of straightening teeth is explained, with an emphasis on cooperation. Various kinds of braces are shown, with ideas about future aids.

SILVERSTEIN, Alvin, and Virginia B. SILVERSTEIN. *The Story of Your Ear*. Gr. 5–9. Illus. by Susan Gaber. Coward, 1981. 64 pp. $6.99. Nonfiction.
The authors describe the structure of the ear and how it receives sounds and maintains balance. They emphasize avoiding accidents, ear infections, and loud noises and tell of advances in medicine and technology, such as artificial ear bones, hearing aids, and bionic ears.

SILVERSTEIN, Alvin, and Virginia B. SILVERSTEIN. *The Story of Your Mouth*. Gr. 5–9. Illus. by Karen Ackoff. Coward, 1983. 64 pp. $8.00. Nonfiction.
In this introduction to the mouth and its functions, the authors describe activities of eating and speech.

SILVERSTEIN, Alvin, and Virginia B. SILVERSTEIN. *The Sugar Disease: Diabetes*. Gr. 5–6. Lippincott, 1980. 111 pp. $7.95. Nonfiction.
The causes of diabetes, its effects on the body, and the types of treatment available are explained. The history of the disease, from ancient Egypt to today, is told.

SILVERSTEIN, Alvin, and Virginia B. SILVERSTEIN. *The World of Bionics*. Gr. 6–7. Illus. Methuen, 1979. 116 pp. $8.95. Nonfiction.
From research on animals, appliances are developed to aid vision and hearing and to create artificial limbs and organs.

SIMON, Nissa. *Don't Worry, You're Normal: A Teenager's Guide to Self-Health*. Gr. 7 and up. Har-Row, 1982. 192 pp. $8.89; pap. Har-Row, $4.75. Nonfiction.
To encourage teenagers to be aware of and confident in their bodies, the authors give information about growth changes, nutrition, medical problems, sexuality, and emotional concerns. The section on roles and rights of patients emphasizes personal responsibility for health.

SIMON, Norma. *Go Away, Warts!* Gr. 3–4. Illus. by Susan Lexa. A Whitman, 1980. Unp. $7.50. Fiction.
When Freddie's warts bleed, interfering with playing ball, his mother brings him to a doctor. Freddie takes the prescribed

vitamin pills randomly, yet the warts disappear. His misconceptions about warts are countered with facts.

SIMON, Norma. *How Do I Feel?* Gr. ps–2. Illus. by Joe Lasker. A Whitman, 1970. Unp. $8.25. Fiction.
Children have many feelings, including anger, frustration, pride, weariness, and strength.

SIMON, Norma. *We Remember Philip.* Gr. 2–4. Illus. by Ruth Sanderson. A Whitman, 1979. 32 pp. $8.25. Fiction.
After the accidental death of their teacher's son, Sam and his classmates find ways to express their feelings by writing letters to their teacher, telling him their feelings, trying to understand his grief, and planting an oak tree in Philip's memory.

SIMON, Norma. *Why Am I Different?* Gr. 1–2. Illus. by Dora Leder. A Whitman, 1976. 31 pp. $6.95. Nonfiction.
Everyday situations are detailed in which children see themselves as different in family styles, appearance, skills, and wishes. The children feel that being different is all right.

SIMON, Seymour. *About Your Heart.* Gr. 2–3. Illus. by Angeline Culfogienis. McGraw-Hill, 1974. 38 pp. $4.72. Nonfiction.
Experiments show the physical and biological characteristics and functions of the heart and circulatory system.

SIMON, Seymour. *Body Sense, Body Nonsense.* Gr. 4–6. Illus. by Dennis Kendrich. Lippincott, 1981. Unp. $8.89. Nonfiction.
Presenting the sense and nonsense in twenty-two familiar sayings about the body, such as "drafts cause colds," this book clarifies common misconceptions.

SINGER, Marilyn. *It Can't Hurt Forever.* Gr. 5–6. Illus. by Leigh Grant. Har-Row, 1978. 186 pp. $10.89. Fiction.
Ellie has an electrocardiogram and an X ray. She is hospitalized for cardiac catheterization and heart surgery. She learns a great deal about her body and procedures in the hospital as well as about hospital staff and other patients. She is helped by her parents, her humor, and the expression of feelings about her experiences.

SISLOWITZ, Marcel J. *Look! How Your Eyes See.* Gr. 2–3. Illus. by Jim Arnosky. Coward, 1977. 46 pp. $6.99. Nonfiction.
Each part of the eye and its functions are described. An eye examination is detailed and problems described briefly, such as vision impairment, strabismus, and amblyopia. Suggestions are given for healthy eye care.

SKURZYNSKI, Gloria. *Bionic Parts for People: The Real Story of Artificial Organs and Replacement Parts.* Gr. 7–8. Illus. by Frank Schwarz. Four Winds, 1978. 147 pp. $9.95. Nonfiction.
The artificial kidney, eye, ear, heart, arm, and leg are described and illustrated. Disabled people who need them must work to adapt themselves to these aids and appliances.

SLEPIAN, Jan. *The Alfred Summer.* Gr. 5–6. Macmillan, 1980. 119 pp. $8.95. Fiction.
Twelve-year-old Myron builds a boat to sail away from a nagging mother and his sisters' derision, with the help of Alfred, who is mildly retarded, and Lester, who has cerebral palsy.

SLEPIAN, Jan. *Lester's Turn.* Gr. 7–8. Macmillan, 1981. 139 pp. $8.95. Fiction.
Lester, who has cerebral palsy, learns about using, needing, and loving friends when he tries to rescue his friend Alfie, who is retarded and seriously ill in the hospital.

SLOTE, Alfred. *Hang Tough, Paul Mather.* Gr. 5–6. Lippincott, 1973. 156 pp. $10.95; pap. Avon, $1.75. Fiction.
Paul tells his own story while he is hospitalized for terminal leukemia. He recounts examinations and the pain of treatments. He also recalls his effort to join a Little League team, despite his father's and physician's objections. A doctor talks with Paul about illness, fear of death, and the reality of restraint, and helps him to develop courage.

SMITH, Doris Buchanan. *Kelly's Creek.* Gr. 3–7. Illus. by Alan Tiergreen. Har-Row, 1975. 80 pp. $9.95. Fiction.
Nine-year-old Kelly cannot ride a bicycle, catch a football, or write his own name. His learning disability makes it hard for his eyes, hands, and brain to coordinate, but his family, friends, and teacher think he is not trying. He plays by the creek and is finally able to share what he has learned there with someone who cares.

SMITH, Elwood H. *The See and Hear and Smell and Touch Book.* Gr. ps–1. Illus. J Philip O'Hara, 1973. Unp. $4.98. Nonfiction.
Watercolor drawings and brief text introduce children to the five senses.

SMITH, Lucia B. *A Special Kind of Sister.* Gr. 2–3. Illus. by Chuck Hall. HR&W, 1979. Unp. $5.95. Fiction.
A young girl describes her feelings about and activities with her younger brother, who is retarded and has brain damage.

SNELL, Nigel. *Johnny Gets Some Glasses.* Gr. ps–1. Illus. by the author. Hamish Hamilton, 1980. 32 pp. $5.95. Fiction.
When Johnny's vision blurs, he is examined and glasses are fitted.

SNELL, Nigel. *Kate Visits the Doctor.* Gr. ps–1. Illus. by the author. Hamish Hamilton, 1981. 32 pp. $5.95. Fiction.
A doctor gives Kate a physical examination, showing the instruments and procedures.

SNELL, Nigel. *Lucy Loses Her Tonsils.* Gr. ps–1. Illus. by the author. Hamish Hamilton, 1978. Unp. $5.95. Fiction.
A simple story of going to the hospital for a tonsillectomy tells of ice cream and play but also of medicine and anesthesia.

SNELL, Nigel. *Peter Gets a Hearing Aid.* Gr. ps–1. Illus. by the author. Hamish Hamilton, 1980. 32 pp. $5.95. Fiction.
After Peter's hearing is tested and he is examined, he is given a hearing aid to improve his hearing.

SNELL, Nigel. *Tom Visits the Dentist.* Gr. ps–1. Illus. by the author. Hamish Hamilton, 1979. Unp. $5.95. Fiction.
Tom does not want to get the holes in his teeth repaired by the dentist, but he finds it is not uncomfortable. The dentist also shows him how he will make braces for his teeth, and Tom is hopeful about how well he will look.

SNYDER, Anne. *My Name Is Davy, I'm an Alcoholic.* Gr. 7–8. Illus. Holt, 1977. 128 pp. $5.95; pap. New Amer Lib, $1.50. Fiction.
Fifteen-year-old Davy and his girl friend are alcoholics who experience illness, beatings, and shame until she drowns accidentally while drunk. Davy is eventually able to return to Alcoholics Anonymous and start a difficult recovery.

SNYDER, Gerald S. *Human Rights.* Gr. 5–6. Photog. by UNICEF and others. Watts, 1980. 63 pp. $7.90. Nonfiction.
Child-abuse protection and education for the handicapped are among the children's rights and the rights of the disabled included in this discussion.

SNYDER, Gerald S. *Test-Tube Life: Scientific Advance and Moral Dilemma.* Gr. 9 and up. Messner, 1982. 158 pp. $9.29. Nonfiction.
Genetic engineering can produce useful bacteria and medicines (from biologic rather than chemical sources), and can fertilize human ova in a culture dish. Ethical and philosophical beliefs affect the progress of this work.

SOBOL, Harriet Langsam. *The Interns.* Gr. 6–8. Photog. by Patricia Agre. Coward, 1981. 64 pp. $6.96. Nonfiction.
The photographs and narrative illustrate the day-to-day experiences of two pediatric interns at Columbia Presbyterian's Babies Hospital. The importance of internship in medical education is emphasized.

SOBOL, Harriet Langsam. *My Brother Steven Is Retarded.* Gr. 3–6. Photog. by Patricia Agre. Macmillan, 1977. 26 pp. $8.95. Nonfiction.
Eleven-year-old Beth has mixed feelings about her retarded, brain damaged brother, Steven. It is hard to have a brother who is moody and clumsy and does not learn as fast as other children, but she is hurt when the children laugh at him.

SONNET, Sherry. *Smoking.* Gr. 4–6. Illus. Watts, 1977. 64 pp. $7.90. Nonfiction.
The author describes the history of smoking and its effects on the organs of the body, and discourages children from smoking.

SOUTHALL, Ivan. *Head in the Clouds.* Gr. 3–5. Illus. by Richard Kennedy. Macmillan, 1972. 106 pp. $4.95. Fiction.
An accident-prone nine-year-old recovering from a car accident is in a wheelchair and unable to go out. To punish the friends who ignore him, he tries magic spells until one of the spells appears to work.

SPENCE, Eleanor. *The Devil Hole.* Gr. 5–9. Lothrop, 1977. 215 pp. $9.50. Fiction.
Ten-year-old Douglas finally learns to tolerate the demanding and apparently illogical behavior of his autistic younger brother.

SPENCE, Eleanor. *The Nothing Place.* Gr. 6–7. Illus. by Geraldine Spence. Har-Row, 1973. 228 pp. $8.89. Fiction.
Glen has a severe hearing impairment, which he tries to hide in his new school. His friend raises money to buy him a hearing aid, but he is offended. After a teacher talks with his mother, Glen considers the hearing aid and going to special school, and understands his friend's generosity.

SPENCER, Zane, and Jay LEECH. *Cry of the Wolf.* Gr. 4–5. Westminster, 1977. 144 pp. $7.95. Fiction.
Sixteen-year-old Jim is disabled in an accident that kills his father. He must overcome his feelings of loss and guilt in order to help maintain the family ranch.

SPLAVER, Sarah. *Your Handicap—Don't Let It Handicap You.* Gr. 7–8. Messner, 1974. 224 pp. $7.29. Nonfiction.
The author describes visual, auditory, and speech impairment and orthopedic disability. Resources available to handicapped young people are listed, such as career education, personal counseling, and governmental help.

SPOCK, Benjamin McLane. *A Teenager's Guide to Life and Love.* Gr. 9 and up. Pocket Bks, 1971. 174 pp. pap. $1.25. Nonfiction.
The famous pediatrician discusses dating, the use of marijuana and other drugs, and sexuality, including homosexuality, marriage, and pregnancy.

SPRADLEY, Thomas S., and James R. SPRADLEY. *Deaf Like Me.* Gr. 10 and up. Random House, 1978. 281 pp. $11.95. Nonfiction.
A mother and father try to follow expert advice and raise their deaf daughter as a hearing child but find that they can help her more by using sign language and other methods that acknowledge her disability.

STANEK, Muriel. *Don't Hurt Me, Mama.* Gr. 1–3. Illus. A Whitman, 1983. 32 pp. $8.25. Fiction.

When Mama drinks too much and feels no one cares about her, she hits her daughter. The teacher sends the girl to the school nurse, who is able to help her.

STANEK, Muriel. *Growl When You Say R.* Gr. 2–3. Illus. by Phil Smith. A Whitman, 1979. Unp. $6.95. Fiction.
Through the story of a boy who substitutes the "w" for the "r" sound, the book explains how the speech therapist works together with the child and his family to help him correct his articulation errors.

STANEK, Muriel. *Left Right, Left Right.* Gr. k–2. Illus. by Lucy Hawkinson. A Whitman, 1969. 40 pp. $8.25. Fiction.
A young girl (who happens to wear glasses) confuses left and right until her grandmother gives her a ring to wear on her right hand. She does well and realizes she does not need the ring after a while. She gives it to her younger brother to help him learn too.

STANEK, Muriel. *Who's Afraid of the Dark?* Gr. 1–3. Illus. by Helen Cogancherry. A Whitman, 1980. Unp. $7.50. Fiction.
With the help of his family, Kenny learns to cope with his fear of the dark.

STANTON, Elizabeth, and Henry STANTON. *Sometimes I Like to Cry.* Gr. 1–2. Illus. by Richard Leyden. A Whitman, 1978. Unp. $8.25. Fiction.
When Joey cuts his finger, and when his pet hamster dies, he cries. He finds out that people also cry on some happy occasions.

STEEDMAN, Julie. *Emergency Room: An ABC Tour.* Gr. ps–3. Photog. Windy Hill Pr, 1974. 38 pp. pap. $3.95. Nonfiction.
With A for ambulance, C for cast, D for doctor, and X for X ray, this ABC book teaches about a unique part of a medical center. Photos and explanations for each medical word reassure young readers while showing them the reality of an otherwise scary place.

STEFANIK, Alfred T. *Copycat Sam: Developing Ties with a Special Child.* Gr. 1–3. Illus. by Laura Huff. Hum Sci Pr, 1982. Unp. $9.95. Fiction.
Freddie overcomes his irritation about the imitative behavior of a boy who has Down's syndrome, and becomes his friend.

STEIG, William. *Doctor De Soto*. Gr. ps–1. Illus. FS&G, 1982. 32 pp. $11.95. Fiction.
A mouse dentist has to decide what to do when a fox comes to his clinic for treatment.

STEIN, Sara Bonnett. *About Dying: An Open Family Book for Parents and Children Together*. Gr. 1–2. Photog. by Dick Frank. Walker, 1974. 47 pp. $7.95. Fiction.
When his pet bird dies, Eric and his friends are curious. They look at the bird and then bury him. His mother talks with him about death and then about Grandpa's death, how he was buried too, and how people felt afterward. The comments for adult readers are next to the children's story.

STEIN, Sara Bonnett. *About Handicaps: An Open Family Book for Parents and Children Together*. Gr. 1–2. Photog. by Dick Frank. Walker, 1974. 47 pp. $8.95. Fiction.
Matthew is frightened of Joe at first, because Joe does not walk the same way Matthew does. As he learns more about Joe and acknowledges fears about his own imperfections, he becomes more accepting. He also sees a man with a hook, who explains how his artificial arm works. He and his dad talk together about it. Accompanying information for adults further explores how nondisabled children react to disabled peers.

STEIN, Sara Bonnett. *About Phobias: An Open Family Book for Parents and Children Together*. Gr. 2–3. Photog. by Erika Stone. Walker, 1979. 47 pp. $6.95. Fiction.
Phobias are exaggerated fears that may be temporary or long-lasting. A four-year-old's sudden fear of dogs is told in a story. In the accompanying text for parents, analysis and suggestions are given for dealing with such fears.

STEIN, Sara Bonnett. *A Hospital Story: An Open Family Book for Parents and Children Together*. Gr. 1–2. Photog. by Doris Pinney. Walker, 1974. 47 pp. $7.95. Fiction.
With separate texts for adults and children, this simple, direct story shows Jill's hospitalization for tonsillectomy. Throughout, her feelings are a part of the narrative. The accompanying advice for adults helps them respond to children's concerns arising from the story.

STEVENS, Leonard A. *Neurons: Building Blocks of the Brain.* Gr. 7 and up. Illus. by Henry Roth. Har-Row, 1974. 87 pp. $9.95. Non-fiction.
Stories of the scientists who have studied the nervous system inform the reader about the structure, function, and importance of neurons, or nerve cells.

STILLER, Richard. *Your Body Is Trying to Tell You Something: How to Understand Its Signals and Respond to Its Needs.* Gr. 7–8. HarBraceJ, 1979. 128 pp. $7.95. Nonfiction.
The author details the symptoms and treatment of headaches, muscular pain, skin problems, viruses, venereal diseases, and drug and alcohol abuse.

STINE, Jovial Bob, and Jane STINE. *The Sick of Being Sick Book.* Gr. 3–7. Illus. by Carol Nicklaus. Dutton, 1980. 68 pp. $7.95. Fiction.
Jokes, games, and advice such as "how to get the most sympathy from your illness" and "10 things that won't make you feel better" are designed to help children laugh themselves into feeling better.

STOLZ, Mary. *The Edge of Next Year.* Gr. 7–8. Har-Row, 1974. 195 pp. $10.89; pap. Dell, $1.50. Fiction.
A fourteen-year-old boy must adjust to the sudden death of his mother and cope with alienation that has divided his grieving family.

STOLZ, Mary. *In a Mirror.* Gr. 7–12. Dell, 1971. 211 pp. pap. $2.25. Fiction.
A college student resolves her problem of overweight by analyzing people close to her, and by self-analysis.

STORR, Catherine. *Thursday.* Gr. 7–8. Har-Row, 1972. 274 pp. $8.95. Fiction.
Although fifteen-year-old Bea is recovering from infectious mononucleosis, she helps a boy she and her family have befriended named Thursday. He is emotionally ill, and Bea helps his recovery by persistent caring and by believing in him.

STRASSER, Todd. *Angel Dust Blues.* Gr. 7–8. Coward, 1979. 203 pp. $9.95; pap. Dell, $1.75. Fiction.

Once a model high-school student and tennis star, Alex finds an easier, more profitable way of life in drug dealing. When he falls in love for the first time, he must make a difficult choice.

STRASSER, Todd. *Friends Till the End.* Gr. 8–9. Delacorte, 1981. 192 pp. $9.95; pap. Dell, $2.25. Fiction.
When Howie is hospitalized with leukemia, his new friend, David, visits and encourages him.

STWERTKA, Eve, and Albert STWERTKA. *Genetic Engineering.* Gr. 7 and up. Watts, 1982. 96 pp. $7.90. Nonfiction.
The authors discuss the processes of, and controversy about, amniocentesis, genetic counseling, and laboratory conception.

STWERTKA, Eve, and Albert STWERTKA. *Marijuana.* Gr. 7–9. Illus. Watts, 1979. 64 pp. $5.95. Nonfiction.
Marijuana use is widespread. The plant's origin and cultivation and its psychological and physiological effects are described, and laws about its use and sale are detailed.

SULLIVAN, Mary Beth, and Linda BOURKE. *A Show of Hands: Say It in Sign Language.* Gr. 4–8. Illus. by Linda Bourke. Addison-Wesley, 1980. 96 pp. $8.95. Nonfiction.
With illustrated sign language, readers are encouraged to "talk" with their hands.

SULLIVAN, Mary Beth, Alan J. BRIGHTMAN, and Joseph BLATT. *Feeling Free.* Gr. 4–5. Illus. by Marci Davis and Linda Bourke. Photog. by Alan J. Brightman. Addison-Wesley, 1979. 186 pp. $10.95. Nonfiction.
Children share their experiences about what it is like to be different, to be disabled, and to be stared at and questioned by others.

SULLIVAN, Navin. *Controls in Your Body.* Gr. 4–5. Illus. by Anthony Ravielli. Lippincott, 1971. 64 pp. $6.95. Nonfiction.
Various mechanisms in the human body control its growth, movement, breathing, and temperature.

SULLIVAN, Tom, and Gill DEREK. *If You Could See What I Hear.* Gr. 10–12. Illus. Har-Row, 1975. 184 pp. $10.95; pap. New Amer Lib, $2.50. Nonfiction.

A young, blind husband and father recalls his lonely childhood, education, early adulthood, refusals to submit to his disability, and struggles to succeed in sports, music, and life.

SUSSMAN, Alan. *The Rights of Young People: The Basic ACLU Guide to a Young Person's Rights.* Gr. 10 and up. Avon, 1977. 249 pp. pap. $3.50. Nonfiction.
In question-and-answer format this book includes information on medical care, contraception, abortion, pregnancy, child abuse and neglect, rape, and the use of alcohol and tobacco.

TALBOT, Charlene J. *The Great Rat Island Adventure.* Gr. 4–6. Atheneum, 1977. 164 pp. $7.95. Fiction.
Eleven-year-old Joel is overweight. He spends the summer on an island with his father. After several adventures, and being too busy to eat as much as before, Joel loses weight.

TAYLOR, David M., and Maxine A. ROCK. *Gut Reactions: How to Handle Stress and Your Stomach.* Gr. 7 and up. Saunders, 1980. 167 pp. $10.95. Nonfiction.
When a physical examination shows no organic problem even though a person has stomachaches, nausea, or other abdominal symptoms, other factors must be considered. The authors, a gastroenterologist and a science writer, discuss personality factors, the physical effects of stress, and the results of diets and prescription medications.

TENSEN, Gordon. *Youth and Sex: Pleasure and Responsibility.* Gr. 10 and up. Nelson-Hall, 1979. 173 pp. $9.95; pap. Nelson-Hall, $5.95. Nonfiction.
To enable teenagers to make their own decisions, this psychiatrist-author gives plentiful detail on sexuality, pregnancy, abortion, venereal diseases, and contraception.

TERRY, Luther L., and Daniel HORN. *To Smoke or Not To Smoke.* Gr. 7–12. Illus. by Robert Quackenbush. Lothrop, 1969. 64 pp. $8.16. Nonfiction.
A former Surgeon General of the United States explains how smoking habits begin, how to help someone to quit smoking, and how smoking can lead to disease and death.

THAYER, Jane. *Try Your Hand.* Gr. k–3. Illus. by Joel Schick. Morrow, 1979. Unp. $7.44. Nonfiction.
Fourteen challenging riddles make use of the different meanings for the word *hand,* encouraging readers to consider the many kinds of hands that exist.

THOMAS, William E. *The New Boy Is Blind.* Gr. 3–6. Illus. Messner, 1980. 64 pp. $6.79. Fiction.
When Ricky, a fourth-grader who is blind, is mainstreamed into public school, he learns to use a Brailler and sighted guides. He has mobility training. His sighted classmates and his mother learn to encourage Ricky to do things for himself, to build his sense of accomplishment and self-worth.

THOMPSON, Brenda, and Rosemary GIESEN. *Bones and Skeletons.* Gr. 2–3. Illus. by Carole Viner and Rosemary Giesen. Lerner, 1974. Unp. $4.95. Nonfiction.
The various types of human and animal bones and their functions are described and illustrated.

THOMPSON, Paul. *Nutrition.* Gr. 6 and up. Illus. Watts, 1981. 65 pp. $7.40. Nonfiction.
A balanced diet includes carbohydrates, fats, proteins, and minerals. The author describes how the body uses foods and highlights controversies about food processing and pollution, additives, and vitamins.

THRASHER, Crystal. *The Dark Didn't Catch Me.* Gr. 5–9. Atheneum, 1979. 182 pp. pap. $1.95. Fiction.
Seely and her family cope with poverty, moving to a new community, and the accidental death of her younger brother. She maintains hopefulness as she grows and develops.

THYPIN, Marilyn, and Lynne GLASNER. *Health Care for the Wongs: Health Insurance, Choosing a Doctor.* Gr. 5–6. Photog. by Ira Berger. EMC, 1980. 60 pp. $3.95. Fiction.
In this photodramatization, Mr. and Mrs. Wong use the services of a medical clinic for their children, obtain health insurance, and select a family doctor.

TICHY, William. *Poisons, Antidotes and Anecdotes.* Gr. 7 and up. Illus. Sterling, 1977. 192 pp. $8.95. Nonfiction.
The author explains the history of poisons and describes the physiological reactions to them. Poisonous insects, fish, and animals are shown. Syrup of Ipecac, Universal Antidote kits, and protector tops for medicine can help avoid poisoning at home.

TOBIAS, Tobi. *A Day Off.* Gr. 1–2. Illus. by Ray Cruz. Putnam, 1973. Unp. $3.86. Fiction.
A young boy thinks of the advantages of being slightly sick and having to stay home from school.

TOBIAS, Tobi. *The Quitting Deal.* Gr. 1–4. Illus. by Trina Schart Hyman. Viking, 1975. Unp. $8.95; pap. Penguin, $2.25. Fiction.
Because seven-year-old Jenny wants to stop sucking her thumb and her mother wants to stop smoking, they agree to help each other.

TOURÉ, Halima. *Pain.* Gr. 9–12. Illus. Watts, 1981. 88 pp. $7.50. Nonfiction.
The book describes the nervous system, the nature of pain, and how it originates. Psychosomatic pain and cultural emphasis on areas of pain are explained. Pain is alleviated by surgery, drugs, anesthetics, hypnosis, acupuncture, electrical stimulation, and biofeedback.

TRACHTENBERG, Irene. *My Daughter, My Son.* Gr. 10 and up. Summit, 1978. 271 pp. $9.95. Nonfiction.
A mother tells of her two children who developed ulcerative colitis. She describes various treatments, including ileostomy, and the effects of the illness on the family.

TRIER, Carola S. *Exercise: What It Is, What It Does.* Gr. 1–3. Illus. by Tom Huffman. Greenwillow, 1982. 55 pp. $5.71. Nonfiction.
Exercise is important for health. The author presents instructions for simple exercises that are fun to do alone or with a friend.

TRULL, Patti. *On with My Life.* Gr. 5 and up. Putnam, 1983. 160 pp. $9.95. Nonfiction.
When Patti was fifteen years old she had bone cancer and her leg was amputated. Now, fifteen years later, she describes the

hospital, treatments, physical adjustments, and her determination to recover. An occupational therapist, she describes her work with other young cancer patients.

TULLY, Marianne, and Mary-Alice TULLY. *Dread Diseases.* Gr. 6–7. Illus. Watts, 1978. 65 pp. $7.90. Nonfiction.
Each disease is defined, its source noted (if known), and the treatment described. The list includes smallpox, rabies, venereal diseases, genetic diseases, heart disease, diabetes, multiple sclerosis, and cancer.

TULLY, Marianne, and Mary-Alice TULLY. *Facts About the Human Body.* Gr. 4–6. Watts, 1977. 63 pp. $7.90. Nonfiction.
All the systems of the body are described in answer to specific questions such as, "What are tonsils and why do some people have to have them out?"

TULLY, Mary-Alice, and Marianne TULLY. *Heart Disease.* Gr. 6–8. Watts, 1980. 64 pp. $7.90. Nonfiction.
The authors detail the functions of the heart and what happens when it does not work well, as in rheumatic fever, valve damage, and birth malformations.

VALENS, E. G. *A Long Way Up: The Story of Jill Kinmont.* Gr. 7–8. Photog. by Burk Uzzle and others. Har-Row, 1966. 245 pp. $10.95. Nonfiction.
This is the true story of athlete Jill Kinmont, who had a paralyzing accident while training for the Olympic ski team and had to face a new way of life. The author tells how Kinmont's family and a new friend helped her manage both physical and emotional difficulties.

VANDENBURG, Mary Lou. *Help! Emergencies That Could Happen to You and How to Handle Them.* Gr. 4–5. Illus. by R. L. Markham. Lerner, 1975. 71 pp. $3.95. Nonfiction.
Details are given on how to respond to such common emergencies as swimming and skating accidents, animal bites, and fires.

VAN LEEUWEN, Jean. *I Was a 98-Pound Duckling.* Gr. 7–8. Dial, 1972. 102 pp. $6.95; pap. Dell, $1.50. Fiction.
Trying to follow the advice of her girl friend and beauty magazines, a thirteen-year-old girl uses creams and cosmetics to

hide her skin problems, and acts unintelligent on dates. She is also underweight and feels unattractive. One boy, however, is attracted to her despite her appearance and shows interest in her conversation.

VIGNA, Judith. *Gregory's Stitches.* Gr. 1–2. Illus. by the author. A Whitman, 1974. 32 pp. $7.75. Fiction.
Gregory receives six stitches in his forehead after falling off his bicycle. The story of the incident changes as it travels from friend to friend. He becomes a hero and finds that getting stitches is not so terrible after all.

VISSER, Pat. *Feelings from A to Z.* Gr. k–3. Illus. by Rod Ruth. Western Pub, 1979. Unp. $5.77. Fiction.
Young children's feelings change throughout each day. Sometimes Ann feels angry, Ike feels ill, and Pat feels pretty.

VOELCKERS, Ellen. *Girls' Guide to Menstruation.* Gr. 7–8. Illus. Rosen, 1975. 127 pp. $4.80. Nonfiction.
The author explains the menstrual cycle, the female reproductive system, and problems that can occur and how they may be treated.

WAIDLEY, Ericka. *All About Your X-Ray: IVP.* Gr. ps–1. Illus. by Claudia Gillingwater. Ped Proj, 1983. Unp. pap. $1.50. Nonfiction.
An intravenous pyelogram (IVP) is a diagnostic test that includes an X ray picture of the kidneys. In simple terms and with line drawings the test is described and feelings acknowledged.

WAIDLEY, Ericka. *All About Your X-Ray: UGI.* Gr. ps–1. Illus. by Claudia Gillingwater. Ped Proj, 1983. Unp. pap. $1.50. Nonfiction.
An X ray of the upper gastrointestinal tract (UGI) helps the doctor see the child's esophagus, stomach, and intestines. In simple words and with line drawings the test is described and feelings acknowledged.

WALSWORTH, Nancy, and Patricia BRADLEY. *Coping with School Age Motherhood.* Gr. 7–12. Rosen, 1979. 115 pp. $7.97. Nonfiction.
Adolescent single mothers are welcomed into a familylike group in school, where they receive supportive counseling and help in caring for their babies.

WANDRO, Mark, and Joani BLANK. *My Daddy Is a Nurse.* Gr. ps–3. Illus. by Irene Trivas. Addison-Wesley, 1981. 32 pp. $8.95. Fiction.
Men can be nurses and dental hygienists and can do other work once done mostly by women.

WARBURG, Sandol S. *Growing Time.* Gr. k–3. Illus. by Leonard Weisgard. HM, 1969. 44 pp. $8.95; pap. HM, $1.50. Fiction.
A young boy learns about death from his family. When his beloved dog dies, he learns that the spirit of something you really love will live in your heart.

WARD, Brian R. *Birth and Growth.* Gr. 5 and up. Illus. Watts, 1983. 48 pp. $8.90. Nonfiction.
From conception through fetal development, the human reproductive system provides an environment for growth and protection of the developing person.

WARD, Brian R. *Body Maintenance.* Gr. 5 and up. Illus. Watts, 1983. 48 pp. $8.90. Nonfiction.
The body is supported and maintained by water balance through the kidneys, the hormones, the immune system to control infection, and cell repair.

WARD, Brian R. *The Ear and Hearing.* Gr. 4 and up. Illus. Watts, 1981. 48 pp. $8.90. Nonfiction.
Sound is heard by the ear and understood by the brain. Hearing impairments can be diagnosed, and some can be treated.

WARD, Brian R. *The Eye and Seeing.* Gr. 4 and up. Illus. Watts, 1981. 48 pp. $8.90. Nonfiction.
Eye problems such as myopia, hyperopia, and astigmatism can be corrected. Color blindness is a distortion in color recognition caused by a defect in the cone cells in the retina.

WARD, Brian R. *Food and Digestion.* Gr. 4–6. Illus. Watts, 1982. 48 pp. $8.90. Nonfiction.
Eating gives the body energy and helps it grow and be healthy. The digestive system, including the stomach, liver, pancreas, intestines, and other body parts, work together to absorb food into the body.

WARD, Brian R. *Heart and Blood.* Gr. 4–6. Illus. Watts, 1982. 48 pp. $8.90. Nonfiction.
The circulatory and lymph systems carry the blood and other fluids through the body. Malfunctioning causes illnesses that can be diagnosed and treated.

WARD, Brian R. *Hospital.* Gr. 6–7. Illus. Silver, 1977. 47 pp. $11.64. Nonfiction.
The author surveys the work of hospital staff, including that of doctors, nurses, operating room personnel, kitchen workers, medical engineers, outpatient caregivers, physical therapists, and administrators.

WARD, Brian R. *The Lungs and Breathing.* Gr. 4 and up. Illus. Watts, 1982. 48 pp. $8.90. Nonfiction.
The respiratory system includes the nose, mouth, lungs, and diaphragm. Air passing through the larynx produces vocal sounds.

WARD, Brian R. *Touch, Taste and Smell.* Gr. 4 and up. Illus. Watts, 1982. 40 pp. $8.90. Nonfiction.
Taste, touch, and smell are senses that signal many things to the body, including hunger, pain, odors, and temperatures.

WARMBIER, Jenene, and Ellen VASSY. *Hospital Days, Treatment Ways.* Gr. 3 and up. Illus. Natl Canc Inst, 1982 (NIH Publ. No. 82-2085). 28 pp. Single copy free on request. Fiction.
Each of the black-and-white drawings depicts part of the treatment and care for children with cancer. The brief descriptions cover radiation therapy, protection isolation, bone marrow test, chemotherapy, bone scan, and intravenous medication. Play activities, participating in care, and going back to school are included.

WARNER, S. Lucille, and Ann REIT. *Your A-Z Super Problem Solver.* Gr. 7–12. Schol Bk Serv, 1979. 164 pp. pap. $1.50. Nonfiction.
The authors give many helpful suggestions for coping with teenage physical and emotional problems.

WARTSKI, Maureen Crane. *My Brother Is Special.* Westminster, 1979. 138 pp. $7.95; pap. New Amer Lib, $1.50. Fiction.
With determination, Noni helps her brother, who is retarded, become a winner in the Special Olympics.

WARWICK, Dolores. *Learn to Say Goodbye.* Gr. 7–8. FS&G, 1971. 179 pp. $4.50. Fiction.
Lucy and her younger sister, Marcella, live in an orphanage after their alcoholic and psychologically abusive mother loses custody of them. Lucy's internal struggle to find love and security leads her to strength and coping, although she is still bitter, but Marcella is overwhelmed by her losses.

WEART, Edith Lucie. *The Story of Your Blood.* Gr. 5–6. Illus. by Z. Onyshkewych. Coward, 1960. 63 pp. $6.99. Nonfiction.
Realistic illustrations and descriptions inform readers about circulation, the composition of the blood, and transfusions.

WEART, Edith Lucie. *The Story of Your Bones.* Gr. 5–6. Illus. by Jan Fairservis. Coward, 1966. 63 pp. $6.99. Nonfiction.
Detailed anatomy drawings and descriptions inform readers about the function of bones, effects of age, and repair of fractures.

WEART, Edith Lucie. *The Story of Your Brain and Nerves.* Gr. 5–6. Illus. by Alan Tompkins. Coward, 1961. 64 pp. $6.99. Nonfiction.
The brain and nervous system work together in many ways to control the body.

WEART, Edith Lucie. *The Story of Your Respiratory System.* Gr. 4–7. Illus. by Jan Fairservis. Coward, 1964. 62 pp. $6.99. Nonfiction.
Air has a regulated path through the body and a purpose. How the air moves, is cleaned, and helps the body are described with examples and many facts.

WEART, Edith Lucie. *The Story of Your Skin.* Gr. 5–6. Illus. by Jan Fairservis. Coward, 1970. 64 pp. $6.99. Nonfiction.
Included in this discussion of the structure and functioning of the skin are fingerprints, cell layers, moles and warts, hair color, cleanliness, the effects of emotions on the skin, rashes and irritation, fever and temperature regulation, hair and nails.

WEBER, Alfons. *Elizabeth Gets Well.* Trans. from the Swiss by the author. Illus. by Jacqueline Blass. Crowell, 1969. 28 pp. pap. $9.00. Fiction.
Pictures of intravenous set-ups, oxygen tanks, doctors' instru-

ments, operating room, cast saw, and X ray help tell the story of Elizabeth's hospitalization for an appendectomy.

WEINSTEIN, Grace W. *People Study People: The Story of Psychology.* Gr. 7 and up. Dutton, 1979. 136 pp. $8.95. Nonfiction. The author describes and gives examples of psychoanalysis, behaviorism, Piagetian theories, humanism, and psychological research.

WEISS, Joan Talmage. *Home for a Stranger.* Gr. 4–5. HarBraceJ, 1980. 109 pp. $7.95. Fiction. Eleven-year-old Juana is brought to California from a Mexican orphanage for an operation to correct a cleft lip. With the help of a Latino family, she is able to make a transition to a fascinating and frightening world.

WEISS, Malcolm E. *Blindness.* Gr. 6–8. Watts, 1980. 63 pp. $6.45. Nonfiction. There are a number of causes and some cures for blindness. Methods and devices available for guidance and improved vision include Guide Dogs, Braille (fingertip words), and improving one's other senses. Certain laws benefit the handicapped and enable them to attend regular school.

WEISS, Malcolm E. *Seeing Through the Dark: Blind and Sighted—A Vision Shared.* Gr. 5–6. Illus. by Gary Tong. HarBraceJ, 1976. 84 pp. $5.95. Nonfiction. There are many ways of seeing—through the senses, and through imagination, observation, and abstraction. This study of the ability of blind people to learn to observe and interpret with all their senses is illustrated with photographs and diagrams.

WEISS, Malcolm E., and Ann E. WEISS. *The Vitamin Puzzle.* Gr. 3–6. Illus. by Pat de Aloe. Messner, 1976. 96 pp. $6.29. Nonfiction. The authors discuss the development of vitamins and their beneficial effects. Detrimental effects of overdosing can occur, and unknowns about what vitamins do in the body still exist.

WHEAT, Patte, with Leonard L. LIEBER. *Hope for the Children: A Personal History of Parents Anonymous.* Gr. 10 and up. Winston, 1979. 391 pp. $6.95. Nonfiction.

Parents Anonymous is an organization devoted to stopping child abuse by treating abusers and educating the general public.

WHELAN, Gloria. *A Time to Keep Silent.* Gr. 7–12. Putnam, 1979. 127 pp. $7.95. Fiction.
Thirteen-year-old Clair stops talking after her mother's death. In order to heal her emotional wounds, Clair's father leaves his job and begins a new life for them in the back country of northern Michigan.

WHITE, Anne Terry, and Gerald S. LIETZ. *Windows on the World.* Gr. 4–7. Illus. by Ted Schroeder. Garrard, 1965. 80 pp. $5.29. Nonfiction.
Stories and experiments show how the body's senses work, including taste, hearing, smell, sight, and touch.

WHITE, Paul. *Janet at School.* Gr. 2–3. Photog. by Jeremy Finlay. Crowell, 1978. Unp. $9.89. Nonfiction.
Five-year-old Janet, who has spina bifida, goes to school in a wheelchair. She tries many activities with her friends and, despite her disability, has many successes.

WHITNEY, Alma Marshak. *Just Awful.* Gr. 1–2. Illus. by Lillian Hoban. Addison-Wesley, 1971. Unp. $7.95. Fiction.
A six-year-old cuts his finger while playing and is sent to the school nurse for the first time.

WHITNEY, Phyllis. *Nobody Likes Trina.* Gr. 2–6. New Amer Lib, 1976. 144 pp. pap. $1.50. Fiction.
Sandy is new in school and has to choose between making friends by joining in teasing Trina, who is retarded, or refusing to participate and being a loner as Trina is.

WHITNEY, Phyllis. *Secret of the Emerald Star.* Gr. 6–7. Illus. by Alex Stein. Westminster, 1964. 233 pp. $4.95. Fiction.
Thirteen-year-old Robin develops a friendship with her new neighbor, Stella, who is blind. Stella's grandmother objects. She keeps Stella from doing many things. Robin encourages Stella, listens to her feelings about blindness, and learns Braille.

WIBBELSMAN, Charles, and Kathy MCCOY. *The Teenage Body Book*. Gr. 7–12. Illus. Pocket Bks, 1979. 246 pp. pap. $5.95. Nonfiction.
The authors describe the anatomy and psychology of adolescent development, answering questions on physical changes in puberty, how to care for one's body, sexuality, contraception, and venereal diseases.

WILSON, Ron. *How the Body Works*. Gr. 5 and up. Illus. Larousse, 1979. 96 pp. $8.95. Nonfiction.
The author explains the major systems of the body in detail. He also describes hospitals, including mobile units, aids for disabled persons, and spare-parts surgery.

WINDSOR, Patricia. *Diving for Roses*. Gr. 7 and up. Har-Row, 1976. 248 pp. $7.53. Fiction.
Jean meets a young man she grows to love and becomes pregnant, but she refuses to marry him because she must care for her ill mother. When she realizes her mother is alcoholic and needs the help of others, she recognizes she must build a new life for herself and her baby.

WINTHROP, Elizabeth. *A Little Demonstration of Affection*. Gr. 7–8. Har-Row, 1975. 152 pp. $7.95; pap. Dell, $1.25. Fiction.
Charley and his sister Jenny, children of undemonstrative parents, turn to each other for the affection they need, but find they have created new problems.

WINTHROP, Elizabeth. *Marathon Miranda*. Gr. 4–5. Holiday, 1979. 155 pp. $8.95; pap. Bantam, $1.75. Fiction.
Miranda's asthma is a convenient excuse to avoid competition, but she really fears failing. An older woman, an enthusiastic jogger, encourages her to enter the marathon.

WISEMAN, Bernard. *Morris Has a Cold*. Gr. 2–3. Illus. by the author. Dodd, 1978. Unp. $6.95. Fiction.
In this humorous story, Morris the Moose catches a cold and Boris the Bear tries to help him cure it.

WITTY, Margot. *A Day in the Life of an Emergency Room Nurse*. Gr. 4–8. Photog. by Sarah Lewis. Troll, 1981. 32 pp. $6.89. Nonfiction.

Audrey, an emergency room nurse, helps children who are acutely ill or injured by giving them medication, calming them, talking about what is happening to them, and assisting physicians in giving treatment and performing minor surgery. Photographs depict real emergency events.

WOJCIECHOWSKA, Maia. *Tuned Out.* Gr. 7–8. Har-Row, 1968. 125 pp. $8.97; pap. Dell, $1.50. Fiction.
Sixteen-year-old Jim writes in his journal about the summer his older brother, Kevin, comes home from college addicted to drugs. When Kevin is hospitalized for treatment, Jim believes Kevin does not want to see him and feels hurt and abandoned. Finally he is able to visit and finds Kevin has been ill, has learned about himself and the effects of drugs on his body, and will soon come home.

WOLDE, Gunilla. *Betsy and the Chicken Pox.* Gr. ps–3. Illus. Random House, 1975. Unp. $2.95. Fiction.
Betsy feels neglected when her little brother gets chicken pox and lots of attention from their mother and father, but decides it is not fun to be sick when she gets chicken pox too.

WOLDE, Gunilla. *Betsy and the Doctor.* Gr. ps–1. Illus. Random House, 1977. Unp. $5.99. Fiction.
When Betsy falls out of a tree and is rushed to the hospital, she learns that she does not have to be afraid of the doctor.

WOLDE, Gunilla. *Tommy Goes to the Doctor.* Gr. 1–2. Illus. HM, 1972. Unp. $1.25. Fiction.
Tommy learns the procedures of a visit to the doctor's office when he has a routine examination.

WOLF, Bernard. *Anna's Silent World.* Gr. 3–4. Illus. Lippincott, 1977. 48 pp. $10.35. Nonfiction.
Six-year-old Anna has an active life and, because she is deaf, is learning to communicate through speech and lip reading.

WOLF, Bernard. *Connie's New Eyes.* Gr. 7–8. Photog. by the author. Lippincott, 1976. 95 pp. $9.95. Fiction.
Connie is about to begin her first teaching job at a school for handicapped children. Part of the story focuses on the training of a dog to be helpful to a blind person, first in a loving home and

then at The Seeing Eye training center. The other part tells Connie's story of blindness from birth, as she learns to use signals and the harness to direct the dog that was shown in training, and how Connie is able to teach children with various disabilities.

WOLF, Bernard. *Don't Feel Sorry for Paul*. Gr. 5–6. Photog. by the author. Lippincott, 1974. 94 pp. $8.95. Nonfiction.
Paul's hands and feet are incompletely formed. With artificial feet and a two-part hook for a hand he is active, goes to school, and cares for his needs. His family is supportive of his efforts to help himself.

WOLF, Bernard. *Michael and the Dentist*. Gr. ps–3. Photog. by the author. Schol Bk Serv, 1980. 48 pp. $8.05. Fiction.
When Michael goes to the dentist's office he learns about the instruments used to clean and repair his teeth.

WOLFE, Bob, and Diane WOLFE. *Emergency Room*. Gr. 1–5. Photog. by the authors. Carolrhoda, 1983. 32 pp. $7.95. Nonfiction.
Emergency room staff, including paramedics, treat life-threatening injuries as well as broken fingers, burns, viruses, and cuts.

WOLFF, Angelika. *Mom! I Broke My Arm*. Gr. 3–4. Illus. by Leo Glueckselig. Lion, 1969. 43 pp. $5.95. Fiction.
Six-year-old Steven has to wear a cast after his arm breaks.

WOLFF, Angelika. *Mom! I Need Glasses*. Gr. 3–4. Illus. by Dorothy Hill. Lion, 1970. 40 pp. $5.95. Fiction.
Susan's poor vision shows in class and in games, so she is referred to an oculist. The examination is described and depicted in detail. Then the doctor teaches simple anatomy of the eye to Susan and her mother. At the optician's they buy glasses, her "own private windows."

WOLFF, Ruth. *A Crack in the Sidewalk*. Gr. 7–8. John Day, 1965. 281 pp. $6.95. Fiction.
Linsey tells the story of her loving family, especially her younger brother, who is profoundly retarded, and his important place in their family.

WOSMEK, Frances. *A Bowl of Sun.* Gr. 3–4. Illus. by the author. Childrens, 1976. 48 pp. $8.65. Fiction.
A blind girl finds it difficult to cope with a new house, school, and city until a neighbor shows her how to use a potter's wheel. With a new-found joy in creating and living, she makes some of the needed adjustments.

WRIGHT, Betty Ren. *My Sister Is Different.* Gr. 1–3. Illus. Raintree, 1981. 32 pp. $9.98. Fiction.
Carlo struggles with his ambivalent feelings about his retarded sister.

WRIGHT, David. *Deafness.* Gr. 9 and up. Stein & Day, 1975. 213 pp. pap. $1.95. Nonfiction.
The author, deaf since the age of seven, describes his early and continuing determination to overcome as much of the disability as possible, through formal and self-taught education and the development of a personal philosophy.

YOLEN, Jane. *The Mermaid's Three Wisdoms.* Gr. 4 and up. Illus. by Laura Rader. Philomel, 1981. 112 pp. $8.95. Fiction.
A mermaid who cannot speak is seen by a human being, so she is cast out of the sea, with legs instead of a tail, to live as a human. A twelve-year-old girl who cannot hear finds her. The girl and her only friend, an old sea captain, communicate with the mermaid in sign language. When they learn the Three Wisdoms of the sea—patience, the rhythm of life, and that all lives touch—the mermaid is able to return home.

YOLEN, Jane. *The Seeing Stick.* Gr. 2–3. Illus. by Remy Charlip and Demetra Maraslis. Crowell, 1977. Unp. $6.79. Fiction.
All the doctors and magicians in China are unable to cure the emperor's only daughter of her blindness. A poor, wise old wood-carver teaches the beautiful princess to "see" by using her fingers to feel.

YOUNG, Helen. *What Difference Does It Make, Danny?* Gr. 3–6. Illus. by Quentin Blake. Dutton, 1980. 96 pp. $7.95. Fiction.
Danny is bright and good in sports. Managing epilepsy does not trouble him until a teacher becomes fearful of it and bans him

from gymnastics and swimming. Danny retaliates by misbehaving in school—for a while.

YOUNG, John Sacret. *Special Olympics.* Gr. 7 and up. Warner, 1978. 221 pp. pap. $1.95. Fiction.
Matt is a fourteen-year-old trainable mentally retarded boy who cannot talk well and takes care of himself in limited ways. His family works hard to look after his needs. Matt's affection for others and his perseverance motivate him to excel at the Special Olympics.

ZELONKY, Joy. *I Can't Always Hear You.* Gr. 2–3. Illus. by Barbara Bejna and Shirlee Jensen. Raintree, 1980. 30 pp. $7.99. Fiction.
Kim, a young girl whose hearing is impaired, enters a regular school for the first time. She has difficulty adjusting until she learns that every individual has differences.

ZIEGLER, Sandra. *At the Dentist: What Did Christopher See?* Gr. 2–3. Illus. by Mina Gow McLean. Childs World, 1976. 32 pp. $7.95. Fiction.
After he and his sister visit the dentist, Christopher creates an art exhibit reminding people about proper dental care.

ZIEGLER, Sandra. *At the Hospital: A Surprise for Krissy.* Gr. ps–3. Illus. by Mina Gow McLean. Childs World, 1976. 32 pp. $5.95. Fiction.
Hospitalized for a tonsillectomy, Krissy learns about admissions, call lights, wheelchair rides to X ray, and blood tests before surgery. She can wear her own pajamas, makes friends with her roommate, and brings her toy bear (with a face mask) with her to surgery. Her parents' surprise gift is a musical jewelry box. Going home, however, is best.

ZIM, Herbert S. *Blood.* Gr. 3–7. Illus. by Rene Martin. Morrow, 1968. 64 pp. $7.20. Nonfiction.
Blood brings food and oxygen to each body cell and carries away the wastes. The author includes transfusions, the RH factor, anemia, pituitary hormones, leukemia, and hemophilia.

ZIM, Herbert S. *Bones.* Gr. 3–7. Illus. by Rene Martin. Morrow, 1969. 64 pp. $7.20. Nonfiction.
The human skeleton, composed of various sizes and shapes of bones and their joints, gives form to the body. Bones can be repaired if fractured. Minerals give bone its strength and hardness.

ZIM, Herbert S. *Your Brain and How It Works.* Gr. 4–5. Illus. by Rene Martin. Morrow, 1972. 63 pp. $7.20. Nonfiction.
A brain's development and the functioning of each of its parts are complex. Illustrations and simple descriptions in this book help make the information clearer.

ZIM, Herbert S. *Your Skin.* Gr. 4–6. Illus. by Jean Zallinger. Morrow, 1979. 63 pp. $7.75. Nonfiction.
Skin grows in two layers, the epidermis and the dermis. The differences between the skin of males and females are greater than the differences between the skin of people of various races. Skin problems, including allergies, rashes, and many others, can be helped.

ZIM, Herbert S. *Your Stomach and Digestive Tract.* Gr. 4–5. Illus. by Rene Martin. Morrow, 1973. 63 pp. $7.20. Nonfiction.
The process of digestion and the function of the stomach and digestive tract in humans are compared with several other animals.

ZIZMOR, Jonathan, and Diane ENGLISH. *Doctor Zizmor's Guide to Clearer Skin.* Gr. 6–7. Lippincott, 1980. 183 pp. $9.70. Nonfiction.
Diet, environment, and stress have effects on skin problems.

Directory of
Publishers

This directory provides full names and ordering addresses for all publishers of books cited in the Bibliographic Guide. Publishers are listed by the abbreviation or short form used in the text.

A Whitman
  Albert Whitman & Co.
  5747 West Howard St.
  Niles, IL 60648

AAWCH
  Australian Association for the
    Welfare of Children in
    Hospital
  c/o Pediatric Projects Inc.
  Dept. B, PO Box 1880
  Santa Monica, CA 90406

Abingdon
  Abingdon Press
  Customer Service Dept.
  201 Eighth Ave. South
  Nashville, TN 37202

Aboriginal Ed
  Aboriginal Education Resource
    Unit
  30 Ord St.
  Perth WA 6005, Australia

Acad Therapy
  Academic Therapy
  20 Commercial Blvd.
  Novato, CA 94947

ACCH
  Association for the Care of
    Children's Health
  3615 Wisconsin Ave. NW
  Washington, DC 20016

Ace
  Ace Books
  c/o Grosset & Dunlap
  51 Madison Ave.
  New York, NY 10010

Addison-Wesley
  Addison-Wesley Publishing
    Co., Inc.
  Jacob Way
  Reading, MA 01867

Am Heritage
American Heritage Publishing
Co.
10 Rockefeller Plaza
New York, NY 10029

Andre Deutsch
Andre Deutsch
c/o Elsevier-Dutton
2 Park Ave.
New York, NY 10016

Andrew Mountain Pr
Andrew Mountain Press
PO Box 14353
Hartford, CT 06114

Archway
Archway Paperbacks
c/o Pocket Books
1230 Ave. of the Americas
New York, NY 10020

Aronson
Jason Aronson, Inc.
111 Eighth Ave.
New York, NY 10011

Atheneum
Atheneum Publishers
c/o Scribner
Vreeland Ave.
Paterson, NJ 07512

Aurora
Aurora Publishers Inc.
PO Box 120616
Nashville, TN 37212

Avon
Avon Books
959 Eighth Ave.
New York, NY 10019

Ballantine
Ballantine Books, Inc.
c/o Random House, Inc.
400 Hahn Rd.
Westminster, MD 21157

Bantam
Bantam Books, Inc.
414 East Gold Rd.
Des Plaines, IL 60016

Barron
Barron's Educational Series,
Inc.
113 Crossways Park Dr.
Woodbury, NY 11797

Beacon
Beacon Press, Inc.
c/o Harper & Row
Keystone Industrial Park
Scranton, PA 18512

Berkley
Berkley Publishing Corp.
c/o Putnam
200 Madison Ave.
New York, NY 10016

Bodley
The Bodley Head
c/o Merrimack Book Service
99 Main St.
Salem, NH 03079

Bradbury
Bradbury Press
Dist. by Dutton
2 Park Ave.
New York, NY 10016

Bull
Bull Publishing Co.
PO Box 208
Palo Alto, CA 94302

C Franklin Pr
The Chas. Franklin Press
18409 90 Ave. West
Edmonds, WA 98020

Carolrhoda
Carolrhoda Books, Inc.
241 First Ave. North
Minneapolis, MN 55401

Celestial
    Celestial Arts Publishing Co.
    PO Box 7327
    Berkeley, CA 94707

Childrens
    Childrens Press
    1224 West Van Buren St.
    Chicago, IL 60607

Childs World
    Child's World
    PO Box 989
    Elgin, IL 60120

Chosen Bks
    Chosen Books Publishing Co.
    Lincoln, VA 22078

Collier
    Collier
    c/o Macmillan
    Front & Brown Sts.
    Riverside, NJ 08370

Collins
    William Collins Publishers, Inc.
    2080 West 117 St.
    Cleveland, OH 44111

CompCare
    CompCare Publications
    2415 Annapolis Lane
    Minneapolis, MN 55441

Continuum
    Continuum Publishing Co.
    575 Lexington Ave.
    New York, NY 10022

Coward
    Coward-McCann
    390 Murray Hill Parkway
    East Rutherford, NJ 07073

Cranbrook
    Cranbrook Publishing
    2815 Cranbrook
    Ann Arbor, MI 48104

Creative Ed
    Creative Education, Inc.
    PO Box 227
    Mankato, MN 56001

Crowell
    Crowell
    c/o Harper & Row
    Keystone Industrial Park
    Scranton, PA 18512

Crown
    Crown Publishers, Inc.
    One Park Ave.
    New York, NY 10016

David & Charles
    David & Charles, Inc.
    PO Box 57
    North Pomfret, VT 05053

De Vorss
    De Vorss & Co.
    PO Box 550
    Marina Del Rey, CA 90291

Delacorte
    Delacorte Press
    c/o Dell
    One Dag Hammarskjold Plaza
    245 East 47 St.
    New York, NY 10017

Dell
    Dell Publishing Co., Inc.
    One Dag Hammarskjold Plaza
    245 East 47 St.
    New York, NY 10017

Dial
    Dial Press
    One Dag Hammarskjold Plaza
    245 East 47 St.
    New York, NY 10017

Dillon
    Dillon Press, Inc.
    500 South Third St.
    Minneapolis, MN 55415

Dinosaur
Dinosaur Publications Ltd.
c/o Pediatric Projects
Dept. B, PO Box 1880
Santa Monica, CA 90406

Dodd
Dodd, Mead & Co.
79 Madison Ave.
New York, NY 10016

Doubleday
Doubleday & Co., Inc.
501 Franklin Ave.
Garden City, NY 11530

Dutton
E. P. Dutton
2 Park Ave.
New York, NY 10016

Elsevier/Nelson
Elsevier/Nelson
c/o Lodestar Books
2 Park Ave.
New York, NY 10016

EMC
EMC Publishing
300 York Ave.
St. Paul, MN 55101

Enslow
Enslow Publishers
Bloy St. & Ramsey Ave.
Hillside, NJ 07205

Evans
M. Evans & Co., Inc.
c/o Dutton
2 Park Ave.
New York, NY 10016

Everest House
Everest House Books
4 Valentine Pl.
London SE1 8QH, England

Family Comm
Family Communications, Inc.
c/o Pediatric Projects Inc.
Dept. B, PO Box 1880
Santa Monica, CA 90406

Fawcett
Fawcett Book Group
1515 Broadway
New York, NY 10036

Follett
Follett Publishing Co.
1010 West Washington Blvd.
Chicago, IL 60607

Four Winds
Four Winds
c/o Scholastic Book Services
50 West 44 St.
New York, NY 10036

FS&G
Farrar, Straus & Giroux, Inc.
19 Union Square West
New York, NY 10003

Gallaudet
Gallaudet College Press
Kendall Green
Washington, DC 20002

Garrard
Garrard Publishing Co.
1607 North Market St.
Champaign, IL 61820

Glide
New Glide Publications
330 Ellis St.
San Francisco, CA 94102

Golden Pr
Golden Press
c/o Western Publishing
1220 Mound Ave.
Racine, WI 53404

Golden Pr (Sydney)
Golden Press
2-12 Tennyson Rd.
Gladesville NSW 2111,
Australia

Greenwillow
Greenwillow Books
c/o William Morrow
Wilmor Warehouse, 6

Henderson Dr.
West Caldwell, NJ 07006

Grosset & Dunlap
Grosset & Dunlap, Inc.
51 Madison Ave.
New York, NY 10010

H & H Ent
H & H Enterprises, Inc.
PO Box 1070
946 Tennessee
Lawrence, KS 66044

Hai Feng
Hai Feng Publishing Co.
c/o Pediatric Projects
Dept. B, PO Box 1880
Santa Monica, CA 90406

Hamish Hamilton
Hamish Hamilton Children's
   Books Ltd.
c/o David & Charles
PO Box 57
North Pomfret, VT 05053

HarBraceJ
Harcourt Brace Jovanovich, Inc.
757 Third Ave.
New York, NY 10017

Har-Row
Harper & Row, Publishers, Inc.
Keystone Industrial Park
Scranton, PA 18512

Harvey
Harvey House, Publishers
128 West River St.
Chippewa Falls, WI 54729

Hastings
Hastings House, Publishers,
   Inc.
10 East 40 St.
New York, NY 10016

Hawthorn
Hawthorn
c/o Dutton

2 Park Ave.
New York, NY 10016

Hazelden Fdn
Hazelden Foundation
Center City, MN 55012

HM
Houghton Mifflin Co.
Wayside Rd.
Burlington, MA 01803

Holiday
Holiday House, Inc.
18 East 53 St.
New York, NY 10022

Horn Book
The Horn Book, Inc.
Park Square Bldg.
31 St. James Ave.
Boston, MA 02116

HR&W
Holt, Rinehart & Winston, Inc.
383 Madison Ave.
New York, NY 10017

Human Sci Pr
Human Sciences Press, Inc.
c/o Independent Publishers
   Group
14 Vanderventer Ave.
Port Washington, NY 11050

Independence Pr
Independence Press
Div. of Herald House
Drawer HH, 3225 South
   Noland Rd.
Independence, MO 64055

J Philip O'Hara
J Philip O'Hara
20 East Huron St.
Chicago, IL 60611

Jacaranda
The Jacaranda Press
65 Park Rd.
Milton, QLD, Australia

John Day
John Day Co., Inc.
c/o Harper & Row
Keystone Industrial Park
Scranton, PA 18512

Judson
Judson Press
Valley Forge, PA 19481

Knopf
Alfred A. Knopf, Inc.
201 East 50 St.
New York, NY 10022

Larousse
Larousse & Co., Inc.
572 Fifth Ave.
New York, NY 10036

Lawrence Hill
Lawrence Hill & Co.
520 Riverside Ave.
Westport, CT 06880

Lerner
Lerner Publications Co.
241 First Ave. North
Minneapolis, MN 55401

Lion
Lion Books
c/o Sayre Publishing
111 East 39 St.
New York, NY 10016

Lippincott
J. B. Lippincott Co.
2350 Virginia Ave.
Hagerstown, MD 21740

Little
Little, Brown & Co.
200 West St.
Waltham, MA 02154

Lodestar
Lodestar Books
2 Park Ave.
New York, NY 10016

Lothrop
Lothrop, Lee & Shepard Books
c/o William Morrow
Wilmor Warehouse, 6
Henderson Dr.
West Caldwell, NJ 07006

Lyle Stuart
Lyle Stuart, Inc.
120 Enterprise Ave.
Secaucus, NJ 07094

Macdonald
Macdonald Educational Ltd.
Holywell House, Worship St.
London EC2A 2EN, England

McGraw-Hill
McGraw-Hill Book Co.
1221 Ave. of the Americas
New York, NY 10029

McKay
David McKay Co., Inc.
2 Park Ave.
New York, NY 10016

Macmillan
Macmillan Publishing Co., Inc.
Front & Brown Sts.
Riverside, NJ 08370

Marin
Marin Publishing Co.
PO Box 436
San Rafael, CA 94901

Messner
Julian Messner
1230 Ave. of the Americas
New York, NY 10020

Methuen
Methuen Inc.
c/o Transworld Distribution
Services
80 Northfield Ave., Raritan
Center
Edison, NJ 08817

Morrow
William Morrow & Co., Inc.
Wilmor Warehouse
6 Henderson Dr.
West Caldwell, NJ 07006

Natl Canc Inst
National Cancer Institute
Bldg. 31, Rm. 10A18
Bethesda, MD 20205

Natl Textbk
National Textbook Co.
260 North Elmwood
Skokie, IL 60077

NAVH
National Association for
Visually Handicapped
3201 Balboa St.
San Francisco, CA 94121

NAWCH
National Association for the
Welfare of Children in
Hospital
7 Exton St.
London SE1 8UE, England

Nelson
Thomas Nelson, Inc.
PO Box 14100
Nashville, TN 37214

Nelson-Hall
Nelson-Hall Publishers
c/o Thomas Nelson
PO Box 14100
Nashville, TN 37214

New Amer Lib
New American Library
120 Woodbine St.
Bergenfield, NJ 07621

Oxford
Oxford University Press
16-00 Pollitt Dr.
Fair Lawn, NJ 07410

P-H
Prentice-Hall, Inc.
Box 506
Englewood Cliffs, NJ 07632

Pantheon
Pantheon Books
c/o Random House
400 Hahn Rd.
Westminster, MD 21157

Parents
Parents Magazine Press
c/o Elsevier-Dutton
2 Park Ave.
New York, NY 10016

Ped Proj
Pediatric Projects Inc.
Dept. B, PO Box 1880
Santa Monica, CA 90406

Penguin
Penguin Books, Inc.
625 Madison Ave.
New York, NY 10022

Philomel
Philomel
200 Madison Ave., Suite 1405
New York, NY 10016

Platt
Platt & Munk Publishers
Div. of Grosset & Dunlap
51 Madison Ave.
New York, NY 10010

Playspaces
Playspaces International
50 Thayer Rd.
Waltham, MA 02154

Pocket Bks
Pocket Books
1230 Ave. of the Americas
New York, NY 10020

Popular Lib
Popular Library Inc.

c/o CBS Publications
1515 Broadway
New York, NY 10036

Potter
Clarkson N. Potter, Inc.
One Park Ave.
New York, NY 10010

Proj Two
Project Two
PO Box 2163
Edison, NJ 08818

Putnam
G. P. Putnam's Sons
1050 Wall St. West
Lyndhurst, NJ 07071

Raintree
Raintree Childrens Books
205 West Highland Ave.
Milwaukee, WI 53203

Random House
Random House, Inc.
400 Hahn Rd.
Westminster, MD 21157

Regal
Regal Books
c/o G/L Publications
2300 Knoll Dr.
Ventura, CA 93003

Resources
Resources for Children in Hos-
    pitals
PO Box 10
Belmont, MA 02178

Rosen
Richards Rosen Press
29 East 21 St.
New York, NY 10010

Routledge
Routledge & Kegan Paul, Ltd.
9 Park St.
Boston, MA 02108

S G Phillips
S. G. Phillips, Inc.
PO Box 83
Chatham, NY 12037

S&S
Simon & Schuster, Inc.
1230 Ave. of the Americas
New York, NY 10020

Saunders
W. B. Saunders Co.
218 West Washington Square
Philadelphia, PA 19105

Schocken
Schocken Books, Inc.
200 Madison Ave.
New York, NY 10016

Schol Bk Serv
Scholastic Book Services
c/o Scholastic
906 Sylvan Ave.
Englewood Cliffs, NJ 07632

Scholastic
Scholastic, Inc.
906 Sylvan Ave.
Englewood Cliffs, NJ 07632

Scribner
Charles Scribner's Sons
Shipping & Service Center
Vreeland Ave.
Totowa, NJ 07512

Seabury
Seabury Press, Inc.
Seabury Service Center
Somers, CT 06071

Signet
Signet Books
c/o New American Library
120 Woodbine St.
Bergenfield, NJ 07621

Silver
Silver Burdett Co.
250 James St.
Morristown, NJ 07960

Stein & Day
    Stein & Day Publishers
    Scarborough House
    Briarcliff Manor, NJ 10510

Sterling
    Sterling Publishing Co., Inc.
    2 Park Ave.
    New York, NY 10016

Summit
    Summit Books
    c/o Simon & Schuster
    1230 Ave. of the Americas
    New York, NY 10020

Ticknor
    Ticknor & Fields
    383 Orange St.
    New Haven, CT 06511

Tobey
    Tobey Publishing Co., Inc.
    c/o Dell
    One Dag Hammarskjold Plaza
    245 East 47 St.
    New York, NY 10017

Triad Pub FL
    Triad Publishing Co., Inc.
    PO Box 18096
    University Station
    Gainesville, FL 32604

Troll
    Troll Associates
    320 Route 17
    Mahwah, NJ 07430

UCSF
    University of California San
        Francisco Publications
        Office
    Third & Parnassus Sts.
    San Francisco, CA 94143

Vanguard
    Vanguard Press, Inc.
    424 Madison Ave.
    New York, NY 10017

Viking
    Viking Press, Inc.
    c/o Viking/Penguin
    299 Murray Hill Parkway
    East Rutherford, NJ 07073

Walker
    Walker Educational Book Corp.
    720 Fifth Ave.
    New York, NY 10019

Wallaby
    Wallaby Books
    c/o Pocket Books
    1230 Ave. of the Americas
    New York, NY 10020

Wanderer
    Wanderer Books
    c/o Simon & Schuster
    1230 Ave. of the Americas
    New York, NY 10020

Warne
    Frederick Warne & Co.
    2 Park Ave.
    New York, NY 10016

Warner Bks
    Warner Books, Inc.
    Independent News Co.
    75 Rockefeller Plaza
    New York, NY 10019

Watts
    Franklin Watts Inc.
    387 Park Ave. South
    New York, NY 10019

Western Pub
    Western Publishing Co., Inc.
    1220 Mound Ave.
    Racine, WI 53404

Westminster
    Westminster Press
    PO Box 718, Wm. Penn Annex
    Philadelphia, PA 19105

Westview
  Westview Press
  5500 Central Ave.
  Boulder, CO 80301

Windy Hill Pr
  Windy Hill Press
  c/o Pediatric Projects
  Dept. B, PO Box 1880
  Santa Monica, CA 90406

Wingbow Pr
  Wingbow Press
  2940 Seventh St.
  Berkeley, CA 94710

Winston
  Winston Press, Inc.
  c/o CBS Educational Publishing
  430 Oak Grove, Suite 203
  Minneapolis, MN 55403

Title Index

About Dying: An Open Family Book for Parents and Children Together. Stein, Sara Bonnett

About Handicaps: An Open Family Book for Parents and Children Together. Stein, Sara Bonnett

About Me. Moncure, Jane Belk

About Phobias: An Open Family Book for Parents and Children Together. Stein, Sara Bonnett

About Your Heart. Simon, Seymour

Accident. Colman, Hila Crayder

Addiction: Its Causes, Problems and Treatments. Berger, Gilda

Admission to the Feast. Beckman, Gunnel

After the Goat Man. Byars, Betsy

Aim for a Job in a Medical Laboratory. Reynolds, Moira Davison

Alan and Naomi. Levoy, Myron

Alan and the Animal Kingdom. Holland, Isabelle

Alcohol and You. Claypool, Jane

Alcohol: Proof of What? Lee, Essie E.

Alcohol: What It Is, What It Does. Seixas, Judith S.

Alcoholism. Silverstein, Alvin, and Virginia B. Silverstein

Alesia. Greenfield, Eloise, and Alesia Revis

The Alfred Summer. Slepian, Jan

Alice with Golden Hair. Hull, Eleanor

All About Your X-Ray: IVP. Waidley, Ericka

All About Your X-Ray: UGI. Waidley, Ericka

All Grown Up and No Place to Go. Elkind, David

All the Better to Bite With. Doss, Helen Grigsby, and Richard L. Wells

Allergies. Riedman, Sarah Regal

Allergies. Silverstein, Alvin, and Virginia B. Silverstein

Allergies and You. Burns, Sheila L.

The Ambivalence of Abortion. Francke, Linda Bird

Amen, Moses Gardenia. Ferris, Jean

Anatomy for Children. Gold-
smith, Ilse
Andrew Goes for an X-Ray.
NAWCH Research Team
Andrew Goes to the Outpatients.
NAWCH Research Team
Andrew Has a Blood Test.
NAWCH Research Team
Angel Dust Blues. Strasser, Todd
Angela Ambrosia. Fox, Ray Errol
Angie and Me. Jones, Rebecca C.
Anna Joins In. Arnold, Katrin
Anna's Silent World. Wolf,
Bernard
Annie on My Mind. Garden,
Nancy
Apple Is My Sign. Riskind, Mary
Are You in the House Alone?
Peck, Richard
Arthur's Eyes. Brown, Marc
Ask Me No Questions. Schlee,
Ann
Asthma: The Facts. Lane, Donald
At the Dentist: What Did Chris-
topher See? Ziegler, Sandra
At the Hospital: A Surprise for
Krissy. Ziegler, Sandra
At the Mouth of the Luckiest
River. Griese, Arnold A.
Axe-Time, Sword-Time. Corcoran,
Barbara

A Baby in the Family. Althea
A Baby Starts to Grow. Showers,
Paul
Bacteria. Lietz, Gerald S.
Bacteria: How They Affect Other
Living Things. Patent,
Dorothy Hinshaw
The Balancing Girl. Rabe,
Berniece
The Bear's Toothache. McPhail,
David
Beat the Turtle Drum. Greene,
Constance C.
Becky. Hirsch, Karen

Becky's Story. Baznik, Donna
Before You Were a Baby.
Showers, Paul, and Kay
Sperry Showers
Before You Were Three: How You
Began to Walk, Talk, Explore
and Have Feelings. Harris,
Robie H., and Elizabeth Levy
Being Blind. Marcus, Rebecca B.
Belonging. Kent, Deborah
Benjamin Goes to Hospital: An
Introduction to Hospital for
Children and Parents. Lip-
son, Tony, and the staff of
the Royal Alexandra Hospital
for Children
Benjamin Goes to the Dentist:
An Introduction to the Den-
tist for Children and Parents.
Dunn, Graeme
The Berenstain Bears Go to the
Doctor. Berenstain, Stan, and
Jan Berenstain
The Berenstain Bears Visit the
Dentist. Berenstain, Stan, and
Jan Berenstain
Betsy and the Chicken Pox.
Wolde, Gunilla
Betsy and the Doctor. Wolde,
Gunilla
Better Than Aspirin: How to Get
Rid of Emotions That Give
You a Pain in the Neck. Har-
min, Merrill
Between Friends. Garrigue, Sheila
Biological Clocks. Riedman,
Sarah Regal
Bionic Parts for People: The Real
Story of Artificial Organs
and Replacement Parts. Skur-
zynski, Gloria
The Bionic People Are Here.
Freese, Arthur S.
Bionics. Berger, Melvin
Birth and Growth. Ward, Brian R.
Blimp. Cavallaro, Ann
Blind Flight. Milton, Hilary

Blind Outlaw. Rounds, Glen

Blind Sunday. Evans, Jessica

Blindness. Weiss, Malcolm E.

Blissymbolics: Speaking Without Speech. Helfman, Elizabeth S.

Blood. Zim, Herbert S.

Blood and Guts: A Working Guide to Your Own Insides. Allison, Linda

Blubber. Blume, Judy Sussman

The Blue Rose. Klein, Gerda Weissmann

Bobby Visits the Dentist. Roy, Howard L.

Bodies. Brenner, Barbara

The Body Book. Rayner, Claire

The Body Is the Hero. Glasser, Ronald J.

Body Maintenance. Ward, Brian R.

Body Sense, Body Nonsense. Simon, Seymour

Body Talk. Gay, Kathlyn

Body Words: A Dictionary of the Human Body, How It Works, and Some of the Things That Affect It. Daly, Kathleen N.

Bones. Zim, Herbert S.

Bones and Skeletons. Thompson, Brenda, and Rosemary Giesen

Bonnie Jo, Go Home. Eyerly, Jeannette

A Book About Your Skeleton. Gross, Ruth Belov

The Book of Think: Or How to Solve a Problem Twice Your Size. Burns, Marilyn

Borrowing Time: Growing Up with Juvenile Diabetes. Covelli, Pat

A Bowl of Sun. Wosmek, Frances

A Boy Called Hopeless. Melton, David

The Boy Who Could Make Himself Disappear. Platt, Kin

The Boy Who Couldn't Hear. Bloom, Freddy

The Boy Who Drank Too Much. Greene, Shep

The Boy with a Problem: Johnny Learns to Share His Troubles. Fassler, Joan

The Boy with the Special Face. Girion, Barbara

Boys Have Feelings Too: Growing Up Male for Boys. Carlson, Dale Bick

The Brain: Magnificent Mind Machine. Facklam, Margery, and Howard Facklam

Brain Power: Understanding Human Intelligence. Haines, Gail Kay

A Breath of Air and a Breath of Smoke. Marr, John S.

But I'm Ready to Go. Albert, Louise

A Button in Her Ear. Litchfield, Ada Bassett

Cages of Glass, Flowers of Time. Culin, Charlotte

Call Me Amanda. Carlson, Dale Bick

Can I Help How I Feel? Morrison, Carl V., and Dorothy Nafus Morrison

Cancer. Haines, Gail Kay

Cancer. Silverstein, Alvin, and Virginia B. Silverstein

A Cane in Her Hand. Litchfield, Ada Bassett

Captain Hook, That's Me. Litchfield, Ada Bassett

Careers in a Hospital. Schaleben-Lewis, Joy

Caring for the Mentally Ill. Shapiro, Patricia Gottlieb

Cathy. National Association for Visually Handicapped

Child Abuse. Dolan, Edward F., Jr.

The Child Abuse Help Book.

Haskins, James, with Pat
Connolly
Child of the Morning. Corcoran,
Barbara
Children of Vietnam. Lifton,
Betty Jean, and Thomas C.
Fox
*Children with Emerald Eyes:
Histories of Extraordinary
Boys and Girls.* Rothenberg,
Mira
The Chocolate War. Cormier,
Robert
Cindy, a Hearing Ear Dog. Curtis,
Patricia
*The Circulatory System: The
Rivers Within.* Silverstein,
Alvin, and Virginia B. Silver-
stein
Claire and Emma. Peter, Diana
Clear Skin, Healthy Skin.
Nourse, Alan Edward
The Clinic. Kay, Eleanor
*Cloudy with a Chance of
Meatballs.* Barrett, Judith
The Code of Life. Silverstein,
Alvin, and Virginia B. Silver-
stein
*Cold Against Disease: The
Wonders of Cold.* Kavaler,
Lucy
Cold Comfort. Bennett, Hal Zina
*A College Guide for Students
with Disabilities: A Detailed
Directory of Higher Educa-
tion Services, Programs, and
Facilities Accessible to Handi-
capped Students in the United
States.* Gollay, Elinor, and
Alwina Bennett
*Color and People: The Story of
Pigmentation.* Lerner,
Marguerite Rush
Come By Here. Coolidge, Olivia
Come to the Doctor, Harry.
Chalmers, Mary

*Comeback: Six Remarkable
People Who Triumphed over
Disability.* Bowe, Frank
*Coming Home to a Place You've
Never Been Before.* Clements,
Bruce, and Hanna Clements
*Compulsive Overeater: The Basic
Text for Compulsive Over-
eaters.* B. Bill
Conception and Contraception.
Lipke, Jean Coryllel
*Conception, Contraception: A
New Look.* Loebl, Suzanne
Confessions of an Only Child.
Klein, Norma
Connie's New Eyes. Wolf, Bernard
A Contest. Payne, Sherry Newirth
Controlling Your Weight. Ben-
ziger, Barbara
Controls in Your Body. Sullivan,
Navin
Coping with Anger. Gelinas, Paul
J.
Coping with Physical Disability.
Cox-Gedmark, Jan
*Coping with School Age Mother-
hood.* Walsworth, Nancy, and
Patricia Bradley
Coping with Skin Care. Annex-
ton, May, and Brent Schill-
inger
Coping with Venereal Disease.
Edwards, Gabrielle
Coping with Weight Problems.
Gelinas, Paul J.
Coping with Your Emotions.
Gelinas, Paul J.
*Copycat Sam: Developing Ties
with a Special Child.* Ste-
fanik, Alfred T.
The Courage to Live. Kiev, Ari
A Crack in the Sidewalk. Wolff,
Ruth
The Creep. Dodson, Susan
Cry of the Wolf. Spencer, Zane,
and Jay Leech

Cry Softly! The Story of Child Abuse. Hyde, Margaret Oldroyd

Cushla and Her Books. Butler, Dorothy

A Dance to Still Music. Corcoran, Barbara

Danny and His Thumb. Ernst, Kathryn F.

The Dark Didn't Catch Me. Thrasher, Crystal

Darlene. Greenfield, Eloise

David in Silence. Robinson, Veronica

A Day in the Life of an Emergency Room Nurse. Witty, Margot

A Day Off. Tobias, Tobi

A Deaf Child Listened: Thomas Gallaudet, Pioneer in American Education. Neimark, Anne E.

Deaf Like Me. Spradley, Thomas S., and James R. Spradley

Deafness. Hyman, Jane

Deafness. Wright, David

Death: Everyone's Heritage. Landau, Elaine

Death Is a Noun: A View of the End of Life. Langone, John

A December Tale. Sachs, Marilyn

Deenie. Blume, Judy Sussman

Demons at My Door. Morgenroth, Barbara

The Dentist and Me. Schaleben-Lewis, Joy

Dentist's Tools. Lapp, Carolyn

Depression. Olshan, Neal H.

A Dermatologist's Guide to Home Skin Treatment: An Up-to-Date Guide That Explains the Best Available Treatment for Every Com-

mon Skin Problem, from Acne to Warts. Dvorine, William

The Devil Hole. Spence, Eleanor

Diabetes. Riedman, Sarah Regal

The Diabetes Fact Book. Duncan, Theodore G.

Diabetes Without Fear. Goodman, Joseph I., and W. Watts Bigger

Diary of a Frantic Kid Sister. Colman, Hila Crayder

Did I Have a Good Time? Teenage Drinking. Howard, Marion

The Digestive System: How Living Creatures Use Food. Silverstein, Alvin, and Virginia B. Silverstein

Dinah and the Fat Green Kingdom. Holland, Isabelle

Dinkey Hocker Shoots Smack. Kerr, M. E.

Disease Detectives. Berger, Melvin

Diving for Roses. Windsor, Patricia

D.J.'s Worst Enemy. Burch, Robert

DNA: The Ladder of Life. Frankel, Edward

Do Bananas Chew Gum? Gilson, Jamie

Doctor De Soto. Steig, William

Doctor Shawn. Breinburg, Petronella

The Doctor Within. Bennett, Hal Zina

Doctor Zizmor's Guide to Clearer Skin. Zizmor, Jonathan, and Diane English

Doctors and Nurses: What Do They Do? Greene, Carla

Doctor's Boy. Anckarsvärd, Karin

The Doctor's Guide to You and Your Colon: A Candid, Helpful Guide to Our #1 Hid-

den Health Complaint. Plaut,
Martin E.
Does She Know She's There?
Schaefer, Nicola
The Dollar Man. Mazer, Harry
Donna Finds Another Way.
Hawker, Frances, and Lee
Withall
Don't Call Me Fatso. Philips,
Barbara
Don't Feel Sorry for Paul. Wolf,
Bernard
Don't Forget Me, Mommy! Anderson, Kay Wooster
Don't Forget Tom. Larsen, Hanne
Don't Hurt Laurie! Roberts,
Willo Davis
Don't Hurt Me, Mama. Stanek,
Muriel
Don't Worry, Dear. Fassler, Joan
*Don't Worry, You're Normal: A
Teenager's Guide to Self-
Health.* Simon, Nissa
Dread Diseases. Tully, Marianne,
and Mary-Alice Tully
Dreams. Kettelkamp, Larry
A Drop of Blood. Showers, Paul
Drugs and You. Madison, Arnold
Dumb Old Casey Is a Fat Tree.
Bottner, Barbara

The Ear and Hearing. Ward, Brian
R.
The Ear Book. Perkins, Al
Early Disorder. Josephs, Rebecca
*Early Morning Rounds: A Portrait
of a Hospital.* Holmes, Burnham
The Ears of Louis. Greene,
Constance C.
Ebbie. Rice, Eve
The Edge of Next Year. Stolz,
Mary
Elizabeth Gets Well. Weber,
Alfons

Emergency! Beame, Rona
Emergency Room. Wolfe, Bob,
and Diane Wolfe
Emergency Room: An ABC Tour.
Steedman, Julie
Emergency! 10-33 on Channel 11!
Milton, Hilary
The Empty Window. Bunting,
Eve
Endings: A Book About Death.
Bradley, Buff
*The Endocrine System: Hormones
in the Living World.* Silverstein, Alvin, and Virginia B.
Silverstein
Enzymes in Action. Berger,
Melvin
Epidemic! The Story of the Disease Detectives. Archer, Jules
Epilepsy. Silverstein, Alvin, and
Virginia B. Silverstein
Eric. Lund, Doris Herold
Eric Needs Stitches. Marino,
Barbara Pavis
Escape from Nowhere. Eyerly,
Jeannette
ESP. Aylesworth, Thomas G.
*ESP: The Search Beyond the
Senses.* Cohen, Daniel
*ESP: Your Psychic Powers and
How to Test Them.* Akins,
W. R.
*Everybody's a Winner: A Kid's
Guide to New Sports and
Fitness.* Schneider, Tom
*Everything Your Doctor Would
Tell You If He Had the Time.*
Rayner, Claire
*The Excretory System: How Living Creatures Get Rid of
Wastes.* Silverstein, Alvin,
and Virginia B. Silverstein
*Exercise: What It Is, What It
Does.* Trier, Carola S.
*Exploring Careers in Special
Education.* Jones, Marilyn

Exploring the Mind and Brain.
Berger, Melvin
The Eye and Seeing. Ward, Brian
R.
The Eye Book. LeSieg, Theo

*Face Talk, Hand Talk, Body
Talk.* Castle, Sue
Faces. Brenner, Barbara
Facts About the Human Body.
Tully, Marianne, and Mary-
Alice Tully
Far in the Day. Cunningham,
Julia
Fat and Skinny. Balestrino, Philip
Fat Elliot and the Gorilla.
Pinkwater, Manus
*Fat Free: Common Sense for
Young Weight Worriers.*
Gilbert, Sara D.
Fat Jack. Cohen, Barbara
Fears and Phobias. Hyde,
Margaret Oldroyd
Fears and Phobias: Fighting Back.
Olshan, Neal H., and Julie
Dreyer Wang
Feeling Free. Sullivan, Mary Beth,
Alan J. Brightman, and Joseph
Blatt
*Feeling Good: A Book About You
and Your Body.* Gilbert, Sara
D.
Feelings. Allington, Richard L.,
and Kathleen Cowles
Feelings from A to Z. Visser, Pat
*Feelings: Inside You and Outloud
Too.* Polland, Barbara Kay
Find Debbie! Brown, Roy
Find Out by Touching. Showers,
Paul
The First Seeing Eye Dog.
Holmes, Burnham
Follow Your Nose. Showers, Paul
Food and Digestion. Ward, Brian
R.

Food for People. Riedman, Sarah
Regal
Food, Nutrition and You. Peavy,
Linda, and Ursula Smith
The Food You Eat. Marr, John S.
Foot and Feet. Ramirez, Carolyn
The Foot Book. Seuss, Dr.
For Love of Jody. Branscum,
Robbie
The Force Inside You. Goodbody,
Slim
*Fractures, Dislocations and
Sprains.* Nourse, Alan Edward
Frankie Is Staying Back. Roy,
Ron
Freckle Juice. Blume, Judy
Sussman
*Free to Choose: Decision Making
for Young Men.* Mitchell,
Joyce Slayton
Friends Till the End. Strasser,
Todd
From Anna. Little, Jean
*From Cell to Clone: The Story
of Genetic Engineering.*
Facklam, Margery, and
Howard Facklam
*From Pigeons to People: A Look
at Behavior Shaping.* Hall,
Elizabeth
*A Future in Pediatrics: Medical
and Non-Medical Careers in
Child Health Care.* Lee, Mary
Price
*Futurelife: The Biotechnology
Revolution.* Silverstein,
Alvin, and Virginia B. Silver-
stein

Gary Coleman: Medical Miracle.
The Coleman Family and Bill
Davidson
*Gay: What You Should Know
About Homosexuality.* Hunt,
Morton

Genetic Engineering. Stwertka, Eve, and Albert Stwertka

The Genetics Explosion. Silverstein, Alvin, and Virginia B. Silverstein

Germs. Patent, Dorothy Hinshaw

Germs Make Me Sick: A Health Handbook for Kids. Donahue, Parnell, and Helen Capellaro

Get Hooked on Vegetables. Gay, Kathlyn, Martin Gay, and Marla Gay

Getting Along in Your Family. Naylor, Phyllis Reynolds

Getting Clear: Body Work for Women. Rush, Anne Kent

Getting Smarter. First, Julia

Getting Your Own Way: A Guide to Growing Up Assertively. Mihaly, Mary E.

Gift of Gold. Butler, Beverly Kathleen

The Gift of Magic Sleep: Early Experiments in Anesthesia. Shapiro, Irwin

A Girl Like Tracy. Crane, Caroline

The Girl Who Lived on the Ferris Wheel. Moeri, Louise

The Girl Who Wanted Out. Bradbury, Bianca

Girls' Guide to Menstruation. Voelckers, Ellen

Glorious Triumphs: Athletes Who Conquered Adversity. Pizer, Vernon

Glue Fingers. Christopher, Matt

Go Ask Alice. Anonymous

Go Away, Warts! Simon, Norma

Go Tell It to Mrs. Golightly. Cookson, Catherine

Going into Hospital. Althea

Going to Hospital. McLaren, Annabel

Going to the Doctor. Althea

Going to the Doctor. Jessel, Camilla

Going to the Hospital. Greenwald, Arthur, and Barry Head

Going Vegetarian: A Guide for Teen-agers. Fretz, Sada

Good for Me: All About Food in 32 Bites. Burns, Marilyn

Goodby to Bedlam: Understanding Mental Illness and Retardation. Langone, John

The Great American Stomach Book: How Your Digestion Works and What to Do When It Doesn't. Mylander, Maureen

The Great Rat Island Adventure. Talbot, Charlene J.

Greff: The Story of a Guide Dog. Curtis, Patricia

Gregory's Stitches. Vigna, Judith

Growing Time. Warburg, Sandol S.

Growing Up in a Hurry. Madison, Winifred

Growing Up Slim. Bolian, Polly

Growl When You Say R. Stanek, Muriel

Guess Where I've Been! Freney, Rosemary, Lia Kapelis, and Peter Hicks

Gut Reactions: How to Handle Stress and Your Stomach. Taylor, David M., and Maxine A. Rock

Half the Battle. Hall, Lynn

Handbook for Emergencies: Coming Out Alive. Greenbank, Anthony

A Handful of Stars. Girion, Barbara

Hand-Me-Down Dreams. Peacock, Carol Antoinette

Hands Up! Goode, Ruth
Handtalk: An ABC of Finger Spelling and Sign Language. Charlip, Remy, and Mary Beth Sullivan
Hang Tough, Paul Mather. Slote, Alfred
Hanging In: What You Should Know About Psychotherapy. Greenberg, Harvey R.
Happy Birthday, Sam. Hutchins, Pat
Happy Endings Are All Alike. Scoppettone, Sandra
Haunted Summer. Jordan, Hope D.
Having a Hearing Test. Althea
Having an Eye Test. Althea
Having an Operation. Greenwald, Arthur, and Barry Head
He Is Your Brother. Parker, Richard
Head in the Clouds. Southall, Ivan
Head over Wheels. Kingman, Lee
Headache: Understanding, Alleviation. Lance, James W.
Heads You Win, Tails I Lose. Holland, Isabelle
The Healing Arts. Kettelkamp, Larry
Health. Jacobsen, Karen
Health Care for the Wongs: Health Insurance, Choosing a Doctor. Thypin, Marilyn, and Lynne Glasner
The Healthy Habits Handbook. Goodbody, Slim
Hear Your Heart. Showers, Paul
Heart and Blood. Ward, Brian R.
Heart Disease. Tully, Mary-Alice, and Marianne Tully
Heartbeats: Your Body, Your Heart. Silverstein, Alvin, and Virginia B. Silverstein
Help: A Guide to Counseling and

Therapy Without a Hassle. Marks, Jane
Help! Emergencies That Could Happen to You and How to Handle Them. Vandenburg, Mary Lou
Heredity. Dunbar, Robert E.
Heredity. Lipke, Jean Coryllel
A Hero Ain't Nothin' but a Sandwich. Childress, Alice
He's My Baby, Now. Eyerly, Jeannette
He's My Brother. Lasker, Joe
Hey, Dollface. Hautzig, Deborah
Holding Together. Jones, Penelope
Home for a Stranger. Weiss, Joan Talmage
Home Is Where They Take You In. Seabrooke, Brenda
Hope for the Children: A Personal History of Parents Anonymous. Wheat, Patte, with Leonard L. Lieber
Hormones. Nourse, Alan Edward
Horses, Airplanes, and Frogs. Parker, Mark
The Hospital. Azarnoff, Pat, ed.
Hospital. Ward, Brian R.
The Hospital Book. Howe, James
Hospital Days, Treatment Ways. Warmbier, Jenene, and Ellen Vassy
A Hospital: Life in a Medical Center. Deegan, Paul
Hospital Roadmap: A Book to Help Explain the Hospital Experience to Young Children. Elliott, Ingrid Glatz
The Hospital Scares Me. Hogan, Paula, and Kirk Hogan
A Hospital Story: An Open Family Book for Parents and Children Together. Stein, Sara Bonnett
Hotline. Hyde, Margaret Oldroyd
House in the Waves. Hamilton-

Paterson, James
How Did We Find Out About Vitamins? Asimov, Isaac
How Do I Feel? Simon, Norma
How Doctors Diagnose You and How You Can Help. Gibbons, Thomas B.
How It Feels When a Parent Dies. Krementz, Jill
How Many Teeth? Showers, Paul
How the Body Works. Wilson, Ron
How the Doctor Knows You're Fine. Cobb, Vicki
How to Build a Body. May, Julian
How to Eat: Chewing, Tooth Care, and Diet. Fleege, Francis
How to Eat Your ABC's: A Book About Vitamins. Jones, Hettie
How to Really Fool Yourself: Illusions for All Your Senses. Cobb, Vicki
How We Hear: The Story of Hearing. Fryer, Judith
How We Talk: The Story of Speech. Bennett, Merilyn Brottman, and Sylvia Sanders
How You Talk. Showers, Paul
Howie Helps Himself. Fassler, Joan
A Hug Just Isn't Enough. Ferris, Caren
Hughie's Hospital Adventure. Aboriginal Education Resource Unit
The Human Body. Bruun, Ruth Dowling, and Bertel Bruun
The Human Body: Its Structure and Operation. Asimov, Isaac
The Human Eye. Schuman, Benjamin N.
Human Rights. Snyder, Gerald S.
Hunter in the Dark. Hughes, Monica

The Hurried Child: Growing Up Too Fast Too Soon. Elkind, David
Hypnosis: The Wakeful Sleep. Kettelkamp, Larry

I Am Somebody. Greene, Laura
I Can't Always Hear You. Zelonky, Joy
I Can't Talk Like You. Althea
I Feel: A Picture Book of Emotions. Ancona, George
I Have a Sister, My Sister Is Deaf. Peterson, Jeanne Whitehouse
I Have Asthma. Althea
I Have Diabetes. Althea
I Have Feelings. Berger, Terry
I Have Feelings Too. Berger, Terry
I Know a Dentist. Barnett, Naomi
I Never Promised You a Rose Garden. Green, Hannah
I Really Like Myself. Kottler, Dorothy, and Eleanor Willis
I Use a Wheelchair. Althea
I Want to Be Big. Iverson, Genie
I Was a 98-Pound Duckling. Van Leeuwen, Jean
I Wish I Was Sick, Too! Brandenberg, Franz
Ice Castles. Fleischer, Leonore
Ice Cream Isn't Always Good. Newman, Susan
If You Could See What I Hear. Sullivan, Tom, and Derek Gill
I'll Live. Manes, Stephen
I'll Love You When You're More Like Me. Kerr, M. E.
I'll Never Be Fat Again! Livingston, Carole
Immunity: How Our Bodies Resist Disease. Arehart-Treichel, Joan
In a Mirror. Stolz, Mary
Intelligence: What Is It? Cohen,

Daniel
The Interns. Sobol, Harriet
Langsam
It Can't Hurt Forever. Singer,
Marilyn
*Itch, Sniffle and Sneeze: All
About Asthma, Hay Fever
and Other Allergies.* Silver-
stein, Alvin, and Virginia B.
Silverstein
It's a Mile from Here to Glory.
Lee, Robert C.
It's Just Too Much. Okimoto, Jean
Davies
It's Me, Claudia! Newman, Alyse
It's Okay to Look at Jamie.
Frevert, Patricia Dendtler
It's Too Late for Sorry. Hanlon,
Emily
It's Your Body/Es Tu Cuerpo.
Azarnoff, Pat, ed.

Janet at School. White, Paul
Jay and the Marigold. Robinet,
Harriette
Jim Boen: A Man of Opposites.
Redpath, Ann
Johnny Gets Some Glasses. Snell,
Nigel
Jon O.: A Special Boy. Ominsky,
Elaine
Journey. Massie, Robert K., and
Suzanne Massie
Juan's Eighteen-Wheeler Summer.
Place, Marian T., and Charles
G. Preston
*Junk Food, Fast Food, Health
Food: What America Eats
and Why.* Perl, Lila
Just Awful. Whitney, Alma
Marshak
Just Like Always. Sachs,
Elizabeth-Ann
Just Like Everybody Else. Rosen,
Lillian

Kate Visits the Doctor. Snell,
Nigel
Kathleen, Please Come Home.
O'Dell, Scott
Katie's Magic Glasses. Goodsell,
Jane
*Keep Stompin' Till the Music
Stops.* Pevsner, Stella
*Keeping Fit: A Handbook for
Physical Conditioning and
Better Health.* Neff, Fred
Kelly's Creek. Smith, Doris
Buchanan
Kiss the Candy Days Good-Bye.
Dacquino, V. T.
Kitty O'Neill: Daredevil Woman.
Ireland, Karin
Know About Alcohol. Hyde,
Margaret Oldroyd
Kristy's Courage. Friis, Babbis

The Language of Goldfish. Oneal,
Zibby
Larry. National Association for
Visually Handicapped
Lasers: The Miracle Light. Kettel-
kamp, Larry
The Late Great Me. Scoppettone,
Sandra
Learn to Say Goodbye. Warwick,
Dolores
*Learning About Sex: The Con-
temporary Guide for Young
Adults.* Kelly, Gary F.
Learning to Control Stress.
Buckalew, M. W., Jr.
*Learning to Say Good-bye: When
a Parent Dies.* LeShan, Eda J.
The Left-Handed Book. Lindsay,
Rae
Left Right, Left Right. Stanek,
Muriel
*Lefty: The Story of Left-Handed-
ness.* Lerner, Marguerite Rush
Lenses, Spectacles, Eyeglasses

and Contacts: The Story of
    Vision Aids. Kelley, Alberta
Leslie. Sherburne, Zoa
Lester's Turn. Slepian, Jan
Light a Single Candle. Butler,
    Beverly Kathleen
Like It Is: Facts and Feelings
    About Handicaps from Kids
    Who Know. Adams, Barbara
Like, Love, Lust: A View of Sex
    and Sexuality. Langone, John
Like Me. Brightman, Alan
Like Normal People. Meyers,
    Robert
The Lionhearted. Savitz, Harriet
    May
Lisa and Her Soundless World.
    Levine, Edna S.
Lisa, Bright and Dark. Neufeld,
    John
Listen for the Fig Tree. Mathis,
    Sharon Bell
Listen for the Singing. Little, Jean
Listen to Me! Barness, Richard
Listen to Me, I'm Angry. Laiken,
    Deidre S., and Alan J.
    Schneider
A Little Breathing Room. Graber,
    Richard
A Little Demonstration of Affec-
    tion. Winthrop, Elizabeth
The Little Doctor. Chang Mao-
    chiu
Little Though I Be. Low, Joseph
A Little Time. Baldwin, Anne
    Norris
The Littlest Leaguer. Hoff, Syd
Lives at Stake: The Science and
    Politics of Environmental
    Health. Pringle, Laurence
A Long Way Up: The Story of
    Jill Kinmont. Valens, E. G.
A Look at Alcoholism. Anders,
    Rebecca
A Look at Birth. Pursell, Margaret
    Sanford

A Look at Death. Anders,
    Rebecca
A Look at Drug Abuse. Anders,
    Rebecca
A Look at Mental Retardation.
    Anders, Rebecca
A Look at Physical Handicaps.
    Pursell, Margaret Sanford
Look at Your Eyes. Showers,
    Paul
Look How Many People Wear
    Glasses: The Magic of Lenses.
    Brindze, Ruth
Look! How Your Eyes See. Sislo-
    witz, Marcel J.
Look Who's Beautiful! First, Julia
Looking. Allington, Richard L.,
    and Kathleen Cowles
Looking On. Miles, Betty
Loss and How to Cope with It.
    Bernstein, Joanne E.
Lost. Lisker, Sonia O.
The Lottery Rose. Hunt, Irene
Love and Sex and Growing Up.
    Johnson, Corinne Benson, and
    Eric W. Johnson
Love and Sex in Plain Language.
    Johnson, Eric W.
Love Is Like Peanuts. Bates, Betty
Loveletters. Shreve, Susan
    Richards
Lovey: A Very Special Child.
    MacCracken, Mary
Loving Sex for Both Sexes:
    Straight Talk for Teenagers.
    Carlson, Dale Bick
Lucy Loses Her Tonsils. Snell,
    Nigel
The Lungs and Breathing. Ward,
    Brian R.

Madeline. Bemelmans, Ludwig
The Magic Moth. Lee, Virginia
Making Sense of Sex: The New

Facts About Sex and Love for Young People. Kaplan, Helen Singer

The Man Without a Face. Holland, Isabelle

The Mango Tooth. Pomerantz, Charlotte

Marathon Miranda. Winthrop, Elizabeth

Marie Curie. Reid, Robert

Marijuana. Stwertka, Eve, and Albert Stwertka

Matthew's Accident. Collins-Ahlgren, Marianne

May I Cross Your Golden River? Dixon, Paige

MBD: The Family Book About Minimal Brain Dysfunction. Gardner, Richard A.

Me and Einstein: Breaking Through the Barrier. Blue, Rose

Me and Fat Glenda. Perl, Lila

Me Too. Cleaver, Vera, and Bill Cleaver

Medical Center Lab. Berger, Melvin

Medical Tests and You. Klein, Aaron E.

Medicine Show: Conning People and Making Them Like It. Calhoun, Mary

Meditation for Children. Rozman, Deborah A.

Meditation for Young People. Lesh, Terry

Meet Camille and Danille, They're Special Persons: Hearing Impaired. Glazzard, Margaret H.

Meet Danny, He's a Special Person: Multiply Handicapped. Glazzard, Margaret H.

Meet Lance, He's a Special Person: Trainable Mentally Retarded. Glazzard, Margaret H.

Meet Scott, He's a Special Person: Learning Disabled. Glazzard, Margaret H.

Memoirs of a Tall Girl. Ronayne, Eileen

Menstruation. Maddux, Hilary C.

Menstruation: Just Plain Talk. Nourse, Alan Edward

Mental Illness. Berger, Gilda

Mental Retardation. Dunbar, Robert E.

The Mermaid's Three Wisdoms. Yolen, Jane

Mia Alone. Beckman, Gunnel

Michael and the Dentist. Wolf, Bernard

Michelle. Phillips, Carolyn E.

Mind Drugs. Hyde, Margaret Oldroyd, ed.

Mine for Keeps. Little, Jean

Mitch and Amy. Cleary, Beverly

Molly and the Slow Teeth. Ross, Pat

Mom! I Broke My Arm. Wolff, Angelika

Mom! I Need Glasses. Wolff, Angelika

Monocular Mac. Corn, Anne L.

Morris Has a Cold. Wiseman, Bernard

My Brother Is Special. Wartski, Maureen Crane

My Brother Joey Died. McLendon, Gloria H.

My Brother Steven Is Retarded. Sobol, Harriet Langsam

My Daddy Is a Nurse. Wandro, Mark, and Joani Blank

My Daughter, My Son. Trachtenberg, Irene

My Dentist. Rockwell, Harlow

My Doctor. Rockwell, Harlow

My Feet Do. Holzenthaler, Jean

My Five Senses. Aliki

My Friend Jacob. Clifton, Lucille

My Friend Leslie: The Story of a

Handicapped Child. Rosenberg, Maxine B.

My Hands. Aliki

My Name Is Davy, I'm an Alcoholic. Snyder, Anne

My Own Private Sky. Beckman, Delores

My Sister. Hirsch, Karen

My Sister Is Different. Wright, Betty Ren

My Sister's Silent World. Arthur, Catherine

The Mystery of the Boy Next Door. Montgomery, Elizabeth Rider

Natural and Synthetic Poisons. Haines, Gail Kay

Neurons: Building Blocks of the Brain. Stevens, Leonard A.

Never Quit. Cunningham, Glenn, with George X. Sand

The New Boy Is Blind. Thomas, William E.

The New Genetics. Hyde, Margaret Oldroyd

Next Door to Xanadu. Orgel, Doris

Nick Joins In. Lasker, Joe

The Night Gift. McKillip, Patricia

A Night Without Stars. Howe, James

Nine Black American Doctors. Hayden, Robert C., and Jacqueline Harris

No Dragons to Slay. Greenberg, Jan

No Measles, No Mumps for Me. Showers, Paul

No Time to Lose. Kleiman, Gary, and Dody Sandford

Nobody Cares About Me! Roberts, Sarah

Nobody Likes Trina. Whitney, Phyllis

Nobody's Fault? Hermes, Patricia

Not My Daughter: Facing Up to Adolescent Pregnancy. Oettinger, Katherine B., with Elizabeth C. Mooney

The Nothing Place. Spence, Eleanor

Nurse. Anderson, Peggy

Nutrition. Thompson, Paul

Nutritional Survival Manual for the Eighties: A Young People's Guide to "Dietary Goals for the United States." Franz, Barbara, and William Franz

Oh, Boy! Babies! Herzig, Alison C., and Jane L. Mali

Oliver Button Is a Sissy. de Paola, Tomie

On Wings of Love: The United Nations' Declaration of the Rights of the Child. Agostinelli, Maria E.

On with My Life. Trull, Patti

One Fat Summer. Lipsyte, Robert

One Little Girl. Fassler, Joan

One, Two, Three—Ah-Choo! Allen, Marjorie N.

One, Two, Three . . . The Story of Matt, a Feral Child. Craig, Eleanor

The Operation. Anderson, Penny S.

Ordinary People. Guest, Judith

Other Choices for Becoming a Woman. Mitchell, Joyce Slayton

Ouch! All About Cuts and Other Hurts. Gelman, Rita Golden, and Susan Kovacs Buxbaum

Our Bodies, Ourselves: A Book by and for Women. Boston Women's Health Book Collective

Our New Baby: A Picture Story for Parents and Children. Fagerstrom, Grethe, and Gunilla Hansson

Our Remarkable Feet. Krishef, Robert K.

Oxygen Keeps You Alive. Branley, Franklyn M.

Pain. Touré, Halima

A Partnership of Mind and Body: Biofeedback. Kettelkamp, Larry

Passing Through. Gerson, Corinne

A Patch of Blue. Kata, Elizabeth

Patients: The Experience of Illness. Rosenberg, Mark L.

Patrick: Yes You Can. Frevert, Patricia Dendtler

Patty Gets Well. Frevert, Patricia Dendtler

Paul David Silverman Is a Father. Cone, Molly

A Pebble in Newcomb's Pond. Dengler, Marianna

Penny, the Medicine Maker: The Story of Penicillin. Epstein, Sherrie S.

People Study People: The Story of Psychology. Weinstein, Grace W.

People Who Help People. Moncure, Jane Belk

Period. Gardner-Loulan, JoAnn, Bonnie Lopez, and Marcia Quackenbush

Peter Gets a Hearing Aid. Snell, Nigel

The Peter Pan Bag. Kingman, Lee

Phoebe Dexter Has Harriet Peterson's Sniffles. Numeroff, Laura Joffe

Physical Disabilities. Berger, Gilda

Physical Fitness for Young Cham-pions. Antonacci, Robert J., and Jene Barr

Picking Up the Pieces. Bates, Betty

Pickles and Prunes. Moe, Barbara

The Pig-Out Blues. Greenberg, Jan

The Pistachio Prescription. Danziger, Paula

The Planet of Junior Brown. Hamilton, Virginia

Please Don't Say Hello. Gold, Phyllis

Please Don't Tease Me. Madsen, Jane M., with Diane Bockoras

Please Remember Me: A Young Woman's Story of Her Friendship with an Unforgettable Fifteen-Year-Old Boy. Brady, Mari

Poisons, Antidotes and Anecdotes. Tichy, William

Possible Impossibilities: A Look at Parapsychology. Hall, Elizabeth

Private Zone: A Book Teaching Children Sexual Assault Prevention Tools. Dayee, Frances S.

P.S. Write Soon. Rodowsky, Colby F.

Puberty and Adolescence. Lipke, Jean Coryllel

Questions and Answers About Acne. Reeves, John R. T.

Questions and Answers About Alcoholism. Curtis, Robert H.

The Quiet Revolution: The Struggle for the Rights of Disabled Americans. Haskins, James, and J. M. Stifle

The Quitting Deal. Tobias, Tobi

Rachel. Fanshawe, Elizabeth
Radiation: Waves and Particles, Benefits and Risk. Pringle, Laurence
Rape. Horos, Carol V.
Rape: Preventing It, Dealing with the Legal, Medical, and Emotional Aftermath. Bode, Janet
Rape: What Would You Do If . . . ? Booher, Dianna Daniels
The Respiratory System: How Living Creatures Breathe. Silverstein, Alvin, and Virginia B. Silverstein
Richard Scarry's Nicky Goes to the Doctor. Scarry, Richard
The Riddle of Teeth. Hammond, Winifred G.
The Rights of Young People: The Basic ACLU Guide to a Young Person's Rights. Sussman, Alan
The Rose-Colored Glasses: Melanie Adjusts to Poor Vision. Leggett, Linda Rodgers, and Linda Gambee Andrews
Rosie's Hospital Story. Cooper, Elizabeth
A Row of Tigers. Corcoran, Barbara
Run, Don't Walk. Savitz, Harriet May
Run, Shelley, Run! Samuels, Gertrude
Runaway Sugar: All About Diabetes. Silverstein, Alvin, and Virginia B. Silverstein
Rupert Piper and the Boy Who Could Knit. Parkinson, Ethelyn M.

Sadako and the Thousand Paper Cranes. Coerr, Eleanor B.
Sally Can't See. Petersen, Palle

Sanjo. Mayerson, Evelyn
A School for Tommy. Pieper, Elizabeth
Scott Was Here. Ipswitch, Elaine
Second Star to the Right. Hautzig, Deborah
Secret Dreamer, Secret Dreams. Heide, Florence Parry
The Secret in Miranda's Closet. Greenwald, Sheila
Secret of the Emerald Star. Whitney, Phyllis
The See and Hear and Smell and Touch Book. Smith, Elwood H.
See Me More Clearly: Career and Life Planning for Teens with Physical Disabilities. Mitchell, Joyce Slayton
See You Tomorrow, Charles. Cohen, Miriam
"Seeing" in the Dark. Montgomery, Elizabeth Rider
The Seeing Stick. Yolen, Jane
The Seeing Summer. Eyerly, Jeannette
Seeing Through the Dark: Blind and Sighted—A Vision Shared. Weiss, Malcolm E.
Sesame Street Sign Language Fun. Bove, Linda
Seven Black American Scientists. Hayden, Robert C.
Seven Feet Four and Growing. Lee, H. Alton
Sex and Birth Control: A Guide for the Young. Lieberman, E. James, and Ellen Peck
Sex, Love, and the Physically Handicapped. Ayrault, Evelyn West
Sex: Telling It Straight. Johnson, Eric W.
Sex, with Love: A Guide for Young People. Hamilton, Eleanor

Shelley's Day: The Day of a Legally Blind Child. Hall, Candace Catlin

A Show of Hands: Say It in Sign Language. Sullivan, Mary Beth, and Linda Bourke

The Sick Day. MacLachlan, Patricia

Sick in Bed. Rockwell, Anne, and Harlow Rockwell

The Sick of Being Sick Book. Stine, Jovial Bob, and Jane Stine

The Sick Story. Hirsch, Linda

Silent Dancer. Hlibok, Bruce

Silent Sound: The World of Ultrasonics. Knight, David C.

The Silent Voice. Cunningham, Julia

Simon and the Game of Chance. Burch, Robert

Sixth Sense. Kettelkamp, Larry

The Skating Rink. Lee, Mildred Scudder

The Skeletal System: Frameworks for Life. Silverstein, Alvin, and Virginia B. Silverstein

The Skeleton Inside You. Balestrino, Philip

The Skin: Coverings and Linings of Living Things. Silverstein, Alvin, and Virginia B. Silverstein

Skipper. Dixon, Paige

Sleep and Dreams. Lindsay, Rae

Sleep and Dreams. Silverstein, Alvin, and Virginia B. Silverstein

Sleep Is for Everyone. Showers, Paul

Slim Goodbody: The Inside Story. Burstein, John

Slim Goodbody: What Can Go Wrong and How to Be Strong. Burstein, John

Smile! How to Cope with Braces. Betancourt, Jeanne

Smoking. Sonnet, Sherry

Smoking and You. Madison, Arnold

Sniffles. Larranaga, Robert D.

"So You Want to Be a Doctor!" The Realities of Pursuing Medicine as a Career. Bluestone, Naomi

So You're Getting Braces: A Guide to Orthodontics. Silverstein, Alvin, and Virginia B. Silverstein

Something Special Within. Richter, Betts

Sometimes I Like to Cry. Stanton, Elizabeth, and Henry Stanton

Son-Rise. Kaufman, Barry Neil

Sorrow's Song. Callen, Larry

Spare Parts for the Human Body. Nolen, William A.

A Special Kind of Sister. Smith, Lucia B.

Special Olympics. Young, John Sacret

Special Olympics and Paralympics. Henriod, Lorraine

Spectacles. Raskin, Ellen

The Specter. Nixon, Joan Lowery

Speech and Language Disorders. Berger, Gilda

Sports Doc: Medical Advice, Diet, Fitness Tips, and Other Essential Hints for Young Athletes. Donahue, Parnell

Sports for the Handicapped. Allen, Anne

Sports Medicine. Berger, Melvin

Spots Are Special. Galbraith, Kathryn Osebold

Squarehead and Me. Haynes, Henry Louis

S.S. Valentine. Phelan, Terry Wolfe

Step on a Crack. Anderson, Mary Quirk

The Steps to My Best Friend's House. Minshull, Evelyn W.

Sticks and Stones. Hall, Lynn

The Stop Smoking Book for Teens. Casewit, Curtis W.

The Story of Your Blood. Weart, Edith Lucie

The Story of Your Bones. Weart, Edith Lucie

The Story of Your Brain and Nerves. Weart, Edith Lucie

The Story of Your Ear. Silverstein, Alvin, and Virginia B. Silverstein

The Story of Your Eye. Hammond, Winifred

The Story of Your Heart. Limburg, Peter

The Story of Your Mouth. Silverstein, Alvin, and Virginia B. Silverstein

The Story of Your Respiratory System. Weart, Edith Lucie

The Story of Your Skin. Weart, Edith Lucie

Straight from the Siblings: Another Look at the Rainbow. Murray, Gloria, and Gerald G. Jampolsky, eds.

Straight Talk About Love and Sex for Teenagers. Burgess-Kohn, Jane

The Strange but Wonderful Cosmic Awareness of Duffy Moon. Robinson, Jean

Stress and the Art of Biofeedback. Brown, Barbara B.

Stress: Understanding the Tension You Feel at Home, at School and Among Your Friends. Cohen, Daniel

Stress: What It Is, What It Can Do to Your Health, How to Fight Back. McQuade, Walter, and Ann Aikman

Sue Ellen. Hunter, Edith Fisher

The Sugar Disease: Diabetes. Silverstein, Alvin, and Virginia B. Silverstein

Suicide and Young People. Madison, Arnold

Suicide: The Hidden Epidemic. Hyde, Margaret Oldroyd, and Elizabeth Held Forsyth

The Summer of the Swans. Byars, Betsy

A Summer to Die. Lowry, Lois

Surgeon Under the Knife. Nolen, William A.

Surgery: From Stone Scalpel to Laser Beam. Penney, Peggy L.

Susan. Marcus, June Z.

Susan Perl's Human Body Book. McGuire, Leslie

The Swing. Hanlon, Emily

Take Wing. Little, Jean

Talking. Allington, Richard L., and Kathleen Krull

Talking About Death: A Dialogue Between Parent and Child. Grollman, Earl A.

Tangled Butterfly. Bauer, Marion Dane

Taste, Touch and Smell. Adler, Irving, and Ruth Adler

Tasting. Allington, Richard L., and Kathleen Cowles

Teaching Exceptional Children. Anker, Carol Teig

Teacup Full of Roses. Mathis, Sharon Bell

Teen-Age Alcoholism. Haskins, James

The Teenage Body Book. Wibbelsman, Charles, and Kathy McCoy

The Teenage Body Book Guide to Sexuality. McCoy, Kathy

A Teen-Age Guide to Healthy Skin and Hair. Lubowe, Irwin

I., and Barbara Huss

The Teenage Hospital Experience: You Can Handle It! Richter, Elizabeth

Teenage Sexuality: A Survey of Teenage Sexual Behavior. Hass, Aaron

The Teenager and Sex. Milgram, Gail Gleason

A Teenager's Guide to Life and Love. Spock, Benjamin McLane

Tell Me a Mitzi. Segal, Lore

A Test of Love. Powers, Bill

Test-Tube Life: Scientific Advance and Moral Dilemma. Snyder, Gerald S.

That Makes Me Mad. Kroll, Steven

That Was Then, This Is Now. Hinton, S. E.

That's What Friends Are For. Kidd, Ronald

Then Again, Maybe I Won't. Blume, Judy Sussman

There Is a Rainbow Behind Every Dark Cloud. Center for Attitudinal Healing

There's Only One You: The Story of Heredity. Morrison, Velma F.

These Special Children: The Ostomy Book for Parents of Children with Colostomies, Ileostomies and Urostomies. Jeter, Katherine F.

They Triumphed over Their Handicaps. Harries, Joan

Thinking. Allington, Richard L., and Kathleen Krull

This Can Lick a Lollipop: Body Riddles for Kids. Esto Goza Chupando un Caramelo: Las Partes del Cuerpo en Adivinanzas Infantiles. Rothman, Joel

This Is How My Body Works. Heuser, Edith

This Is Your Body. Brandreth, Gyles

Those Traver Kids. Bradbury, Bianca

Three-Legged Race. Crawford, Charles P.

Threshold: Straight Answers to Teenagers' Questions About Sex. Mintz, Thomas, and Lorelie Miller Mintz

Thursday. Storr, Catherine

Thursday's Child. Poole, Victoria

A Tide Flowing. Phipson, Joan

A Time to Be Born. Bell, David

A Time to Keep Silent. Whelan, Gloria

To Be Me. Hazen, Barbara Shook

To Catch an Angel: Adventures in the World I Cannot See. Russell, Robert

To Elvis, with Love. Canada, Lena

To Smoke or Not to Smoke. Terry, Luther L., and Daniel Horn

To Walk on Two Feet. Cook, Marjorie

Tom and Bear: The Training of a Guide Dog Team. McPhee, Richard

Tom Visits the Dentist. Snell, Nigel

Tommy Goes to the Doctor. Wolde, Gunilla

Too Short Fred. Meddaugh, Susan

Too Young to Die. Klagsbrun, Francine

The Tooth Book. Nourse, Alan Edward

Touch of Light: The Story of Louis Braille. Neimark, Anne E.

Touch, Taste and Smell. Ward, Brian R.

Touching. Allington, Richard L., and Kathleen Cowles

Trace Elements: How They Help and Harm Us. Arehart-Treichel, Joan

Tracy. Mack, Nancy

Triumph! Conquering Your Physical Disability. Hayman, LeRoy

Trouble with Explosives. Kelley, Sally

The Truth About Drugs. Austrian, Geoffrey

Try Your Hand. Thayer, Jane

Trying Hard to Hear You. Scoppettone, Sandra

Tuned Out. Wojciechowska, Maia

The Turkey's Nest. Prince, Alison

Twelve Is Too Old. Mann, Peggy

Twenty-Eight Days. Elgin, Kathleen, and John F. Osterritter

Twins: The Story of Multiple Births. Cole, Joanna, and Madeleine Edmondson

Twins: The Story of Twins. Lerner, Marguerite Rush

Two, Four, Six, Eight: A Book About Legs. Kessler, Ethel, and Leonard Kessler

Ulcers. Eisenberg, Michael

The Unchosen. Gilbert, Nan

Under the Influence. Butterworth, W. E.

Underneath I'm Different. Rabinowich, Ellen

Understanding Body Talk. Aylesworth, Thomas G.

The Unmaking of Rabbit. Greene, Constance C.

Up Day, Down Day. Hann, Jacquie

The Ups and Downs of Drugs. Elgin, Kathleen, and John F. Osterritter

Use Your Brain. Showers, Paul

Vaccines and Viruses. Rosenberg, Nancy, and Louis Z. Cooper

VD: A Doctor's Answers. Sgroi, Suzanne M.

VD: Facts You Should Know. Blanzaco, Andre

VD: The Silent Epidemic. Hyde, Margaret Oldroyd

VD: Venereal Disease and What You Should Do About It. Johnson, Eric W.

Viruses. Nourse, Alan Edward

Viruses: Life's Smallest Enemies. Knight, David C.

A Visit to the Dentist. Packard, Mary

Visiting the Dentist. Althea

The Vitamin Puzzle. Weiss, Malcolm E., and Ann E. Weiss

Vitamins. Nourse, Alan Edward

Waiting for Johnny Miracle. Bach, Alice

Walk with Your Eyes. Brown, Marcia

The War on Villa Street. Mazer, Harry

Watching the New Baby. Samson, Joan

A Way of His Own. Dyer, Thomas A.

A Way of Love, a Way of Life: A Young Person's Introduction to What It Means to Be Gay. Hanckel, Frances, and John Cunningham

We Remember Philip. Simon, Norma

We Were Hooked: Thirteen Young Ex-Addicts Tell About Their Experiences with Heroin, LSD, Speed, and Other Drugs and How They Kicked the Habit. Flender, Harold

Wearing a Cast. Greenwald, Arthur, and Barry Head

Welcome Home, Jellybean. Shyer, Marlene F.

We're Going to the Doctor. Roy, Howard L.

What Are You Using? A Birth Control Guide for Teen-Agers. Balis, Andrea

What Difference Does It Make, Danny? Young, Helen

What Do You Do in Quicksand? Ruby, Lois

What Do You Do When Your Mouth Won't Open? Pfeffer, Susan Beth

What Every Kid Should Know. Kalb, Jonah, and David Viscott

What Happens in Therapy? Gilbert, Sara D.

What Happens to a Hamburger? Showers, Paul

What If They Knew? Hermes, Patricia

What If You Couldn't? . . . A Book About Special Needs. Kamien, Janet

What Is Genetics? Bornstein, Jerry, and Sandy Bornstein

What Makes Me Feel This Way? Growing Up with Human Emotions. LeShan, Eda J.

What to Do If You or Someone You Know Is Under 18 and Pregnant. Richards, Arlene Kramer, and Irene Willis

What to Do When There's No One but You. Gore, Harriet Margolis

What to Eat and Why: The Science of Nutrition. Fodor, R. V.

What's a Body to Do? Odor, Ruth S.

Wheelchair Champions: A History of Wheelchair Sports. Savitz, Harriet May

When My Dad Died: A Child's

View of Death. Hammond, Janice Marie

When My Mommy Died: A Child's View of Death. Hammond, Janice Marie

When People Die. Bernstein, Joanne E., and Stephen V. Gullo

Where's Your Head? Psychology for Teenagers. Carlson, Dale Bick

Who Am I? Who Are You?: Coping with Friends, Feelings, and Other Teenage Dilemmas. London, Kathy, and Frank Caparulo

Who Cares About Espie Sanchez? Dunnahoo, Terry

The Whole World of Hands. Berger, Gilda, and Melvin Berger

Who's Afraid of the Dark? Stanek, Muriel

Who's Running Your Life? A Look at Young People's Rights. Archer, Jules

Why Am I Different? Simon, Norma

Why Am I Going to the Hospital? A Helpful Guide to a New Experience. Ciliotta, Claire, and Carole Livingston

Why Am I So Miserable If These Are the Best Years of My Life? A Survival Guide for the Young Woman. Eagan, Andrea B.

Why Are Some People Left-Handed? Haislet, Barbara

Why Are They Starving Themselves? Understanding Anorexia Nervosa and Bulimia. Landau, Elaine

Why Did He Die? Harris, Audrey

Why Have the Birds Stopped Singing? Sherburne, Zoa

Why I Cough, Sneeze, Shiver, Hiccup, and Yawn. Berger, Melvin

Why Me? The Story of Jenny.
Dizenzo, Patricia
*Why You Feel Down and What
You Can Do About It: A Psy-
chotherapist Tells Everything
You Want to Know About
Teenage Depression.* Myers,
Irma, and Arthur Myers
*Why You Feel Hot, Why You Feel
Cold: Your Body's Tempera-
ture.* Berry, James R.
*Why Your Stomach Hurts: A
Handbook of Digestion and
Nutrition.* Null, Gary, and
Steve Null
*Will the Real Monday Please
Stand Up.* Reynolds, Pamela
Will to Live. Franks, Hugh
William. Hunt, Irene
*Wilma: The Story of Wilma Ru-
dolph.* Rudolph, Wilma, as
told to Bud Greenspan
Wilted. Kropp, Paul
Wind Rose. Dragonwagon,
Crescent
Windows on the World. White,
Anne Terry, and Gerald S.
Lietz
*Winners: Eight Special Young
People.* Siegel, Dorothy
Schainman
Winning. Brancato, Robin
*With a Little Help from My
Friends.* Hawker, Frances, and
Lee Withall
The Wobbly Tooth. Cooney,
Nancy Evans
*The Woman Doctor's Diet for
Teen-Age Girls.* Edelstein,
Barbara
*The Wonderful Story of How You
Were Born.* Gruenberg, Sid-
onie M.
The World of Ben Lighthart.
Haar, Jaap ter
The World of Bionics. Silverstein,

Alvin, and Virginia B. Silver-
stein
The World of Ellen March.
Eyerly, Jeannette
World of Her Own. Levinson,
Nancy

X-Rays and Gamma Rays.
Halacy, Daniel B., Jr.

*You and Leukemia: A Day at a
Time.* Baker, Lynn S., in col-
laboration with Charles G.
Roland and Gerald S.
Gilchrist
*You and Your Body: A Book of
Experiments to Perform on
Yourself.* Klein, Aaron E.
*You Can't Catch Diabetes from a
Friend.* Kipnis, Lynne, and
Susan Adler
*You Can't Make a Move Without
Your Muscles.* Showers, Paul
You Can't Put Braces on Spaces.
Richter, Alice Numeroff,
and Laura Joffe Numeroff
*You Don't Say: How People
Communicate Without
Speech.* Pizer, Vernon
You Go Away. Corey, Dorothy
*You Have a Right: A Guide for
Minors.* Englebardt, Leland S.
*The Young Person's Guide to
Love.* Hunt, Morton
Young, Sober and Free. Marshall,
Shelly
Your A-Z Super Problem Solver.
Warner, S. Lucille, and Ann
Reit
Your Blood and Its Cargo. Kalina,
Sigmund
*Your Body Is Trying to Tell You
Something: How to Under-
stand Its Signals and Re-*

spond to Its Needs. Stiller,
Richard
Your Body's Defenses. Knight,
David C.
Your Brain and How It Works.
Zim, Herbert S.
Your Busy Brain. McNamara,
Louise Greep, and Ada
Bassett Litchfield
Your Career in Nursing. Searight,
Mary
Your Ears. Adler, Irving, and Ruth
Adler
Your Eyes. Adler, Irving, and Ruth
Adler
*Your Future: A Guide for the
Handicapped Teenager.* Fein-
gold, S. Norman, and Norma
R. Miller
*Your Future in a Paramedic
Career.* Keyes, Fenton
*Your Future in Occupational
Therapy Careers.* Shuff,
Frances
Your Future in Social Work.
Keyes, Fenton

*Your Handicap—Don't Let It
Handicap You.* Splaver, Sarah
Your Immune System. Nourse,
Alan Edward
*Your Muscles—And Ways to
Exercise Them.* Cosgrove,
Margaret
Your Nerves and Their Messages.
Kalina, Sigmund
Your New Kidney. Burton,
Adrianne
Your Skin. Zim, Herbert S.
Your Skin and Mine. Showers,
Paul
Your Skin Holds You In. Doss,
Helen Grigsby
*Your Stomach and Digestive
Tract.* Zim, Herbert S.
Your Turn, Doctor. Robison,
Deborah, and Carla Perez
Your Weight. Eagles, Douglas A.
*You're Somebody Special on a
Horse.* Brown, Fern
*Youth and Sex: Pleasure and
Responsibility.* Tensen, Gor-
don

Subject Guide

This guide contains eight major groupings of subjects, each followed by a descriptive summary and a listing of areas that may be related to that particular grouping. These lists can help to identify subject headings, so that the user who is interested in "Aids/Appliances," for instance, will note 17 possible subjects listed under that grouping. Actual titles of books can be found in the Subject Index.

Aids/Appliances

An external device becomes an extension of the child's body and can therefore influence ideas and feelings about self. Such devices can restore a sense of body dependability that was lost when the child became disabled. These subject headings can lead the reader to books about aids that are used by disabled children, or appliances that assist in body function, mobility, and locomotion.

Artificial body parts   Hearing aids
Bliss symbols   Hearing Ear Dog
Brace, body   Hook
Braces, leg   Seeing Eye Dog
Braces, teeth   Sign language
Cast   Signed English
Contact lenses   Vision aids
Glasses   Wheelchair
Guide Dog

Body

Children may hear diagnoses and feel treatments on parts of their bodies they never knew existed. The names for some body parts may not be in

189

their vocabularies. External parts can be seen and named but inner, unseen parts can be more mysterious and magical. These subject headings will lead the reader to books about parts of the body, its anatomy, physiology, systems, functions, and stages.

Adolescence	Heredity
Baby	Hormones
Bilingual — Spanish/English	Immune system
Biorhythms	Intelligence
Birth	Left-handed
Blood	Legs
Body	Menstruation
Body language	Metabolism
Brain	Mouth
Circulatory system	Muscular system
Communication	Nervous system
Conception	Nose
Death	Nutrition
Digestion	Oxygen
Dioxyribonucleic acid	Perception
Dreams	Physical fitness
Ears	Pregnancy
Endocrine system	Reproductive system
Enzymes	Respiratory system
Excretory system	Senses
Eyes	Skeletal system
Face	Skin
Feet	Sleep
Freckles	Smell
Gastrointestinal tract	Speech
Growth	Stomach
Hair	Taste
Hands	Teeth
Health	Touch
Hearing	Twins
Heart	Vision
Height	Weight control

Diagnosis

Determining the source and nature of a condition, disease, impairment, or illness usually involves the use of instruments as well as interaction between adults and children. Children seldom have a chance to see an instrument in use, to note its relatively small size and safety and to understand its purpose. Illustrations, stories, and facts can be used to relieve stress and provide information and reassurance about the diagnostic process. These subject headings can lead the reader to books about the machinery, instruments, and methods used in diagnosis.

Blood test	Electroencephelography
Cardiac catheterization	Emergency
Communication	Intravenous pyelogram
Computerized axial tomography	Laboratory test
Dentist's office	Ultrasound
Doctor's office	X ray
Electrocardiography	

Disability

It helps to know you are not the only one, in fact that some people, even fictional characters, have it worse. It can be inspiring to see that, even with severe disabling conditions, the human spirit can survive and that sometimes the human body can overcome limitations. Children can identify with the people in stories, gaining some understanding of themselves through the experiences of others. They can also learn about disability and illness and what is being done to help.

The World Health Organization differentiates between "impairment," referring to abnormalities of body structure and appearance, with organ or system dysfunctions; "disability," referring to the consequences of impairment in function and activity; and "handicap," referring to the disadvantages experienced by the impaired or disabled individual, including interaction with and adaptation to the surroundings. These subject headings can lead the reader to books of fact and fiction about conditions and diseases that may result in impairment, disability, or handicap.

Acne	Burns
Acquired immune deficiency	Cancer
syndrome	Cataract
Addiction	Cerebral palsy
Alcohol use and abuse	Chicken pox
Allergy	Child abuse/Neglect
Amblyopia	Cholera
Amputation	Chronic illness
Amyotrophic lateral sclerosis	Cleft lip/palate
Anorexia nervosa	Cold, common
Arthritis	Communication disability
Asthma	Cystic fibrosis
Attitudes toward disabled	Deafness
Autism	Depression
Behavior disorder	Diabetes
Blindness	Digestion disorder
Brain injury	Disability
Bulimia	Disabled in school

Disabled in sports
Down's syndrome
Drug use and abuse
Dyslexia
Emotional illness
Enuresis
Epilepsy
Foot disability
Freckles
Friendship with disabled
Glaucoma
Handicap
Hearing impairment
Heart disease
Hemophilia
Hodgkin's disease
Illness
Infection
Injury
Kidney disease
Kleptomania
"Lazy eye"
Learning disability
Leg disability
Legionnaire's disease
Leukemia
Leukocytoclastic angiitis
Loss
Lou Gehrig's disease
Measles
Mental illness
Minimal brain dysfunction
Mononucleosis

Multiple handicap
Multiple sclerosis
Mumps
Muscular dystrophy
Mute
Paralysis
Phenylketonuria
Poisoning
Psychosomatic illness
Rape
Retardation
Rights
Schizophrenia
Scoliosis
Sexual abuse/Molestation
Sexual assault
Sexually transmitted disease
Sibling of ill, disabled
Sickle cell anemia
Skin conditions
Smoking
Speech impairment
Spina bifida
Spinal disability
Stomach disorder
Stuttering
Suicide/Suicide attempt
Ulcer
Upper respiratory infection
Venereal disease
Vision impairment
Warts

Feelings

How does it feel to be small, to be different, to be disabled? The expression of such feelings in true stories or fiction may help ill or disabled children to acknowledge and express their own emotions. Able-bodied children may also understand better what disabled classmates, friends, or siblings are feeling, and explore their emotions about health, illness, and disability as well. These subject headings can lead the reader to books that describe or depict a variety of feelings.

Alcohol use and abuse
Anger

Appearance
Attitudes toward disability

Body language
Child life specialist
Communication
Crying
Death
Depression
Disability
Dreams
Drug use and abuse
Emergency
Emotional illness
Emotional support
Fear and phobia
Feelings
Friendship with disabled
Handicap
Hypnosis
Kleptomania

Loss
Love
Medical play
Pain
Parapsychology
Psychiatrist
Psychologist
Psychosomatic illness
Psychotherapy
Rights
Schizophrenia
Self-care
Self-esteem
Separation
Sexuality
Social worker
Special education
Stress

Roles and Relationships

Books on this topic reflect the trend to more sex instruction at an earlier age, classes in family life education, and more public discussion of lifestyle. There are books about conception but also about responsibility. There are books about disturbing issues of sexual abuse and assault but also about varied forms of loving relationships. A recent interest in books for children is the effect of their siblings on children who have health or mental health problems. These subject headings will lead the reader to books about sex roles and human relationships.

Abortion
Adolescence
Adolescent married parent
Adolescent single father
Adolescent single mother
Adolescent, single pregnant
Attitudes toward disability
Baby
Birth
Birth control
Body language
Child abuse/Neglect
Conception
Contraception
Death of child

Death of friend
Death of parent
Death of self
Death of sibling
Disabled in school
Disabled in sports
Drug use and abuse
Dreams
Emotional illness
Friendship with disabled
Loss
Love
Medical play
Parapsychology
Psychiatrist

Psychologist
Rape
Rights
Separation
Sex roles
Sexual abuse/Molestation

Sexual assault
Sexuality
Sexually transmitted disease
Sibling of ill, disabled
Social worker
Twins

Signs and Symptoms

How do children, parents, or doctors know when there is illness? A sign is a difference from normal bodily functioning that can be measured. A symptom, usually perceived and reported by the patient, is a felt change in the body, usually uncomfortable and unwelcome, that may indicate illness. However, children ordinarily do not recognize and describe their symptoms well and do not seek medical help. Instead, their parents note differences and bring the child to the medical setting or apply home remedies. These subject headings can lead the reader to books that help children recognize and understand signs and symptoms they may have heard about or experienced.

Accident
Acne
Addiction
Alcohol use and abuse
Appearance
Bacteria
Bedwetting
Behavior disorder
Body language
Child abuse/Neglect
Disability
Emergency
Epidemic
Fear and phobia
Foot disability
Germs
Hair loss
Handicap
Health
Hearing impairment

Illness
Infection
Injury
Learning disability
Left-handed
Leg disability
Pain
Poisoning
Sexual abuse/Molestation
Smoking
Speech impairment
Stress
Stuttering
Suicide/Suicide attempt
Thumbsucking
Upper respiratory infection
Virus
Vision impairment
Warts

Treatment

The use of instruments, medications, chemicals, therapeutic procedures, and patient-directed healing methods to avoid illness, restore body functions, or reduce disability is considered to be treatment. It can be confusing to children, not only because treatment may be unfamiliar but also because the methods can appear to be unrelated to the illness. How does an injection in the buttocks, for example, help a sore throat? Or a blood transfusion help the stomachache of sickle cell anemia? Or how does not eating before surgery help in removing tonsils? These subject headings can lead the reader to books that describe treatments in stories and factual accounts.

Abortion	Laser therapy
Amputation	Medication
Anesthesia	Meditation
Artificial body parts	Nutrition
Bilingual—Spanish/English	Occupational therapy
Biofeedback	Orthodontics
Bionics	Physical fitness
Chemotherapy	Physical therapist
Cryogenics	Psychotherapy
Dentist's office	Radiation therapy
Doctor's office	Recreation therapist
Emotional support	Self-care
Exercise	Sleep
First aid	Special education
Healing	Special Olympics/Paralympics
Hearing aids	Stitches
Hospitalization	Surgery
Hypnosis	Vaccination
Injection	Vision aids
Intensive care	Vitamins
Intravenous therapy	Weight control

Subject Index

Subjects are listed alphabetically, with titles under each subject in alphabetical order of author's last name. Consult the Bibliographic Guide for full bibliographic information for each title. Consult the Subject Guide to ascertain areas related to a particular group of subjects.

Abortion

Beckman, Gunnel. *Mia Alone*
Eyerly, Jeannette. *Bonnie Jo, Go Home*
Francke, Linda Bird. *The Ambivalence of Abortion*
Langone, John. *Death Is a Noun: A View of the End of Life*
Madison, Winifred. *Growing Up in a Hurry*
Oettinger, Katherine B., with Elizabeth C. Mooney. *Not My Daughter: Facing Up to Adolescent Pregnancy*
Powers, Bill. *A Test of Love*
Richards, Arlene Kramer, and Irene Willis. *What to Do If You or Someone You Know Is Under 18 and Pregnant*
Tensen, Gordon. *Youth and Sex: Pleasure and Responsibility*

Accident

Bates, Betty. *Picking Up the Pieces*
Bradbury, Bianca. *The Girl Who Wanted Out*
Brancato, Robin. *Winning*
Butterworth, W. E. *Under the Influence*
Collins-Ahlgren, Marianne. *Matthew's Accident*
Colman, Hila Crayder. *Accident*
Cook, Marjorie. *To Walk on Two Feet*
Coolidge, Olivia. *Come By Here*
Eyerly, Jeannette. *The World of Ellen March*
Fleischer, Leonore. *Ice Castles*
Friis, Babbis. *Kristy's Courage*
Gore, Harriet Margolis. *What to Do When There's No One but You*

Greene, Constance C. *Beat the Turtle Drum*

Greenfield, Eloise, and Alesia Revis. *Alesia*

Guest, Judith. *Ordinary People*

Haar, Jaap ter. *The World of Ben Lighthart*

Hermes, Patricia. *Nobody's Fault*

Kingman, Lee. *Head over Wheels*

Jordan, Hope D. *Haunted Summer*

Lee, Robert C. *It's a Mile from Here to Glory*

Leggett, Linda Rodgers, and Linda Gambee Andrews. *The Rose-Colored Glasses: Melanie Adjusts to Poor Vision*

Milton, Hilary. *Emergency! 10-33 on Channel 11!*

Neufeld, John. *Lisa, Bright and Dark*

O'Dell, Scott. *Kathleen, Please Come Home*

Place, Marian T., and Charles G. Preston. *Juan's Eighteen-Wheeler Summer*

Scoppettone, Sandra. *Trying Hard to Hear You*

Sherburne, Zoa. *Leslie*

Snyder, Anne. *My Name Is Davy, I'm an Alcoholic*

Southall, Ivan. *Head in the Clouds*

Spencer, Zane, and Jay Leech. *Cry of the Wolf*

Valens, E. G. *A Long Way Up: The Story of Jill Kinmont*

Acne

See also Skin conditions.

Dvorine, William. *A Dermatologist's Guide to Home Skin Treatment: An Up-to-Date Guide That Explains the Best Available Treatment for Every Common Skin Problem, from Acne to Warts*

Lubowe, Irwin I., and Barbara Huss. *A Teen-Age Guide to Healthy Skin and Hair*

Nourse, Alan Edward. *Clear Skin, Healthy Skin*

Reeves, John R. T. *Questions and Answers About Acne*

Acquired Immune Deficiency Syndrome (AIDS)

See also Venereal disease.

Edwards, Gabrielle. *Coping with Venereal Disease*

Addiction

See also Alcohol use and abuse; Drug use and abuse.

Berger, Gilda. *Addiction: Its Causes, Problems and Treatments*

Adolescence

See also Adolescent married parent; Adolescent single father; Adolescent single mother; Adolescent, single pregnant.

Albert, Louise. *But I'm Ready to Go*

Balis, Andrea. *What Are You Using? A Birth Control Guide for Teenagers*

Berger, Melvin. *Exploring the Mind and Brain*

Burgess-Kohn, Jane. *Straight Talk About Love and Sex for Teenagers*

Carlson, Dale Bick. *Boys Have Feelings Too: Growing Up Male for Boys*

Carlson, Dale Bick. *Loving Sex for Both Sexes: Straight Talk for Teenagers*

Carlson, Dale Bick. *Where's Your Head? Psychology for Teenagers*

Casewit, Curtis W. *The Stop Smoking Book for Teens*

Eagan, Andrea B. *Why Am I So Miserable If These Are the Best Years of My Life?: A Survival Guide for the Young Woman*

Edelstein, Barbara. *The Woman Doctor's Diet for Teen-Age Girls*

Elkind, David. *All Grown Up and No Place to Go*

Feingold, S. Norman, and Norma R. Miller. *Your Future: A Guide for the Handicapped Teenager*

Fretz, Sada. *Going Vegetarian: A Guide for Teen-agers*

Gilbert, Sara D. *Feeling Good: A Book About You and Your Body*

Gollay, Elinor, and Alwina Bennett. *A College Guide for Students with Disabilities: A Detailed Directory of Higher Education Services, Programs and Facilities Accessible to Handicapped Students in the United States*

Greenfield, Eloise, and Alesia Revis. *Alesia*

Hass, Aaron. *Teenage Sexuality: A Survey of Teenage Sexual Behavior*

Haskins, James. *Teen-Age Alcoholism*

Howard, Marion. *Did I Have a Good Time? Teenage Drinking*

Hyde, Margaret Oldroyd. *Hotline*

Kaplan, Helen Singer. *Making*

Sense of Sex: The New Facts About Sex and Love for Young People

Kelley, Gary F. *Learning About Sex: The Contemporary Guide for Young Adults*

Lipke, Jean Coryllel. *Puberty and Adolescence*

London, Kathy, and Frank Caparulo. *Who Am I? Who Are You?: Coping with Friends, Feelings, and Other Teenage Dilemmas*

Lubowe, Irwin I., and Barbara Huss. *A Teen-Age Guide to Healthy Skin and Hair*

McCoy, Kathy. *The Teenage Body Book Guide to Sexuality*

Milgram, Gail Gleason. *The Teenager and Sex*

Mintz, Thomas, and Lorelie Miller Mintz. *Threshold: Straight Answers to Teenagers' Questions About Sex*

Mitchell, Joyce Slayton. *See Me More Clearly: Career and Life Planning for Teens with Physical Disabilities*

Myers, Irma, and Arthur Myers. *Why You Feel Down and What You Can Do About It: A Psychotherapist Tells Everything You Want to Know About Teenage Depression*

Oettinger, Katherine B., with Elizabeth C. Mooney. *Not My Daughter: Facing Up to Adolescent Pregnancy*

Richter, Elizabeth. *The Teenage Hospital Experience: You Can Handle It!*

Simon, Nissa. *Don't Worry, You're Normal: A Teenager's Guide to Self-Health*

Spock, Benjamin McLane. *A*

*Teenager's Guide to Life and
Love*
Wibbelsman, Charles, and Kathy
McCoy. *The Teenage Body
Book*

Adolescent Married Parent

Cone, Molly. *Paul David Silverman Is a Father*

Adolescent Single Father

Eyerly, Jeannette. *He's My Baby,
Now*
Peacock, Carol Antoinette. *Hand-
Me-Down Dreams*
Ruby, Lois. *What Do You Do in
Quicksand?*
Windsor, Patricia. *Diving for
Roses*

Adolescent Single Mother

Eyerly, Jeannette. *He's My Baby,
Now*
Hunt, Irene. *William*
Peacock, Carol Antoinette. *Hand-
Me-Down Dreams*
Prince, Alison. *The Turkey's Nest*
Walsworth, Nancy, and Patricia
Bradley. *Coping with School
Age Motherhood*
Windsor, Patricia. *Diving for
Roses*

Adolescent, single
pregnant

See also Abortion.

Bates, Betty. *Love Is Like Peanuts*
Beckman, Gunnel. *Mia Alone*
Eyerly, Jeannette. *Bonnie Jo, Go
Home*
Madison, Winifred. *Growing Up
in a Hurry*

O'Dell, Scott. *Kathleen, Please
Come Home*
Oettinger, Katherine B., with
Elizabeth C. Mooney. *Not My
Daughter: Facing Up to
Adolescent Pregnancy*
Peacock, Carol Antoinette. *Hand-
Me-Down Dreams*
Powers, Bill. *A Test of Love*
Prince, Alison. *The Turkey's Nest*
Richards, Arlene Kramer, and
Irene Willis. *What to Do If
You or Someone You Know
Is Under 18 and Pregnant*
Shreve, Susan Richards. *Love-
letters*
Windsor, Patricia. *Diving for
Roses*

Alcohol Use and Abuse

Anders, Rebecca. *A Look at
Alcoholism*
Berger, Gilda. *Addiction: Its
Causes, Problems and
Treatments*
Butterworth, W. E. *Under the
Influence*
Childress, Alice. *A Hero Ain't
Nothin' but a Sandwich*
Claypool, Jane. *Alcohol and You*
Curtis, Robert H. *Questions and
Answers About Alcoholism*
Greene, Shep. *The Boy Who
Drank Too Much*
Haskins, James. *Teen-Age
Alcoholism*
Howard, Marion. *Did I Have
a Good Time?: Teenage
Drinking*
Hyde, Margaret Oldroyd. *Know
About Alcohol*
Hyde, Margaret Oldroyd. *Mind
Drugs*
Lee, Essie E. *Alcohol, Proof of
What?*

Madison, Arnold. *Drugs and You*
Marshall, Shelly. *Young, Sober and Free*
Mitchell, Joyce Slayton. *Free to Choose: Decision Making for Young Men*
Naylor, Phyllis Reynolds. *Getting Along in Your Family*
Peacock, Carol Antoinette. *Hand-Me-Down Dreams*
Scoppettone, Sandra. *The Late Great Me*
Seabrooke, Brenda. *Home Is Where They Take You In*
Seixas, Judith S. *Alcohol: What It Is, What It Does*
Silverstein, Alvin, and Virginia B. Silverstein. *Alcoholism*
Snyder, Anne. *My Name Is Davy, I'm an Alcoholic*
Stolz, Mary. *The Edge of Next Year*
Warwick, Dolores. *Learn to Say Goodbye*

Allergy

Allen, Marjorie N. *One, Two, Three—Ah-Choo!*
Beckman, Delores. *My Own Private Sky*
Burns, Sheila L. *Allergies and You*
First, Julia. *Look Who's Beautiful*
Larranaga, Robert D. *Sniffles*
Lubowe, Irwin I., and Barbara Huss. *A Teen-Age Guide to Healthy Skin and Hair*
Morrison, Velma F. *There's Only One You: The Story of Heredity*
Nourse, Alan Edward. *Your Immune System*
Riedman, Sarah Regal. *Allergies*
Silverstein, Alvin, and Virginia B. Silverstein. *Allergies*
Silverstein, Alvin, and Virginia B. Silverstein. *Itch, Sniffle and*

Sneeze: All About Asthma, Hay Fever and Other Allergies

Amblyopia

Althea. *Having an Eye Test*

Amputation

See also Artificial body parts; Bionics; Surgery, transplant.

Cook, Marjorie. *To Walk on Two Feet*
Harries, Joan. *They Triumphed over Their Handicaps*
Lifton, Betty Jean, and Thomas C. Fox. *Children of Vietnam*
Phillips, Carolyn E. *Michelle*
Pizer, Vernon. *Glorious Triumphs: Athletes Who Conquered Adversity*
Trull, Patti. *On with My Life*

Amyotrophic Lateral Sclerosis (ALS)

Dixon, Paige. *May I Cross Your Golden River?*

Anesthesia

See also Surgery.

Anderson, Penny S. *The Operation*
Kettelkamp, Larry. *Hypnosis: The Wakeful Sleep*
Shapiro, Irwin. *The Gift of Magic Sleep: Early Experiments in Anesthesia*
Snell, Nigel. *Lucy Loses Her Tonsils*

Anger

Gelinas, Paul J. *Coping with Anger*
Kroll, Steven. *That Makes Me Mad!*
Laiken, Deidre S., and Alan J. Schneider. *Listen to Me, I'm Angry*
Nixon, Joan Lowery. *The Specter*

Anorexia Nervosa

See also Weight control.

Hautzig, Deborah. *Second Star to the Right*
Josephs, Rebecca. *Early Disorder*
Landau, Elaine. *Why Are They Starving Themselves? Understanding Anorexia Nervosa and Bulimia*

Appearance

Beckman, Delores. *My Own Private Sky*
Friis, Babbis. *Kristy's Courage*
Girion, Barbara. *The Boy with the Special Face*
Greene, Constance C. *The Ears of Louis*
Madsen, Jane M., with Diane Bockoras. *Please Don't Tease Me*
Newman, Alyse. *It's Me, Claudia*
Simon, Norma. *Go Away, Warts!*
Stein, Sara Bonnett. *About Handicaps: An Open Family Book for Parents and Children Together*
Van Leeuwen, Jean. *I Was a 98-Pound Duckling*

Arthritis

Jones, Rebecca C. *Angie and Me*
Madsen, Jane M., with Diane Bockoras. *Please Don't Tease Me*
Nourse, Alan Edward. *Your Immune System*

Artificial Body Parts

Berger, Melvin. *Bionics*
Freese, Arthur S. *The Bionic People Are Here*
Litchfield, Ada Bassett. *Captain Hook*
Nolen, William A. *Spare Parts for the Human Body*
Silverstein, Alvin, and Virginia B. Silverstein. *Futurelife: The Biotechnology Revolution*
Skurzynski, Gloria. *Bionic Parts for People: The Real Story of Artificial Organs and Replacement Parts*
Wolf, Bernard. *Don't Feel Sorry for Paul*

Asthma

Althea. *I Have Asthma*
Danziger, Paula. *The Pistachio Prescription*
Lane, Donald J. *Asthma: The Facts*
McLaren, Annabel, ed. *Going to Hospital*
Silverstein, Alvin, and Virginia B. Silverstein. *Itch, Sniffle and Sneeze: All About Asthma, Hay Fever and Other Allergies*
Winthrop, Elizabeth. *Marathon Miranda*

Attitudes Toward Disabled

Albert, Louise. *But I'm Ready to Go*
Althea. *I Can't Talk Like You*
Althea. *I Use a Wheelchair*
Anderson, Kay Wooster. *Don't Forget Me, Mommy*
Arthur, Catherine. *My Sister's Silent World*
Bach, Alice. *Waiting for Johnny Miracle*
Baldwin, Anne Morris. *A Little Time*
Berger, Gilda. *Physical Disabilities*
Butler, Beverly Kathleen. *Gift of Gold*
Butler, Beverly Kathleen. *Light a Single Candle*
Butler, Dorothy. *Cushla and Her Books*
Cook, Marjorie. *To Walk on Two Feet*
Corn, Anne L. *Monocular Mac*
Eyerly, Jeannette. *The Seeing Summer*
Frevert, Patricia Dendtler. *It's Okay to Look at Jamie*
Friis, Babbis. *Kristy's Courage*
Girion, Barbara. *A Handful of Stars*
Greene, Constance C. *The Ears of Louis*
Greene, Constance C. *The Unmaking of Rabbit*
Griese, Arnold A. *At the Mouth of the Luckiest River*
Hanlon, Emily. *It's Too Late for Sorry*
Levine, Edna S. *Lisa and Her Soundless World*
Lasker, Joe. *Nick Joins In*
Levinson, Nancy. *World of Her Own*

Madsen, Jane M., with Diane Bockoras. *Please Don't Tease Me*
Marcus, June Z. *Susan*
Sobol, Harriet Langsam. *My Brother Steven Is Retarded*
Whitney, Phyllis. *Nobody Likes Trina*

Audiologist

See also Deafness; Hearing impairment.

Althea. *Having a Hearing Test*
Litchfield, Ada Bassett. *A Button in Her Ear*

Autism

Gold, Phyllis. *Please Don't Say Hello*
Kaufman, Barry Neil. *Son-Rise*
Parker, Richard. *He Is Your Brother*
Rothenberg, Mira. *Children with Emerald Eyes: Histories of Extraordinary Boys and Girls*
Spence, Eleanor. *The Devil Hole*

Baby

See also Adolescent married parent; Adolescent single father; Adolescent single mother.

Althea. *A Baby in the Family*
Banish, Roslyn. *I Want to Tell You About My Baby*
Bell, David. *A Time to Be Born*
Cone, Molly. *Paul David Silverman Is a Father*
Eyerly, Jeannette. *He's My Baby, Now*
Fagerstrom, Grethe, and Gunilla Hansson. *Our New Baby: A*

Picture Story for Parents and Children
Herzig, Alison C., and Jane L. Mali. *Oh, Boy! Babies!*
Klein, Norma. *Confessions of an Only Child*
Samson, Joan. *Watching the New Baby*
Showers, Paul. *A Baby Starts to Grow*

Back Disability

See also Spinal disability.

Crawford, Charles. *Three-Legged Race*

Bacteria

See also Germs.

Lietz, Gerald S. *Bacteria*
Patent, Dorothy Hinshaw. *Bacteria: How They Affect Other Living Things*
Patent, Dorothy Hinshaw. *Germs*

Bedwetting

Fassler, Joan. *Don't Worry, Dear*

Behavior Disorder

See also Autism; Brain injury; Minimal brain dysfunction.

Adams, Barbara. *Like It Is: Facts and Feelings About Handicaps from Kids Who Know*
Craig, Eleanor. *One, Two, Three . . . The Story of Matt, a Feral Child*
Gold, Phyllis. *Please Don't Say Hello*
Hall, Elizabeth. *From Pigeons to*

People: A Look at Behavior Shaping
Hinton, S. E. *That Was Then, This Is Now*
Langone, John. *Goodby to Bedlam: Understanding Mental Illness and Retardation*
Lasker, Joe. *He's My Brother*
Shyer, Marlene F. *Welcome Home, Jellybean*
Spence, Eleanor. *The Devil Hole*

Bilingual — Spanish/ English

Azarnoff, Pat, ed. *The Hospital*
Azarnoff, Pat, ed. *It's Your Body/ Es Tu Cuerpo*
Rothman, Joel. *This Can Lick a Lollipop: Body Riddles for Kids. Esto Goza Chupando un Caramelo: Las Partes del Cuerpo en Adivinanzas Infantiles*

Biofeedback

Brown, Barbara B. *Stress and the Art of Biofeedback*
Facklam, Margery, and Howard Facklam. *The Brain: Magnificent Mind Machine*
Kettelkamp, Larry. *A Partnership of Mind and Body: Biofeedback*
Lesh, Terry. *Meditation for Young People*

Bionics

Berger, Melvin. *Bionics*
Freese, Arthur S. *The Bionic People Are Here*
Nolen, William A. *Spare Parts for the Human Body*

Silverstein, Alvin, and Virginia B. Silverstein. *Futurelife: The Biotechnology Revolution*

Silverstein, Alvin, and Virginia B. Silverstein. *The World of Bionics*

Skurzynski, Gloria. *Bionic Parts for People: The Real Story of Artificial Organs and Replacement Parts*

Biorhythms

Riedman, Sarah Regal. *Biological Clocks*

Birth

See also Baby; Reproductive system.

Althea. *A Baby in the Family*

Dragonwagon, Crescent. *Wind Rose*

Fagerstrom, Grethe, and Gunilla Hansson. *Our New Baby: A Picture Story for Parents and Children*

Pursell, Margaret Sanford. *A Look at Birth*

Showers, Paul, and Kay Sperry Showers. *Before You Were a Baby*

Ward, Brian R. *Birth and Growth*

Birth Control

See Contraception.

Blindness

See also Guide Dog; Seeing Eye Dog; Surgery, eye; Vision impairment.

Bowe, Frank. *Comeback: Six Remarkable People Who Triumphed over Disability*

Butler, Beverly Kathleen. *Gift of Gold*

Butler, Beverly Kathleen. *Light a Single Candle*

Cohen, Miriam. *See You Tomorrow, Charles*

Cookson, Catherine. *Go Tell It to Mrs. Golightly*

Coolidge, Olivia. *Come By Here*

Evans, Jessica. *Blind Sunday*

Eyerly, Jeannette. *The Seeing Summer*

Fleischer, Leonore. *Ice Castles*

Frevert, Patricia Dendtler. *Patrick: Yes You Can*

Haar, Jaap ter. *The World of Ben Lighthart*

Hall, Candace Catlin. *Shelley's Day: The Day of a Legally Blind Child*

Hall, Lynn. *Half the Battle*

Hunt, Irene. *William*

Kamien, Janet. *What If You Couldn't . . . ? A Book About Special Needs*

Kata, Elizabeth. *A Patch of Blue*

Kent, Deborah. *Belonging*

Kleiman, Gary, and Sandford Dody. *No Time to Lose*

Litchfield, Ada Bassett. *A Cane in Her Hand*

Little, Jean. *Listen for the Singing*

McPhee, Richard. *Tom and Bear: Training of a Guide Dog Team*

Marcus, Rebecca B. *Being Blind*

Mathis, Sharon Bell. *Listen for the Fig Tree*

Milton, Hilary. *Blind Flight*

Montgomery, Elizabeth Rider. *"Seeing" in the Dark*

Neimark, Anne E. *Touch of Light: The Story of Louis Braille*

Parker, Mark. *Horses, Airplanes, and Frogs*
Petersen, Palle. *Sally Can't See*
Russell, Robert. *To Catch an Angel: Adventures in the World I Cannot See*
Siegel, Dorothy Schainman. *Winners: Eight Special Young People*
Sullivan, Tom, and Derek Gill. *If You Could See What I Hear*
Thomas, William E. *The New Boy Is Blind*
Weiss, Malcolm E. *Blindness*
Weiss, Malcolm E. *See Through the Dark: Blind and Sighted—A Vision Shared*
Whitney, Phyllis A. *Secret of the Emerald Star*
Wolf, Bernard. *Connie's New Eyes*
Wosmek, Frances. *A Bowl of Sun*
Yolen, Jane. *The Seeing Stick*

Blindness—Animal

Rounds, Glen. *Blind Outlaw*

Bliss Symbols

See also Communication disability.

Hawker, Frances, and Lee Withall. *Donna Finds Another Way*
Helfman, Elizabeth S. *Blissymbolics: Speaking Without Speech*
Pizer, Vernon. *You Don't Say: How People Communicate Without Speech*

Blood

See also Circulatory system.

Allison, Linda. *Blood and Guts: A Working Guide to Your Own Insides*
Kalina, Sigmund. *Your Blood and Its Cargo*
Showers, Paul. *A Drop of Blood*
Ward, Brian R. *Heart and Blood*
Weart, Edith Lucie. *The Story of Your Blood*
Zim, Herbert S. *Blood*

Blood Test

NAWCH Research Team. *Andrew Has a Blood Test*
Showers, Paul. *A Drop of Blood*

Body

Allison, Linda. *Blood and Guts: A Working Guide to Your Own Insides*
Asimov, Isaac. *The Human Body: Its Structure and Operation*
Azarnoff, Pat, ed. *It's Your Body/ Es Tu Cuerpo*
Berry, James. *Why You Feel Hot, Why You Feel Cold: Your Body's Temperature*
Boston Women's Health Book Collective. *Our Bodies, Ourselves: A Book by and for Women.*
Brandreth, Gyles. *This Is Your Body*
Brenner, Barbara. *Bodies*
Bruun, Ruth Dowling, and Bertel Bruun. *The Human Body*
Burstein, John. *Slim Goodbody: The Inside Story*
Daly, Kathleen N. *Body Words: A Dictionary of the Human Body, How It Works, and Some of the Things That Affect It*

Eagan, Andrea B. *Why Am I So Miserable If These Are the Best Years of My Life?: A Survival Guide for the Young Woman*

Glasser, Ronald J. *The Body Is the Hero*

Goldsmith, Ilse. *Anatomy for Children*

Heuser, Edith. *This Is How My Body Works*

Klein, Aaron E. *You and Your Body: A Book of Experiments to Perform on Yourself*

Knight, David C. *Your Body's Defenses*

McCoy, Kathy. *The Teenage Body Book Guide to Sexuality*

McGuire, Leslie. *Susan Perl's Human Body Book*

May, Julian. *How to Build a Body*

Odor, Ruth S. *What's a Body to Do?*

Rayner, Claire. *The Body Book*

Rayner, Claire. *Everything Your Doctor Would Tell You If He Had the Time*

Rothman, Joel. *This Can Lick a Lollipop: Body Riddles for Kids. Esto Goza Chupando un Caramelo: Las Partes del Cuerpo en Adivinanzas Infantiles*

Simon, Seymour. *Body Sense, Body Nonsense*

Sullivan, Navin. *Controls in Your Body*

Tully, Marianne, and Mary-Alice Tully. *Facts About the Human Body*

Ward, Brian R. *Body Maintenance*

Wibbelsman, Charles, and Kathy McCoy. *The Teenage Body Book*

Wilson, Ron. *How the Body Works*

Body Language

Aylesworth, Thomas G. *Understanding Body Talk*

Castle, Sue. *Face Talk, Hand Talk, Body Talk*

Gay, Kathlyn. *Body Talk*

Bones

See Skeletal system.

Brace, body

See also Scoliosis.

Blume, Judy Sussman. *Deenie*

Braces, leg

Blume, Judy Sussman. *Deenie*

Frevert, Patricia Dendtler. *It's Okay to Look at Jamie*

Hawker, Frances, and Lee Withall. *With a Little Help from My Friends*

Massie, Robert, and Suzanne Massie. *Journey*

Rodowsky, Colby F. *P.S. Write Soon*

Savitz, Harriet May. *The Lionhearted*

Braces, teeth

Betancourt, Jeanne. *Smile! How to Cope with Braces*

First, Julia. *Look Who's Beautiful!*

Gilson, Jamie. *Do Bananas Chew Gum?*

Okimoto, Jean Davies. *It's Just Too Much*

Richter, Alice, and Laura Joffe Numeroff. *You Can't Put Braces on Spaces*

Silverstein, Alvin, and Virginia B. Silverstein. *So You're Getting Braces: A Guide to Orthodontics*

Brain

See also Intelligence.

Berger, Melvin. *Exploring the Mind and Brain*
Facklam, Margery, and Howard Facklam. *The Brain: Magnificent Mind Machine*
Haines, Gail Kay. *Brain Power: Understanding Human Intelligence*
McNamara, Louise Greep, and Ada Bassett Litchfield. *Your Busy Brain*
Showers, Paul. *Use Your Brain*
Stevens, Leonard A. *Neurons: Building Blocks of the Brain*
Weart, Edith Lucie. *The Story of Your Brain and Nerves*
Zim, Herbert S. *Your Brain and How It Works*

Brain Injury

See also Minimal brain dysfunction.

Albert, Louise. *But I'm Ready to Go*
Bates, Betty. *Love Is Like Peanuts*
Corcoran, Barbara. *Axe-Time, Sword-Time*
Craig, Eleanor. *One, Two, Three . . . The Story of Matt, a Feral Child*
Larsen, Hanne. *Don't Forget Tom*
Melton, David. *A Boy Called Hopeless*
Schaefer, Nicola. *Does She Know That She's Here?*
Smith, Lucia B. *A Special Kind of Sister*

Sobol, Harriet Langsam. *My Brother Steven Is Retarded*
Wolff, Ruth. *A Crack in the Sidewalk*

Bulimia

See also Weight control.

Landau, Elaine. *Why Are They Starving Themselves? Understanding Anorexia Nervosa and Bulimia*

Burns

See also Surgery, plastic.

Cunningham, Glenn, with George X. Sand. *Never Quit*
Holland, Isabelle. *The Man Without a Face*
Howe, James. *A Night Without Stars*
Lifton, Betty Jean, and Thomas C. Fox. *Children of Vietnam*

Cancer

See also Chemotherapy; Hair loss; Hodgkin's disease; Leukemia; Radiation therapy.

Brady, Mari. *Please Remember Me: A Young Woman's Story of Her Friendship with an Unforgettable Fifteen-Year-Old Boy*
Center for Attitudinal Healing. *There Is a Rainbow Behind Every Dark Cloud*
Greenberg, Jan. *No Dragons to Slay*
Haines, Gail Kay. *Cancer*
Hyde, Margaret Oldroyd. *The New Genetics*
Ipswitch, Elaine. *Scott Was Here*
Knight, David C. *Viruses, Life's Smallest Enemies*

Lowry, Lois. *A Summer to Die*
Lubowe, Irwin I., and Barbara
Huss. *A Teen-Age Guide to
Healthy Skin and Hair*
Lund, Doris Herold. *Eric*
Manes, Stephen. *I'll Live*
Murray, Gloria, and Gerald G.
Jampolsky, eds. *Straight from
the Siblings: Another Look at
the Rainbow*
Nixon, Joan Lowery. *The Specter*
Pizer, Vernon. *Glorious Tri-
umphs: Athletes Who Con-
quered Adversity*
Silverstein, Alvin, and Virginia B.
Silverstein. *Cancer*
Trull, Patti. *On with My Life*
Warmbier, Jenene, and Ellen
Vassy. *Hospital Days, Treat-
ment Ways*

Cardiac Catheterization

See also Circulatory system;
Surgery, heart ; X Ray

Singer, Marilyn. *It Can't Hurt
Forever*

Careers in Health, Mental Health, Special Education

Anker, Carol Teig. *Teaching Ex-
ceptional Children: A Special
Career*
Bluestone, Naomi. *"So You Want
to Be a Doctor?" The Reali-
ties of Pursuing Medicine as
a Career*
Feingold, S. Norman, and Norma
R. Miller. *Your Future: A
Guide for the Handicapped
Teenager*
Jones, Marilyn. *Exploring Careers
in Special Education*
Keyes, Fenton. *Your Future in a
Paramedic Career*

Keyes, Fenton. *Your Future in
Social Work*
Lee, Mary Price. *A Future in
Pediatrics: Medical and Non-
Medical Careers in Child
Health Care*
Mitchell, Joyce Slayton. *See Me
More Clearly: Career and
Life Planning for Teens with
Physical Disabilities*
Reynolds, Moira Davison. *Aim
for a Job in a Medical Lab-
oratory*
Schaleben-Lewis, Joy. *Careers in
a Hospital*
Searight, Mary. *Your Career in
Nursing*
Shuff, Frances. *Your Future in
Occupational Therapy
Careers*

Cast

Balestrino, Philip. *The Skeleton
Inside You*
Blume, Judy Sussman. *Deenie*
Frevert, Patricia Dendtler. *It's
Okay to Look at Jamie*
Graber, Richard. *A Little
Breathing Room*
Greenwald, Arthur, and Head,
Barry. *Wearing a Cast*
Wolff, Angelika. *Mom! I Broke
My Arm*

Cataract

See also Vision impairment.

Hunt, Irene. *William*

Cerebral Palsy

See also Bliss symbols; Communication disability.

Canada, Lena. *To Elvis, with
Love*
Fassler, Joan. *Howie Helps Him-
self*

Gerson, Corinne. *Passing Through*
Hawker, Frances, and Lee Withall.
Donna Finds Another Way
Little, Jean. *Mine for Keeps*
Mack, Nancy. *Tracy*
Payne, Sherry Newirth. *A Contest*
Robinet, Harriette G. *Jay and the Marigold*
Slepian, Jan. *The Alfred Summer*
Slepian, Jan. *Lester's Turn*
Stein, Sara Bonnett. *About Handicaps: An Open Family Book for Parents and Children Together*

Chemotherapy

See also Cancer; Leukemia.

Bach, Alice. *Waiting for Johnny Miracle*
Center for Attitudinal Healing. *There Is a Rainbow Behind Every Dark Cloud*
Frevert, Patricia Dendtler. *Patty Gets Well*
Hughes, Monica. *Hunter in the Dark*
Lund, Doris Herold. *Eric*
Murray, Gloria, and Gerald G. Jampolsky, eds. *Straight from the Siblings: Another Look at the Rainbow*
Phillips, Carolyn E. *Michelle*
Silverstein, Alvin, and Virginia B. Silverstein. *Cancer*
Warmbier, Jenene, and Ellen Vassy. *Hospital Days, Treatment Ways*

Chicken Pox

Galbraith, Kathryn Osebold. *Spots Are Special*
Nourse, Alan Edward. *Viruses*
Wolde, Gunilla. *Betsy and the Chicken Pox*

Child Abuse/Neglect

See also Rights.

Anderson, Mary Quirk. *Step on a Crack*
Bradbury, Bianca. *Those Traver Kids*
Coolidge, Olivia. *Come By Here*
Cormier, Robert. *The Chocolate War*
Culin, Charlotte. *Cages of Glass, Flowers of Time*
Dolan, Edward F., Jr. *Child Abuse*
Dunnahoo, Terry. *Who Cares About Espie Sanchez?*
Graber, Richard. *A Little Breathing Room*
Green, Hannah. *I Never Promised You a Rose Garden*
Haskins, James, with Pat Connolly. *The Child Abuse Help Book*
Hunt, Irene. *The Lottery Rose*
Hyde, Margaret Oldroyd. *Cry Softly! The Story of Child Abuse*
Kata, Elizabeth. *A Patch of Blue*
MacCracken, Mary. *Lovey: A Very Special Child*
Mazer, Harry. *The War on Villa Street*
Moeri, Louise. *The Girl Who Lived on the Ferris Wheel*
Newman, Susan. *Ice Cream Isn't Always Good*
Peacock, Carol Antoinette. *Hand-Me-Down Dreams*
Roberts, Willo Davis. *Don't Hurt Laurie!*
Sachs, Marilyn. *A December Tale*
Samuels, Gertrude. *Run, Shelley, Run!*
Schlee, Ann. *Ask Me No Questions*
Seabrooke, Brenda. *Home Is Where They Take You In*

Stanek, Muriel. *Don't Hurt Me, Mama*

Warwick, Dolores. *Learn to Say Goodbye*

Wheat, Patte, with Leonard L. Lieber. *Hope for the Children: A Personal History of Parents Anonymous*

Child Life Specialist

See also Hospitalization.

Howe, James. *The Hospital Book*

Cholera

Schlee, Ann. *Ask Me No Questions*

Chronic Illness

Adams, Barbara. *Like It Is: Facts and Feelings About Handicaps from Kids Who Know*

Berger, Gilda. *Physical Disabilities*

Burstein, John. *Slim Goodbody: What Can Go Wrong and How to Be Strong*

Cox-Gedmark, Jan. *Coping with Physical Disability*

Cunningham, Glenn, with George X. Sand. *Never Quit*

Donahue, Parnell, and Helen Capellaro. *Germs Make Me Sick: A Health Handbook for Kids*

Harries, Joan. *They Triumphed over Their Handicaps*

Hayman, LeRoy. *Triumph! Conquering Your Physical Disability*

Kamien, Janet. *What If You*

Couldn't . . . ? *A Book About Special Needs*

Mitchell, Joyce Slayton. *See Me More Clearly: Career and Life Planning for Teens with Physical Disabilities*

Pursell, Margaret Sanford. *A Look at Physical Handicaps*

Siegel, Dorothy Schainman. *Winners: Eight Special Young People*

Splaver, Sarah. *Your Handicap— Don't Let It Handicap You*

Stiller, Richard. *Your Body Is Trying to Tell You Something: How to Understand Its Signals and Respond to Its Needs*

Sullivan, Mary Beth, Alan J. Brightman, and Joseph Blatt. *Feeling Free*

Tully, Marianne, and Mary-Alice Tully. *Dread Diseases*

Circulatory System

See also Blood; Cardiac catheterization; Surgery, heart.

Kalina, Sigmund. *Your Blood and Its Cargo*

Silverstein, Alvin, and Virginia B. Silverstein. *Circulatory Systems: The Rivers Within*

Weart, Edith Lucie. *The Story of Your Blood*

Cleft Lip/Palate

See also Surgery, cleft lip.

Holland, Isabelle. *Heads You Win, Tails I Lose*

McKillip, Patricia. *The Night Gift*

Rosenberg, Maxine B. *My Friend Leslie: The Story of a Handicapped Child*

Thrasher, Crystal. *The Dark Didn't Catch Me*
Weiss, Joan Talmage. *Home for a Stranger*

Clinic

Johnson, Eric W. *Venereal Disease and What You Should Do About It*
Kay, Eleanor. *The Clinic*
NAWCH Research Team. *Andrew Goes to the Outpatients*
Thypin, Marilyn, and Lynne Glasner. *Health Care for the Wongs: Health Insurance, Choosing a Doctor*

Cold, common

See also Upper respiratory infection (URI).

Bennett, Hal Zina. *Cold Comfort*
Hann, Jacquie. *Up Day, Down Day*
Hirsch, Linda. *The Sick Story*
Numeroff, Laura Joffe. *Phoebe Dexter Has Harriet Peterson's Sniffles*
Segal, Lore. *Tell Me a Mitzi*

Cold, common—Animal

Berenstain, Stan, and Jan Berenstain. *The Berenstain Bears Go to the Doctor*
Wiseman, Bernard. *Morris Has a Cold*

Communication

See also Body language; Speech.

Allington, Richard L., and Kathleen Krull. *Talking*

Communication Disability

See also Bliss symbols; Mute; Speech impairment.

Althea. *I Can't Talk Like You*
Berger, Gilda. *Speech and Language Disorders*
Christopher, Matt. *Glue Fingers*
Fassler, Joan. *Don't Worry, Dear*
Friis, Babbis. *Kristy's Courage*
Greene, Constance C. *The Unmaking of Rabbit*
Heide, Florence Parry. *Secret Dreamer, Secret Dreams*
Helfman, Elizabeth S. *Blissymbolics: Speaking Without Speech*
Holland, Isabelle. *Alan and the Animal Kingdom*
Lee, Mildred Scudder. *The Skating Rink*
Madison, Winifred. *Growing Up in a Hurry*
Pfeffer, Susan Beth. *What Do You Do When Your Mouth Won't Open?*
Pizer, Vernon. *You Don't Say: How People Communicate Without Speech*
Young, John Sacret. *Special Olympics*

Computerized Axial Tomography (CAT scan)

Girion, Barbara. *A Handful of Stars*
Howe, James. *The Hospital Book*

Conception

See also Reproductive system.

Dragonwagon, Crescent. *Wind Rose*

Gruenberg, Sidonie M. *The Wonderful Story of How You Were Born*

Lipke, Jean Coryllel. *Conception and Contraception*

Loebl, Suzanne. *Conception, Contraception: A New Look*

Pursell, Margaret Sanford. *A Look at Birth*

Showers, Paul, and Kay Sperry Showers. *Before You Were a Baby*

Snyder, Gerald S. *Test-Tube Life: Scientific Advance and Moral Dilemma*

Stwertka, Eve, and Albert Stwertka. *Genetic Engineering*

Contact Lenses

See also Vision aids; Vision impairment.

Kelley, Alberta. *Lenses, Spectacles, Eyeglasses and Contacts: The Story of Vision Aids*

Contraception

See also Reproductive system; Venereal disease.

Balis, Andrea. *What Are You Using? A Birth Control Guide for Teen-Agers*

Hamilton, Eleanor. *Sex, with Love: A Guide for Young People*

Lieberman, E. James, and Ellen Peck. *Sex and Birth Control: A Guide for the Young*

Lipke, Jean Coryllel. *Conception and Contraception*

Loebl, Suzanne. *Conception, Contraception: A New Look*

McCoy, Kathy. *The Teenage Body Book Guide to Sexuality*

Tensen, Gordon. *Youth and Sex: Pleasure and Responsibility*

Crying

Stanton, Elizabeth, and Henry Stanton. *Sometimes I Like to Cry*

Cryogenics

Kavaler, Lucy. *Cold Against Disease: The Wonders of Cold*

Cystic Fibrosis

Arnold, Katrin. *Anna Joins In*

Hyde, Margaret Oldroyd. *The New Genetics*

Morrison, Velma F. *There's Only One You: the Story of Heredity*

Deafness

See also Hearing aids; Hearing impairment; Sign language; Signed English.

Arthur, Catherine. *My Sister's Silent World*

Bloom, Freddy. *The Boy Who Couldn't Hear*

Bowe, Frank. *Comeback: Six Remarkable People Who Triumphed over Disability*

Coolidge, Olivia. *Come By Here*

Corcoran, Barbara. *A Dance to Still Music*

Dixon, Paige. *Skipper*

Ferris, Caren. *A Hug Just Isn't Enough*

Hanlon, Emily. *The Swing*

Harries, Joan. *They Triumphed over Their Handicaps*
Hirsch, Karen. *Becky*
Hlibok, Bruce. *Silent Dancer*
Hyman, Jane. *Deafness*
Ireland, Karin. *Kitty O'Neill: Daredevil Woman*
Levine, Edna S. *Lisa and Her Soundless World*
Levinson, Nancy. *World of Her Own*
Montgomery, Elizabeth Rider. *The Mystery of the Boy Next Door*
Neimark, Anne E. *A Deaf Child Listened: Thomas Gallaudet, Pioneer in American Education*
Peter, Diana. *Claire and Emma*
Peterson, Jeanne Whitehouse. *I Have a Sister, My Sister Is Deaf*
Riskind, Mary. *Apple Is My Sign*
Robinson, Veronica. *David in Silence*
Rosen, Lillian. *Just Like Everybody Else*
Siegel, Dorothy Schainman. *Winners: Eight Special Young People*
Spradley, Thomas S., and James R. Spradley. *Deaf Like Me*
Sullivan, Mary Beth, and Linda Bourke. *A Show of Hands: Say It in Sign Language*
Wolf, Bernard. *Anna's Silent World*
Wright, David. *Deafness*
Yolen, Jane. *The Mermaid's Three Wisdoms*

Death of Child

Anonymous. *Go Ask Alice*
Beckman, Gunnel. *Admission to the Feast*

Brady, Mari. *Please Remember Me: A Young Woman's Story of Her Friendship with an Unforgettable Fifteen-Year-Old Boy*
Coerr, Eleanor B. *Sadako and the Thousand Paper Cranes*
Ipswitch, Elaine. *Scott Was Here*
Langone, John. *Death Is a Noun: A View of the End of Life*
Lee, Virginia. *The Magic Moth*
Lifton, Betty Jean, and Thomas C. Fox. *Children of Vietnam*
Lund, Doris Herold. *Eric*
McLendon, Gloria H. *My Brother Joey Died*
Scoppettone, Sandra. *Trying Hard to Hear You*
Simon, Norma. *We Remember Philip*
Slote, Alfred. *Hang Tough, Paul Mather*

Death of Friend

Bradbury, Bianca. *The Girl Who Wanted Out*
Bunting, Eve. *The Empty Window*
Coerr, Eleanor B. *Sadako and the Thousand Paper Cranes*
Jones, Rebecca C. *Angie and Me*
Kingman, Lee. *The Peter Pan Bag*
Moe, Barbara. *Pickles and Prunes*
Scoppettone, Sandra. *Trying Hard to Hear You*
Simon, Norma. *We Remember Philip*
Slepian, Jan. *Lester's Turn*
Snyder, Anne. *My Name Is Davy, I'm an Alcoholic*

Death of Parent

Corcoran, Barbara. *A Row of Tigers*

Cormier, Robert. *The Chocolate War*

Jones, Penelope. *Holding Together*

Hammond, Janice Marie. *When My Dad Died: A Child's View of Death*

Hammond, Janice Marie. *When My Mommy Died: A Child's View of Death*

Hanlon, Emily. *The Swing*

Hunt, Irene. *William*

Krementz, Jill. *How It Feels When a Parent Dies*

LeShan, Eda J. *Learning to Say Goodbye: When a Parent Dies*

Manes, Stephen. *I'll Live*

Minshull, Evelyn W. *The Steps to My Best Friend's House*

Spencer, Zane, and Jay Leech. *Cry of the Wolf*

Stolz, Mary. *The Edge of Next Year*

Whelan, Gloria. *A Time to Keep Silent*

Death of Self

See also Suicide/suicide attempt.

Beckman, Gunnel. *Admission to the Feast*

Center for Attitudinal Healing. *There Is a Rainbow Behind Every Dark Cloud*

Hyde, Margaret Oldroyd. *Suicide: The Hidden Epidemic*

Klagsbrun, Francine. *Too Young to Die: Youth and Suicide*

Lowry, Lois. *A Summer to Die*

Madison, Arnold. *Suicide and Young People*

Death of Sibling

Burch, Robert. *Simon and the Game of Chance*

Dixon, Paige. *Skipper*

Dunnahoo, Terry. *Who Cares About Espie Sanchez?*

Gerson, Corinne. *Passing Through*

Greene, Constance C. *Beat the Turtle Drum*

Guest, Judith. *Ordinary People*

Hermes, Patricia. *Nobody's Fault?*

Klein, Norma. *Confessions of an Only Child*

Lowry, Lois. *A Summer to Die*

McLendon, Gloria H. *My Brother Joey Died*

Mathis, Sharon Bell. *Teacup Full of Roses*

Thrasher, Crystal. *The Dark Didn't Catch Me*

Dentist's Office

See also Braces, teeth; Surgery, oral; Teeth.

Althea. *Visiting the Dentist*

Barnett, Naomi. *I Know a Dentist*

Cooney, Nancy E. *The Wobbly Tooth*

Doss, Helen, with Richard L. Wells. *All the Better to Bite With*

Dunn, Graeme. *Benjamin Goes to the Dentist: An Introduction to the Dentist for Children and Parents*

Fleege, Francis. *How to Eat: Chewing, Tooth Care, and Diet*

Lapp, Carolyn. *Dentist's Tools*

Nourse, Alan Edward. *The Tooth Book*

Packard, Mary. *A Visit to the Dentist*

Rockwell, Harlow. *My Dentist*

Ross, Pat. *Molly and the Slow Teeth*

Roy, Howard L. *Bobby Visits the Dentist*

Schaleben-Lewis, Joy. *The Dentist and Me*
Snell, Nigel. *Tom Visits the Dentist*
Wolf, Bernard. *Michael and the Dentist*
Ziegler, Sandra. *At the Dentist: What Did Christopher See?*

Dentist's Office — Animal

Berenstain, Stan, and Jan Berenstain. *The Berenstain Bears Visit the Dentist*
McPhail, David. *The Bear's Toothache*
Steig, William. *Doctor De Soto*

Depression

See also Suicide/suicide attempt.

Berger, Gilda. *Mental Illness*
Burch, Robert. *Simon and the Game of Chance*
Hamilton, Virginia. *The Planet of Junior Brown*
Kiev, Ari. *The Courage to Live*
Myers, Irma, and Arthur Myers. *Why You Feel Down and What You Can Do About It: A Psychotherapist Tells Everything You Want to Know About Teenage Depression*
Neufeld, John. *Lisa, Bright and Dark*
Olshan, Neal H. *Depression*

Diabetes

See also Endocrine system.

Althea. *I Have Diabetes*
Covelli, Pat. *Borrowing Time: Growing Up with Juvenile Diabetes*
Duncan, Theodore G. *The Diabetes Fact Book*
Dacquino, V. T. *Kiss the Candy Days Good-bye*
Goodman, Joseph I., and W. Watts Bigger. *Diabetes Without Fear*
Kipnis, Lynne, and Susan Adler. *You Can't Catch Diabetes from a Friend*
Kleiman, Gary, and Dody Sandford. *No Time to Lose*
Riedman, Sarah Regal. *Diabetes*
Silverstein, Alvin, and Virginia B. Silverstein. *Runaway Sugar: All About Diabetes*
Silverstein, Alvin, and Virginia B. Silverstein. *The Sugar Disease: Diabetes*

Digestion

See also Nutrition.

Marr, John S. *The Food You Eat*
Mylander, Maureen. *The Great American Stomach Book: How Your Digestion Works and What to Do When It Doesn't*
Null, Gary, and Steve Null. *Why Your Stomach Hurts: A Handbook of Digestion and Nutrition*
Showers, Paul. *What Happens to a Hamburger?*
Silverstein, Alvin, and Virginia B. Silverstein. *The Digestive System: How Living Creatures Use Food*
Ward, Brian R. *Food and Digestion*
Zim, Herbert S. *Your Stomach and Digestive Tract*

Digestion Disorder

See also Nutrition.

Mylander, Maureen. *The Great American Stomach Book: How Your Digestion Works and What to Do When It Doesn't*
Null, Gary, and Steve Null. *Why Your Stomach Hurts: A Handbook of Digestion and Nutrition*

Dioxyribonucleic Acid (DNA)

See also Genetics.

Bornstein, Jerry, and Sandy Bornstein. *What Is Genetics?*
Dunbar, Robert E. *Heredity*
Facklam, Margery, and Howard Facklam. *From Cell to Clone: The Story of Genetic Engineering*
Frankel, Edward. *DNA: The Ladder of Life*
Silverstein, Alvin, and Virginia B. Silverstein. *The Code of Life*
Silverstein, Alvin, and Virginia B. Silverstein. *The Genetics Explosion*

Disability

Anker, Carol Teig. *Teaching Exceptional Children: A Special Career*
Bates, Betty. *Picking Up the Pieces*
Berger, Gilda. *Physical Disabilities*
Bowe, Frank. *Comeback: Six Remarkable People Who Triumphed over Disability*

Cox-Gedmark, Jan. *Coping with Physical Disability*
Dixon, Paige. *Skipper*
Gollay, Elinor, and Alwina Bennett. *The College Guide for Students with Disabilities: A Detailed Directory of Higher Education Services, Programs, and Facilities Accessible to Handicapped Students in the United States*
Greenfield, Eloise, and Alesia Revis. *Alesia*
Haskins, James, and J. M. Stifle. *The Quiet Revolution: The Struggle for the Rights of Disabled Americans*
Hayman, LeRoy. *Triumph! Conquering Your Physical Disability*
Mitchell, Joyce Slayton. *See Me More Clearly: Career and Life Planning for Teens with Physical Disabilities*

Disabled in School

Althea. *I Can't Talk Like You*
Arnold, Katrin. *Anna Joins In*
Bradbury, Bianca. *The Girl Who Wanted Out*
Butler, Beverly Kathleen. *Light a Single Candle*
Cohen, Miriam. *See You Tomorrow, Charles*
Fanshawe, Elizabeth. *Rachel*
Fassler, Joan. *Howie Helps Himself*
Glazzard, Margaret H. *Meet Camille and Danille, They're Special Persons: Hearing Impaired*
Glazzard, Margaret H. *Meet Scott, He's a Special Person: Learning Disabled*
Kent, Deborah. *Belonging*

Lasker, Joe. *Nick Joins In*
Levinson, Nancy. *A World of Her Own*
Litchfield, Ada Bassett. *Captain Hook, That's Me*
Little, Jean. *Mine for Keeps*
Lund, Doris Herold. *Eric*
Montgomery, Elizabeth Rider. *"Seeing" in the Dark*
Payne, Sherry Newirth. *A Contest*
Phelan, Terry Wolfe. *The S.S. Valentine*
Pieper, Elizabeth. *A School for Tommy*
Rabe, Berniece. *The Balancing Girl*
Savitz, Harriet May. *The Lionhearted*
Savitz, Harriet May. *Run, Don't Walk*
Thomas, William E. *The New Boy Is Blind*
Zelonky, Joy. *I Can't Always Hear You*

Disabled in Sports

See also Exercise; Physical fitness; Sports medicine.

Allen, Anne. *Sports for the Handicapped*
Althea. *I Have Asthma*
Antonacci, Robert J., and Jene Barr. *Physical Fitness for Young Champions*
Brown, Fern G. *You're Somebody Special on a Horse*
Cunningham, Glenn, with George X. Sand. *Never Quit*
Fleischer, Leonore. *Ice Castles*
Ireland, Karin. *Kitty O'Neill, Daredevil Woman*
Lee, Robert C. *It's a Mile from Here to Glory*
Lund, Doris Herold. *Eric*

Pizer, Vernon. *Glorious Triumphs: Athletes Who Conquered Adversity*
Rudolph, Wilma, as told to Bud Greenspan. *Wilma! The Story of Wilma Rudolph*
Savitz, Harriet May. *The Lionhearted*
Savitz, Harriet May. *Wheelchair Champions: A History of Wheelchair Sports*
Slote, Alfred. *Hang Tough, Paul Mather*
Wartski, Maureen Crane. *My Brother Is Special*
Wolf, Bernard. *Don't Feel Sorry for Paul*
Young, Helen. *What Difference Does It Make, Danny?*

Doctor's Office

See also Physician.

Althea. *Going to the Doctor*
Cobb, Vicki. *How the Doctor Knows You're Fine*
Gardner-Loulan, JoAnn, Bonnie Lopez, and Marcia Quackenbush. *Period*
Gibbons, Thomas B. *How Doctors Diagnose You and How You Can Help*
Greene, Carla. *Doctors and Nurses: What Do They Do?*
Hayden, Robert C., and Jacqueline Harris. *Nine Black American Doctors*
Holmes, Burnham. *Early Morning: Portrait of a Hospital*
Jessel, Camilla. *Going to the Doctor*
Moncure, Jane Belk. *People Who Help People*
Rockwell, Harlow. *My Doctor*

Snell, Nigel. *Kate Visits the Doctor*
Thypin, Marilyn, and Lynne Glasner. *Health Care for the Wongs: Health Insurance, Choosing a Doctor*
Wolde, Gunilla. *Tommy Goes to the Doctor*

Doctor's Office — Animal

Berenstain, Stan, and Jan Berenstain. *The Berenstain Bears Go to the Doctor*
Chalmers, Mary. *Come to the Doctor, Harry*
Roy, Howard L. *We're Going to the Doctor*
Scarry, Richard. *Richard Scarry's Nicky Goes to the Doctor*

Down's Syndrome

Anderson, Kay Wooster. *Don't Forget Me, Mommy!*
Baldwin, Anne Norris. *A Little Time*
Garrigue, Sheila. *Between Friends*
Mayerson, Evelyn. *Sanjo*
Ominsky, Elaine. *Jon O.: A Special Boy*
Stefanik, Alfred T. *Copycat Sam: Developing Ties with a Special Child*

Dreams

See also Sleep.

Anderson, Mary Quirk. *Step on a Crack*
Kettelkamp, Larry. *Dreams*
Lindsay, Rae. *Sleep and Dreams*
Robison, Deborah, and Carla Perez. *Your Turn, Doctor*

Showers, Paul. *Sleep Is for Everyone*
Silverstein, Alvin, and Virginia B. Silverstein. *Sleep and Dreams*

Drug Use and Abuse

Anders, Rebecca. *A Look at Drug Abuse*
Anonymous. *Go Ask Alice*
Austrian, Geoffrey. *The Truth About Drugs*
Barness, Richard. *Listen to Me!*
Berger, Gilda. *Addiction: Its Causes, Problems and Treatments*
Butterworth, W. E. *Under the Influence*
Childress, Alice. *A Hero Ain't Nothin' but a Sandwich*
Dunnahoo, Terry. *Who Cares About Espie Sanchez?*
Elgin, Kathleen, and John F. Osterritter. *The Ups and Downs of Drugs*
Eyerly, Jeannette. *Escape from Nowhere*
Flender, Harold, as told to. *We Were Hooked: Thirteen Young Ex-Addicts Tell About Their Experiences with Heroin, LSD, Speed, and Other Drugs and How They Kicked the Habit*
Hinton, S. E. *That Was Then, This Is Now*
Harries, Joan. *They Triumphed over Their Handicaps*
Holland, Isabelle. *Heads You Win, Tails I Lose*
Hyde, Margaret Oldroyd, ed. *Mind Drugs*
Kingman, Lee. *The Peter Pan Bag*
Madison, Arnold. *Drugs and You*

Mathis, Sharon Bell. *Teacup Full of Roses*
Mitchell, Joyce Slayton. *Free to Choose: Decision Making for Young Men*
Mitchell, Joyce Slayton. *Other Choices for Becoming a Woman*
O'Dell, Scott. *Kathleen, Please Come Home*
Peacock, Carol Antoinette. *Hand-Me-Down Dreams*
Reynolds, Pamela. *Will the Real Monday Please Stand Up*
Sherburne, Zoa. *Leslie*
Spock, Benjamin McLane. *A Teenager's Guide to Life and Love*
Strasser, Todd. *Angel Dust Blues*
Stwertka, Albert, and Eve Stwertka. *Marijuana*
Wojciechowska, Maia. *Tuned Out*

Dyslexia

See also Learning disability.

Blue, Rose. *Me and Einstein: Breaking Through the Reading Barrier*
Gilson, Jamie. *Do Bananas Chew Gum?*
Haynes, Henry Louis. *Squarehead and Me*
Pevsner, Stella. *Keep Stompin' Till the Music Stops*

Ears

See also Hearing.

Adler, Irving, and Ruth Adler. *Your Ears*
Fryer, Judith. *How We Hear: The Story of Hearing*
Greene, Constance C. *The Ears of Louis*
Greene, Constance C. *The Unmaking of Rabbit*
Newman, Alyse. *It's Me, Claudia!*

Perkins, Al. *Ear Book*
Silverstein, Alvin, and Virginia B. Silverstein. *The Story of Your Ear*
Ward, Brian R. *The Ear and Hearing*

Electrocardiography (ECG)

See also Heart disease; Surgery, heart.

Howe, James. *The Hospital Book*
Silverstein, Alvin, and Virginia B. Silverstein. *Heartbeats: Your Body, Your Heart*
Singer, Marilyn. *It Can't Hurt Forever*

Electroencephalography (EEG)

See also Brain; Epilepsy.

Girion, Barbara. *A Handful of Stars*

Emergency

See also Paramedic.

Beame, Rona. *Emergency!*
Ciliotta, Claire, and Carole Livingston. *Why Am I Going to the Hospital: A Helpful Guide to a New Experience*
Gore, Harriet Margolis. *What to Do When There's No One but You*
Greenbank, Anthony. *A Handbook for Emergencies: Coming Out Alive*
Mann, Peggy. *Twelve Is Too Old*
Marino, Barbara Pavis. *Eric Needs Stitches*
Milton, Hilary. *Emergency! 10-33 on Channel 11!*
Steedman, Julie. *Emergency Room: An ABC Tour*
Vandenburg, Mary Lou. *Help! Emergencies That Could*

Happen to You and How to Handle Them
Vigna, Judith. *Gregory's Stitches*
Witty, Margot. *A Day in the Life of an Emergency Room Nurse*
Wolde, Gunilla. *Betsy and the Doctor*
Wolfe, Bob, and Diane Wolfe. *Emergency Room*

Emotional Illness

See also Autism; Depression; Kleptomania; Psychiatrist; Psychologist; Psychotherapy; Schizophrenia; Social Worker.

Bauer, Marion Dane. *Tangled Butterfly*
Berger, Gilda. *Mental Illness*
Carlson, Dale Bick. *Call Me Amanda*
Carlson, Dale Bick. *Where's Your Head? Psychology for Teenagers*
Cavallaro, Ann. *Blimp*
Clements, Hanna, and Bruce Clements. *Coming Home to a Place You've Never Been Before*
Craig, Eleanor. *One, Two, Three ... The Story of Matt, a Feral Child*
Dengler, Marianna. *A Pebble in Newcomb's Pond*
Green, Hannah. *I Never Promised You a Rose Garden*
Hamilton, Virginia. *The Planet of Junior Brown*
Hamilton-Paterson, James. *House in the Waves*
Heide, Florence Parry. *Secret Dreamer, Secret Dreams*
Kiev, Ari. *The Courage to Live*
Kingman, Lee. *The Peter Pan Bag*
Langone, John. *Goodbye to Bed-*

lam: Understanding Mental Illness and Retardation
Levoy, Myron. *Alan and Naomi*
Lifton, Betty Jean, and Thomas C. Fox. *Children of Vietnam*
MacCracken, Mary. *Lovey: A Very Special Child*
McKillip, Patricia. *The Night Gift*
Minshull, Evelyn W. *The Steps to My Best Friend's House*
Morgenroth, Barbara. *Demons at My Door*
Neufeld, John. *Lisa, Bright and Dark*
Olshan, Neal H. *Depression*
Oneal, Zibby. *The Language of Goldfish*
Platt, Kin. *The Boy Who Could Make Himself Disappear*
Rabinowich, Ellen. *Underneath I'm Different*
Rothenberg, Mira. *Children with Emerald Eyes: Histories of Extraordinary Boys and Girls*
Shapiro, Patricia Gottlieb. *Caring for the Mentally Ill*
Shreve, Susan Richards. *Love-letters*
Shyer, Marlene F. *Welcome Home, Jellybean*
Storr, Catherine. *Thursday*
Whelan, Gloria. *A Time to Keep Silent*

Emotional Support

See also Attitudes toward disabled; Friendship with disabled; Psychotherapy.

Anderson, Mary Quirk. *Step on a Crack*
Burns, Marilyn. *The Book of Think: Or How to Solve a Problem Twice Your Size*
Blume, Judy Sussman. *Then Again, Maybe I Won't*

Carlson, Dale Bick. *Where's Your Head? Psychology for Teenagers*
Clements, Hanna, and Bruce Clements. *Coming Home to a Place You've Never Been Before*
Eagan, Andrea B. *Why Am I So Miserable If These Are the Best Years of My Life?: A Survival Guide for the Young Woman*
Elkind, David. *All Grown Up and No Place to Go*
Fassler, Joan. *The Boy with a Problem: Johnny Learns to Share His Troubles*
Fleischer, Leonore. *Ice Castles*
Frevert, Patricia Dendtler. *Patty Gets Well*
Gilbert, Sara D. *What Happens in Therapy*
Greenberg, Jan. *No Dragons to Slay*
Hawker, Frances, and Lee Withall. *With a Little Help from My Friends*
Hogan, Paula, and Kirk Hogan. *The Hospital Scares Me*
Hyde, Margaret Oldroyd. *Hotline*
LeShan, Eda. *What Makes Me Feel This Way: Growing Up with Human Emotions*
London, Kathy, and Frank Caparulo. *Who Am I? Who Are You? Coping with Friends, Feelings, and Other Teenage Dilemmas*
Marks, Jane. *Help: A Guide to Counseling and Therapy Without a Hassle*
Mihaly, Mary E. *Getting Your Own Way: Growing Up Assertively*
Morrison, Carl V., and Dorothy Nafus Morrison. *Can I Help How I Feel?*

Myers, Irma, and Arthur Myers. *Why You Feel Down and What You Can Do About It: A Psychotherapist Tells Everything You Want to Know About Teenage Depression*
Simon, Norma. *How Do I Feel?*
Simon, Norma. *Why Am I Different?*
Warner, S. Lucille, and Ann Reit. *Your A-Z Super Problem Solver*

Emotions

See Feelings.

Endocrine System

See also Diabetes.

Nourse, Alan Edward. *Hormones*
Silverstein, Alvin, and Virginia B. Silverstein. *The Endocrine System: Hormones in the Living World*

Enuresis

See Bedwetting.

Environment

Pringle, Laurence. *Lives at Stake: The Science and Politics of Environmental Health*

Enzymes

See also Digestion.

Berger, Melvin. *Enzymes in Action*

Epidemic

Archer, Jules. *Epidemic! The Story of the Disease Detectives*
Berger, Melvin. *Disease Detectives*

Epilepsy

See also Brain; Electroencephalography. (EEG)

Corcoran, Barbara. *Child of the Morning*
Girion, Barbara. *A Handful of Stars*
Hermes, Patricia. *What If They Knew?*
Sherburne, Zoa. *Why Have the Birds Stopped Singing?*
Silverstein, Alvin, and Virginia B. Silverstein. *Epilepsy*
Young, Helen. *What Difference Does It Make, Danny?*

Excretory System

Plaut, Martin E. *The Doctor's Guide to You and Your Colon: A Candid, Helpful Guide to Our #1 Hidden Health Complaint*
Silverstein, Alvin, and Virginia B. Silverstein. *The Excretory System*

Exercise

See also Disabled in sports; Physical fitness; Sports medicine.

Bennett, Hal Zina. *The Doctor Within*

Benziger, Barbara. *Controlling Your Weight*
Bolian, Polly. *Growing Up Slim*
Cosgrove, Margaret. *Your Muscles —And Ways to Exercise Them*
Goodbody, Slim. *The Force Inside You*
Jacobsen, Karen. *Health*
McLaren, Annabel, ed. *Going to Hospital*
Maddux, Hilary C. *Menstruation*
Odor, Ruth S. *What's a Body to Do?*
Riedman, Sarah Regal. *Diabetes*
Rush, Anne Kent. *Getting Clear: Body Work for Women*
Schneider, Tom. *Everybody's a Winner: A Kid's Guide to New Sports and Fitness*
Trier, Carola S. *Exercise: What It Is, What It Does*

Extrasensory Perception

See Parapsychology.

Eyes

See also Vision.

Adler, Irving, and Ruth Adler. *Your Eyes*
Brown, Marcia. *Walk with Your Eyes*
Hammond, Winifred. *The Story of Your Eye*
LeSieg, Theo. *The Eye Book*
Schuman, Benjamin N. *The Human Eye*
Showers, Paul. *Look at Your Eyes*
Sislowitz, Marcel J. *Look! How Your Eyes See*
Ward, Brian R. *The Eye and Seeing*

Face

Brenner, Barbara. *Faces*
Castle, Sue. *Face Talk, Hand Talk, Body Talk*
Girion, Barbara. *The Boy with the Special Face*

Fear and Phobia

See also Doctor's office—animal; Feelings.

Anderson, Penny S. *The Operation*
Hyde, Margaret Oldroyd. *Fears and Phobias*
Olshan, Neal H., and Julie Dreyer Wang. *Fears and Phobias: Fighting Back*
Pfeffer, Susan B. *What Do You Do When Your Mouth Won't Open?*
Stanek, Muriel. *Who's Afraid of the Dark?*
Stein, Sara Bonnett. *About Phobias: An Open Family Book for Parents and Children Together*

Feelings

Adams, Barbara. *Like It Is: Facts and Feelings About Handicaps from Kids Who Know*
Allington, Richard L., and Kathleen Cowles. *Feelings*
Ancona, George. *I Feel: A Picture Book of Emotions*
Banish, Roslyn. *I Want to Tell You About My Baby*
Berger, Terry. *I Have Feelings*
Berger, Terry. *I Have Feelings Too*
Carlson, Dale Bick. *Boys Have Feelings Too*
Center for Attitudinal Healing.

There Is a Rainbow Behind Every Dark Cloud
Gelinas, Paul J. *Coping with Anger*
Gelinas, Paul J. *Coping with Your Emotions*
Gilbert, Sara D. *Feeling Good: A Book About You and Your Body*
Howe, James. *The Hospital Book*
Kroll, Steven. *That Makes Me Mad*
LeShan, Eda J. *What Makes Me Feel This Way? Growing Up with Human Emotions*
Marino, Barbara Pavis. *Eric Needs Stitches*
Morrison, Carl V., and Dorothy Nafus Morrison. *Can I Help How I Feel?*
Polland, Barbara. *Inside You and Outloud Too*
Simon, Norma. *How Do I Feel?*
Simon, Norma. *Why Am I Different?*
Splaver, Sarah. *Your Handicap—Don't Let It Handicap You*
Stanton, Elizabeth, and Henry Stanton. *Sometimes I Like to Cry*
Visser, Pat. *Feelings from A to Z*

Feet

See also Foot disability.

Cook, Marjorie. *To Walk on Two Feet*
Holzenthaler, Jean. *My Feet Do*
Krishef, Robert K. *Our Remarkable Feet*
Ramirez, Carolyn. *Foot and Feet*
Seuss, Dr. *The Foot Book*

First Aid

See also Emergency.

Gore, Harriet Margolis. *What to Do When There's No One but You*

Foot Disability

Griese, Arnold A. *At the Mouth of the Luckiest River*

Freckles

Blume, Judy Sussman. *Freckle Juice*
Girion, Barbara. *The Boy with the Special Face*

Friendship with Disabled

See also Disabled in school.

Bates, Betty. *Picking Up the Pieces*
Clifton, Lucille. *My Friend Jacob*
Crawford, Charles P. *Three-Legged Race*
Eyerly, Jeannette. *The Seeing Summer*
Garrigue, Sheila. *Between Friends*
Haynes, Henry Louise. *Squarehead and Me*
Kidd, Ronald. *That's What Friends Are For*
Levinson, Nancy. *World of Her Own*
Parker, Mark. *Horses, Airplanes, and Frogs*
Robinson, Veronica. *David in Silence*
Rosen, Lillian. *Just Like Everybody Else*
Rosenberg, Maxine B. *My Friend Leslie: The Story of a Handicapped Child*

Roy, Ron. *Frankie Is Staying Back*
Slepian, Jan. *The Alfred Summer*
Slepian, Jan. *Lester's Turn*
Stefanik, Alfred T. *Copycat Sam: Developing Ties with a Special Child*
Stein, Sara Bonnett. *About Handicaps: An Open Family Book for Parents and Children Together*
Strasser, Todd. *Friends Till the End*
Whitney, Phyllis. *Secret of the Emerald Star*

Gastrointestinal Tract

See also Digestion; Excretory system.

Plaut, Martin E. *The Doctor's Guide to You and Your Colon: A Candid, Helpful Guide to Our #1 Hidden Health Complaint*
Waidley, Ericka. *All About Your X-Ray: UGI*

Genetics

See also Dioxyribonucleic acid (DNA).

Bornstein, Jerry, and Sandy Bornstein. *What Is Genetics?*
Dunbar, Robert E. *Heredity*
Facklam, Howard, and Margery Facklam. *From Cell to Clone: The Story of Genetic Engineering*
Hyde, Margaret Oldroyd. *The New Genetics*
Lipke, Jean Coryllel. *Heredity*
Morrison, Velma Ford. *There's*

Only One You: The Story of
Heredity
Silverstein, Alvin, and Virginia B.
Silverstein. The Code of Life
Silverstein, Alvin, and Virginia B.
Silverstein. The Genetics Ex-
plosion
Stwertka, Eve, and Albert
Stwertka. Genetic Engineer-
ing
Tully, Marianne, and Mary-Alice
Tully. Dread Diseases

Germs

See also Bacteria.

Donahue, Parnell, and Helen
Capellaro. Germs Make Me
Sick: A Health Handbook for
Kids
Lietz, Gerald S. Bacteria
Patent, Dorothy Hinshaw. Germs

Glasses

See also Vision aids; Vision impairment.

Althea. Having an Eye Test
Brindze, Ruth. Look How Many
People Wear Glasses: The
Magic of Lenses
First, Julia. Getting Smarter
Goodsell, Jane. Katie's Magic
Glasses
Hall, Candace Catlin. Shelley's
Day: The Day of a Legally
Blind Child
Kelley, Alberta. Lenses,
Spectacles, Eyeglasses and
Contacts: The Story of Vision
Aids
Kropp, Paul. Wilted
Leggett, Linda Rodgers, and Linda
Gambee Andrews. The Rose-

Colored Glasses: Melanie Ad-
justs to Poor Vision
Litchfield, Ada Bassett. A Cane
in Her Hand
Little, Jean. From Anna
National Association for Visually
Handicapped. Cathy
Raskin, Ellen. Spectacles
Snell, Nigel. Johnny Gets Some
Glasses
Stanek, Muriel. Left Right, Left
Right
Wolff, Angelika. Mom! I Need
Glasses

Glasses – Animal

Brown, Marc. Arthur's Eyes

Glaucoma

See also Blindness; Vision impairment.

Butler, Beverly Kathleen. Gift of
Gold
Frevert, Patricia Dendtler.
Patrick: Yes You Can

Growth

Harris, Robie H., and Elizabeth
Levy. Before You Were Three:
How You Began to Walk,
Talk, Explore and Have Feel-
ings
Hutchins, Pat. Happy Birthday,
Sam
Iverson, Genie. I Want to Be Big
Lee, H. Alton. Seven Feet Four
and Growing
Mihaly, Mary E. Getting Your
Own Way: A Guide to Grow-
ing Up Assertively
Showers, Paul. A Baby Starts to
Grow

Warburg, Sandol S. *Growing Time*

Ward, Brian R. *Birth and Growth*

Guide Dog

See also Seeing Eye Dog.

Butler, Beverly Kathleen. *Light a Single Candle*

Curtis, Patricia. *Greff: The Story of a Guide Dog*

McPhee, Richard. *Tom and Bear: The Training of a Guide Dog Team*

Weiss, Malcolm E. *Blindness*

Hair

Lubowe, Irwin I., and Barbara Huss. *A Teen-Age Guide to Healthy Skin and Hair*

Hair Loss

See also Cancer: Chemotherapy; Leukemia; Loss; Radiation therapy.

Center for Attitudinal Healing. *There Is a Rainbow Behind Every Dark Cloud*

Warmbier, Jenene, and Ellen Vassy. *Hospital Days, Treatment Ways*

Handicap

Adams, Barbara. *Like It Is: Facts and Feelings About Handicaps from Kids Who Know*

Allen, Anne. *Sports for the Handicapped*

Anker, Carol Teig. *Teaching Exceptional Children: A Special Career*

Feingold, S. Norman, and Norma

R. Miller. *Your Future: A Guide for the Handicapped Teenager*

Glazzard, Margaret H. *Meet Danny, He's a Special Person: Multiply Handicapped*

Harries, Joan. *They Triumphed over Their Handicaps*

Pursell, Margaret Sanford. *A Look at Physical Handicaps*

Rosenberg, Maxine B. *My Friend Leslie: The Story of a Handicapped Child*

Splaver, Sarah. *Your Handicap— Don't Let It Handicap You*

Stein, Sara Bonnett. *About Handicaps: An Open Family Book for Parents and Children Together*

Hands

Aliki. *My Hands*

Berger, Gilda, and Melvin Berger. *The Whole World of Hands*

Castle, Sue. *Face Talk, Hand Talk, Body Talk*

Goode, Ruth. *Hands Up!*

Thayer, Jane. *Try Your Hand*

Healing

Bennett, Hal Zina. *The Doctor Within*

Burstein, John. *Slim Goodbody: What Can Go Wrong and How to Be Strong*

Kavaler, Lucy. *Cold Against Disease: The Wonders of Cold*

Kettelkamp, Larry. *The Healing Arts*

Nourse, Alan Edward. *Fractures, Dislocations and Sprains*

Health

Donahue, Parnell, and Helen Capellaro. *Germs Make Me Sick: A Health Handbook for Kids*

Jacobsen, Karen. *Health*

Lubowe, Irwin I., and Barbara Huss. *A Teen-Age Guide to Healthy Skin and Hair*

Perl, Lila. *Junk Food, Fast Food, Health Food: What America Eats and Why*

Plaut, Martin E. *The Doctor's Guide to You and Your Colon: A Candid, Helpful Guide to Our #1 Hidden Health Complaint*

Simon, Nissa. *Don't Worry, You're Normal: A Teenager's Guide to Self-Health*

Thypin, Marilyn, and Lynne Glasner. *Health Care for the Wongs: Health Insurance, Choosing a Doctor*

Hearing

See also Ears.

Adler, Irving, and Ruth Adler. *Your Ears*

Fryer, Judith. *How We Hear: The Story of Hearing*

Ward, Brian R. *The Ear and Hearing*

Hearing Aids

See also Deafness; Hearing impairment.

Althea. *Having a Hearing Test*

Arthur, Catherine. *My Sister's Silent World*

Collins-Ahlgren, Marianne. *Matthew's Accident*

Hyman, Jane. *Deafness*

Levine, Edna S. *Lisa and Her Soundless World*

Litchfield, Ada Bassett. *A Button in Her Ear*

Peter, Diana. *Claire and Emma*

Silverstein, Alvin, and Virginia B. Silverstein. *The Story of Your Ear*

Snell, Nigel. *Peter Gets a Hearing Aid*

Spence, Eleanor. *The Nothing Place*

Zelonky, Joy. *I Can't Always Hear You*

Hearing Ear Dog

See also Deafness.

Curtis, Patricia. *Cindy, a Hearing Ear Dog*

Hearing Impairment

See also Deafness; Hearing aids.

Althea. *Having a Hearing Test*

Fryer, Judith. *How We Hear: The Story of Hearing*

Glazzard, Margaret H. *Meet Camille and Danille, They're Special Persons: Hearing Impaired*

Kamien, Janet. *What If You Couldn't . . .? A Book About Special Needs*

Litchfield, Ada Bassett. *A Button in Her Ear*

Rosenberg, Maxine B. *My Friend Leslie: The Story of a Handicapped Child*

Spence, Eleanor. *The Nothing Place*

Wolf, Bernard. *Anna's Silent World*

Yolen, Jane. *The Mermaid's Three Wisdoms*
Zelonky, Joy. *I Can't Always Hear You*

Heart

See also Circulatory system.

Limburg, Peter. *The Story of Your Heart*
Showers, Paul. *Hear Your Heart*
Simon, Seymour. *About Your Heart*
Silverstein, Alvin, and Virginia B. Silverstein. *Heartbeats: Your Body, Your Heart*
Ward, Brian R. *The Heart and Blood*

Heart Disease

See also Cardiac catheterization; Electrocardiography (ECG); Surgery, heart.

Lee, Virginia. *The Magic Moth*
Limburg, Peter. *The Story of Your Heart*
Singer, Marilyn. *It Can't Hurt Forever*
Tully, Marianne, and Mary-Alice Tully. *Heart Disease*

Height

Beckman, Delores. *My Own Private Sky*
Greene, Constance C. *The Unmaking of Rabbit*
Hoff, Syd. *The Littlest Leaguer*
Iverson, Genie. *I Want to Be Big*
Lee, H. Alton. *Seven Feet Four and Growing*
Lee, Robert C. *It's a Mile from Here to Glory*

Low, Joseph. *Little Though I Be*
Meddaugh, Susan. *Too Short Fred*
Robinson, Jean. *The Strange but Wonderful Cosmic Awareness of Duffy Moon*
Ronayne, Eileen. *Memoirs of a Tall Girl*
Van Leeuwen, Jean. *I Was a 98-Pound Duckling*

Hemophilia

See also Braces, leg; Circulatory system.

Hyde, Margaret Oldroyd. *The New Genetics*
Massie, Robert, and Suzanne Massie. *Journey*
Morrison, Velma F. *There's Only One You: The Story of Heredity*
Siegel, Dorothy Schainman. *Winners: Eight Special Young People*

Heredity

See also Genetics.

Cole, Joanna, and Madeleine Edmondson. *Twins: The Story of Multiple Births*
Dunbar, Robert E. *Heredity*
Frankel, Edward. *DNA: The Ladder of Life*
Lipke, Jean Coryllel. *Heredity*
Morrison, Velma F. *There's Only One You: The Story of Heredity*

Hodgkin's Disease

See also Cancer.

Ipswitch, Elaine. *Scott Was Here*
Nixon, Joan Lowery. *The Specter*

Hook

Litchfield, Ada Bassett. *Captain Hook: That's Me*
Stein, Sara Bonnett. *About Handicaps: An Open Family Book for Parents and Children Together*
Wolf, Bernard. *Don't Feel Sorry for Paul*

Hormones

See also Endocrine system.

Nourse, Alan Edward. *Hormones*

Hospital School

Hawker, Frances, and Lee Withall. *With a Little Help from My Friends*

Hospitalization

Aboriginal Education Resource Unit. *Hughie's Hospital Adventure*
Althea. *Going into Hospital*
Anderson, Penny S. *The Operation*
Azarnoff, Pat, ed. *The Hospital*
Azarnoff, Pat, ed. *It's Your Body/ Es Tu Cuerpo*
Baznik, Donna. *Becky's Story*
Bell, David. *A Time to Be Born*
Blume, Judy Sussman. *Deenie*
Ciliotta, Claire, and Carole Livingston. *Why Am I Going to the Hospital? A Helpful Guide to a New Experience*
The Coleman Family and Bill Davidson. *Gary Coleman: Medical Miracle*
Cooper, Elizabeth. *Rosie's Hospital Story*

Crawford, Charles P. *Three-Legged Race*
Deegan, Paul. *A Hospital: Life in a Medical Center*
Elliott, Ingrid Glatz. *Hospital Roadmap: A Book to Help Explain the Hospital Experience to Young Children*
Eyerly, Jeannette. *Bonnie Jo, Go Home*
Eyerly, Jeannette. *The World of Ellen March*
Fox, Ray Errol. *Angela Ambrosia*
Freney, Rosemary, Lia Kapelis, and Peter Hicks. *Guess Where I've Been!*
Greenwald, Arthur, and Barry Head. *Going to the Hospital*
Hall, Lynn. *Sticks and Stones*
Hautzig, Deborah. *Second Star to the Right*
Hinton, S.E. *That Was Then, This Is Now*
Hogan, Paula, and Kirk Hogan. *The Hospital Scares Me*
Holmes, Burnham. *Early Morning Rounds: A Portrait of a Hospital*
Howe, James. *A Night Without Stars*
Howe, James. *The Hospital Book*
Jones, Rebecca C. *Angie and Me*
Lee, Robert C. *It's a Mile from Here to Glory*
Lipson, Tony, and the staff of the Royal Alexandra Hospital for Children. *Benjamin Goes to Hospital: An Introduction to Hospital for Children and Parents*
McLaren, Annabel, ed. *Going to Hospital*
Moe, Barbara. *Pickles and Prunes*
Nixon, Joan Lowery. *The Specter*
Phelan, Terry Wolfe. *The S.S. Valentine*
Poole, Victoria. *Thursday's Child*

Richter, Elizabeth. *The Teenage Hospital Experience: You Can Handle It!*

Roberts, Willo. *Don't Hurt Laurie!*

Rosenberg, Mark L. *Patients: The Experience of Illness*

Sachs, Elizabeth-Ann. *Just Like Always*

Singer, Marilyn. *It Can't Hurt Forever*

Slepian, Jan. *Lester's Turn*

Stein, Sara Bonnett. *A Hospital Story: An Open Family Book for Parents and Children Together*

Strasser, Todd. *Friends Till the End*

Ward, Brian R. *Hospital*

Weber, Alfons. *Elizabeth Gets Well*

Ziegler, Sandra. *At the Hospital: A Surprise for Krissy*

Hypnosis

Kettelkamp, Larry. *Hypnosis: The Wakeful Sleep*

Illness

See also Cold, common; Psychosomatic illness; Upper respiratory infection.

Burstein, John. *Slim Goodbody: What Can Go Wrong and How to Be Strong*

Hann, Jacquie. *Up Day, Down Day*

Hirsch, Linda. *The Sick Story*

Jessel, Camilla. *Going to the Doctor*

Knight, David C. *Your Body's Defenses*

Little, Jean. *Mine for Keeps*

MacLachlan, Patricia. *The Sick Day*

Numeroff, Laura Joffe. *Phoebe Dexter Has Harriet Peterson's Sniffles*

Payne, Sherry Newirth. *A Contest*

Rockwell, Anne, and Harlow Rockwell. *Sick in Bed*

Rosenberg, Mark L. *Patients: The Experience of Illness*

Segal, Lore. *Tell Me a Mitzi*

Snyder, Anne. *My Name Is Davy, I'm an Alcoholic*

Stine, Jovial Bob, and Jane Stine. *The Sick of Being Sick Book*

Tobias, Tobi. *A Day Off*

Illness — Animal

Brandenberg, Franz. *I Wish I Was Sick, Too!*

Roberts, Sarah. *Nobody Cares About Me!*

Immune System

See also Acquired immune deficiency syndrome (AIDS); Vaccination.

Arehart-Treichel, Joan. *Immunity: How Our Bodies Resist Disease*

Glasser, Ronald J. *The Body Is the Hero*

Haines, Gail Kay. *Cancer*

Knight, David C. *Your Body's Defenses*

Nourse, Alan Edward. *Your Immune System*

Ward, Brian R. *Body Maintenance*

Infection

See also Upper respiratory infection (URI).

Donahue, Parnell, and Helen Capellaro. *Germs Make Me Sick: A Health Handbook for Kids*

Injection

See also Hospitalization; Immune system; Intravenous pyelogram; Intravenous therapy; Surgery.

Dunn, Graeme. *Benjamin Goes to the Dentist: An Introduction to the Dentist for Children and Parents*
Rockwell, Anne, and Harlow Rockwell. *Sick in Bed.*

Injury

See also Accident; Brain injury; Emergency.

Bates, Betty. *Picking Up the Pieces*
Burch, Robert. *D.J.'s Worst Enemy*
Cooper, Elizabeth. *Rosie's Hospital Story*
Gelman, Rita Golden, and Susan Kovacs Buxbaum. *Ouch! All About Cuts and Other Hurts*
Hinton, S.E. *That Was Then, This Is Now*
Hogan, Paula, and Kirk Hogan. *The Hospital Scares Me*
Jordan, Hope D. *Haunted Summer*
Lee, Robert C. *It's a Mile from Here to Glory*
Lifton, Betty Jean, and Thomas C. Fox. *Children of Vietnam*
Nourse, Alan Edward. *Fractures, Dislocations and Sprains*
Place, Marian T., and Charles G. Preston. *Juan's Eighteen-Wheeler Summer*
Whitney, Alma Marshak. *Just Awful*
Wolff, Angelika. *Mom! I Broke My Arm*

Intelligence

Allington, Richard L., and Kathleen Krull. *Thinking*
Berger, Melvin. *Bionics*
Berger, Melvin. *Exploring the Mind and Brain*
Cohen, Daniel. *Intelligence: What Is It?*
Haines, Gail Kay. *Brain Power: Understanding Human Intelligence*
Haynes, Henry Louis. *Squarehead and Me*
Low, Joseph. *Little Though I Be*
Showers, Paul. *Use Your Brain*

Intensive Care

See also Surgery.

Bell, David. *A Time to Be Born*

Intravenous Pyelogram (IVP)

See also X ray.

Frevert, Patricia Dendtler. *It's Okay to Look at Jamie*
Waidley, Ericka. *All About Your X-Ray: IVP*

Intravenous Therapy (IV)

See also Hospitalization; Surgery

Althea. *Going into Hospital*
Weber, Alfons. *Elizabeth Gets Well*

Kidney Disease

See also Surgery, transplant.

Burton, Adrianne. *Your New Kidney*

The Coleman Family and Bill
Davidson. *Gary Coleman:
Medical Miracle*
Kleiman, Gary, and Sandford
Dody. *No Time to Lose*

Kleptomania

See also Emotionally ill.

Carlson, Dale Bick. *Call Me
Amanda*

Laboratory Test

See also Hospitalization.

Berger, Melvin. *Medical Center
Lab*
Cobb, Vicki. *How the Doctor
Knows You're Fine*
Klein, Aaron E. *Medical Tests
and You*
Reynolds, Moira Davison. *Aim
for a Job in a Medical Lab*

Laser Therapy

Kettelkamp, Larry. *Lasers: The
Miracle Light*
Penny, Peggy L. *Surgery: From
Stone Scalpel to Laser Beam*

"Lazy eye"

See Amblyopia.

Learning Disability

See also Communication disability; Dyslexia.

Albert, Louise. *But I'm Ready to
Go*
Berger, Melvin. *Exploring the
Mind and Brain*

Cleary, Beverly. *Mitch and Amy*
Corcoran, Barbara. *Axe-Time,
Sword-Time*
Gilson, Jamie. *Do Bananas Chew
Gum!*
Glazzard, Margaret H. *Meet Scott,
He's a Special Person: Learning Disabled*
Gold, Phyllis. *Please Don't Say
Hello*
Lasker, Joe. *He's My Brother*
Roy, Ron. *Frankie Is Staying
Back*
Smith, Doris Buchanan. *Kelly's
Creek*
Stanek, Muriel. *Left Right, Left
Right*

Left-handed

Berger, Gilda, and Melvin Berger.
The Whole World of Hands
Goode, Ruth. *Hands Up!*
Lerner, Marguerite Rush. *Lefty:
The Story of Left-Handedness*
Haislet, Barbara. *Why Are Some
People Left-Handed!*
Lindsay, Rae. *The Left-Handed
Book*

Leg Disability

Cooper, Elizabeth. *Rosie's
Hospital Story*
Dyer, Thomas A. *A Way of His
Own*
Rudolph, Wilma, as told to Bud
Greenspan. *Wilma: The Story
of Wilma Rudolph*

Legionnaire's Disease

Berger, Melvin. *Disease
Detectives*

Legs

Kessler, Ethel, and Leonard
Kessler. *Two, Four, Six,
Eight: A Book About Legs*

Leukemia

See also Cancer; Chemotherapy;
Hair loss; Radiation therapy.

Baker, Lynn S., in collaboration
with Charles G. Roland and
Gerald S. Gilchrist. *You and
Leukemia: A Day at a Time*
Beckman, Gunnel. *Admission to
the Feast*
Center for Attitudinal Healing.
*There Is a Rainbow Behind
Every Dark Cloud*
Coerr, Eleanor B. *Sadako and the
Thousand Paper Cranes*
Fox, Ray Errol. *Angela Ambrosia*
Frevert, Patricia Dendtler. *Patty
Gets Well*
Hughes, Monica. *Hunter in the
Dark*
Kidd, Ronald. *That's What
Friends Are For*
Lowry, Lois. *A Summer to Die*
Lund, Doris Herold. *Eric*
Moe, Barbara. *Pickles and Prunes*
Siegel, Dorothy Schainman.
*Winners: Eight Special Young
People*
Slote, Alfred. *Hang Tough, Paul
Mather*
Strasser, Todd. *Friends Till the
End*

Leukocytoclastic Angiitis

Madsen, Jane M., with Diane
Bockoras. *Please Don't Tease
Me*

Loss

See also Hair loss.

Bernstein, Joanne E. *Loss and
How to Cope with It*
Corey, Dorothy. *You Go Away*
Pomerantz, Charlotte. *The Mango
Tooth*
Rice, Eve. *Ebbie*
Showers, Paul. *How Many Teeth?*
Snell, Nigel. *Lucy Loses Her
Tonsils*
Warwick, Dolores. *Learn to Say
Goodbye*

Lou Gehrig's Disease

See Amyotrophic lateral sclerosis.

Love

Althea. *A Baby in the Family*
Ayrault, Evelyn West. *Sex, Love,
and the Physically Handi-
capped*
Bates, Betty. *Love Is Like Peanuts*
Burgess-Kohn, Jane. *Straight Talk
About Love and Sex for
Teenagers*
Carlson, Dale Bick. *Loving Sex
for Both Sexes: Straight Talk
for Teenagers*
Garden, Nancy. *Annie on My
Mind*
Gruenberg, Sidonie M. *The
Wonderful Story of How You
Were Born*
Hamilton, Eleanor. *Sex, with
Love: A Guide for Young
People*
Hanckel, Frances, and John Cun-
ningham. *A Way of Love, A
Way of Life: A Young*

Person's Introduction to
What It Means to Be Gay
Hunt, Morton. *The Young
Person's Guide to Love*
Johnson, Corinne Benson, and
Eric W. Johnson. *Love and
Sex and Growing Up*
Johnson, Eric W. *Love and Sex in
Plain Language*
Kaplan, Helen Singer. *Making
Sense of Sex: The New Facts
About Sex and Love for
Young People*
Langone, John. *Like, Love, Lust:
A View of Sex and Sexuality*
Powers, Bill. *A Test of Love*
Richter, Betts. *Something Special
Within*
Scoppettone, Sandra. *Happy
Endings Are All Alike*
Shreve, Susan Richards.
Loveletters
Spock, Benjamin McLane. *A
Teenager's Guide to Life and
Love*
Wolff, Ruth. *A Crack in the
Sidewalk*

Measles

See also Immune system.

Showers, Paul. *No Measles, No
Mumps for Me*

Medical Play

Althea. *Going to the Doctor*
Azarnoff, Pat, ed. *The Hospital*
Breinburg, Petronella. *Doctor
Shawn*
Chang Mao-chiu. *The Little
Doctor*
Dunn, Graeme. *Benjamin Goes to
the Dentist: An Introduction*
to the Dentist for Children
and Parents
Freney, Rosemary, Lia Kapelis,
and Peter Hicks. *Guess
Where I've Been!*
Greenwald, Arthur, and Barry
Head. *Having an Operation*
Packard, Mary. *A Visit to the
Dentist*
Robison, Deborah, and Carla
Perez. *Your Turn, Doctor*

Medical Transport

See also Emergency.

Aboriginal Education Resource
Unit. *Hughie's Hospital
Adventure*
Beame, Rona. *Emergency!*
Steedman, Julie. *Emergency
Room: An ABC Tour*

Medication

See also Chemotherapy; Doctor's
office; Hospitalization; Illness.

Calhoun, Mary. *Medicine Show:
Conning People and Making
Them Like It*
The Coleman Family and Bill
Davidson. *Gary Coleman:
Medical Miracle*
Corcoran, Barbara. *Child of the
Morning*
Eisenberg, Michael. *Ulcers*
Epstein, Sherrie S. *Penny, the
Medicine Maker: The Story of
Penicillin*
Girion, Barbara. *A Handful of
Stars*
Greenwald, Arthur, and Barry
Head. *Having an Operation*
Haines, Gail Kay. *Cancer*
Hawker, Frances, and Lee Withall.

With a Little Help from My
Friends
Jessel, Camilla. *Going to the
Doctor*
Larsen, Hanne. *Don't Forget Tom*
McLaren, Annabel, ed. *Going to
Hospital*
Riedman, Sarah Regal. *Diabetes*
Snell, Nigel. *Lucy Loses Her
Tonsils*

Meditation

Lesh, Terry. *Meditation for Young
People*
Rozman, Deborah A. *Meditation
for Children*

Menstruation

See also Reproductive system.

Elgin, Kathleen, and John F.
Osterritter. *Twenty-Eight
Days*
Gardner-Loulan, JoAnn, Bonnie
Lopez, and Marcia Quacken-
bush. *Period*
Lipke, Jean Coryllel. *Puberty and
Adolescence*
Maddux, Hilary C. *Menstruation*
Nourse, Alan Edward.
Menstruation: Just Plain Talk
Voelckers, Ellen. *Girl's Guide to
Menstruation*

Mental Illness

See Emotional illness.

Metabolism

See also Endocrine system;
Weight control.

Balestrino, Philip. *Fat and Skinny*

Minimal Brain
Dysfunction (MBD)

See also Brain injury; Learning
disability.

Gardner, Richard A. *MBD: The
Family Book About Minimal
Brain Dysfunction*
Langone, John. *Goodby to
Bedlam. Understanding Men-
tal Illness and Retardation*

Mononucleosis

Nourse, Alan Edward. *Viruses*
Storr, Catherine. *Thursday*

Mouth

Silverstein, Alvin, and Virginia B.
Silverstein. *The Story of Your
Mouth*

Multiple Handicap

Berger, Gilda. *Physical
Disabilities*
Bowe, Frank. *Comeback: Six
Remarkable People Who
Triumphed over Disability*
Butler, Dorothy. *Cushla and Her
Books*
Glazzard, Margaret H. *Meet
Danny, He's a Special Person:
Multiply Handicapped*
Madsen, Jane M., with Diane
Bockoras. *Please Don't Tease
Me*
Rosenberg, Maxine B. *My Friend
Leslie: The Story of a Handi-
capped Child*

Multiple Sclerosis

Tully, Marianne, and Mary-Alice
Tully. *Dread Diseases*

Mumps

See also Immune system.

Showers, Paul. *No Measles, No Mumps for Me*

Muscular Dystrophy

Franks, Hugh. *Will to Live*
Morrison, Velma F. *There's Only One You: The Story of Heredity*

Muscular System

See also Exercise; Physical fitness.

Cosgrove, Margaret. *Your Muscles —And Ways to Exercise Them*
Showers, Paul. *You Can't Make a Move Without Your Muscles*

Mute

See also Communication disability.

Callen, Larry. *Sorrow's Song*
Cunningham, Julia. *Far in the Day*
Cunningham, Julia. *The Silent Voice*
Heide, Florence Parry. *Secret Dreamer, Secret Dreams*
Rounds, Glen. *Blind Outlaw*
Whelan, Gloria. *A Time to Keep Silent*

Nervous System

Berger, Melvin. *Why I Cough, Sneeze, Shiver, Hiccup, and Yawn*
Kalina, Sigmund. *Your Nerves and Their Messages*

Stevens, Leonard A. *Neurons: Building Blocks of the Brain*
Touré, Halima. *Pain*
Weart, Edith Lucie. *The Story of Your Brain and Nerves*

Nose

Showers, Paul. *Follow Your Nose*

Nurse, emergency room

See also Emergency.

Witty, Margot. *A Day in the Life of an Emergency Room Nurse*

Nurse, hospital

See also Hospitalization.

Anderson, Peggy. *Nurse*
Greene, Carla. *Doctors and Nurses: What Do They Do?*
Searight, Mary. *Your Career in Nursing*
Wandro, Mark, and Joani Blank. *My Daddy is a Nurse*

Nurse, school

See also Child abuse/neglect; Injury.

Stanek, Muriel. *Don't Hurt Me, Mama*
Whitney, Alma Marshak. *Just Awful*

Nutrition

See also Digestion; Vitamins; Weight control.

Althea. *Going to the Doctor*
Arehart-Treichel, Joan. *Trace*

Elements: How They Help and Harm Us
Balestrino, Philip. *Fat and Skinny*
Barrett, Judith. *Cloudy with a Chance of Meatballs*
Bennett, Hal Zina. *The Doctor Within*
Benziger, Barbara. *Controlling Your Weight*
Bolian, Polly. *Growing Up Slim*
Burns, Marilyn. *Good for Me: All About Food in 32 Bites*
Dengler, Marianna. *A Pebble in Newcomb's Pond*
Doss, Helen Grigsby, and Richard L. Wells. *All the Better to Bite With*
Edelstein, Barbara. *The Woman Doctor's Diet for Teen-Age Girls*
Fleege, Francis. *How to Eat: Chewing, Tooth Care, and Diet*
Fodor, R.V. *What to Eat and Why: The Science of Nutrition*
Franz, Barbara, and William Franz. *Nutritional Survival Manual for the Eighties: A Young People's Guide to "Dietary Goals for the United States."*
Fretz, Sada. *Going Vegetarian: A Guide for Teen-agers*
Gay, Kathlyn, Martin Gay, and Marla Gay. *Get Hooked on Vegetables*
Gilbert, Sara D. *Fat Free: Common Sense for Young Weight Worriers*
Goodbody, Slim. *The Healthy Habits Handbook*
Gruenberg, Sidonie M. *The Wonderful Story of How You Were Born*
Jacobsen, Karen. *Health*

Jones, Hettie. *How to Eat Your ABC's: A Book About Vitamins*
Maddux, Hilary C. *Menstruation*
Marr, John S. *The Food You Eat*
Neff, Fred. *Keeping Fit: A Handbook for Physical Conditioning and Better Health*
Null, Gary, and Steve Null. *Why Your Stomach Hurts: A Handbook of Digestion and Nutrition*
Odor, Ruth S. *What's a Body to Do?*
Peavy, Linda, and Ursula Smith. *Food, Nutrition and You.*
Perl, Lila. *Junk Food, Fast Food, Health Food: What America Eats and Why*
Riedman, Sarah Regal. *Diabetes*
Riedman, Sarah Regal. *Food for People*
Thompson, Paul. *Nutrition*

Occupational Therapy

Shuff, Frances. *Your Future in Occupational Therapy*
Trull, Patti. *On with My Life*

Orthodontics

See also Braces, teeth; Dentist's office.

Betancourt, Jeanne. *Smile! How to Cope with Braces*
Nourse, Alan Edward. *The Tooth Book*
Silverstein, Alvin, and Virginia B. Silverstein. *So You're Getting Braces: A Guide to Orthodontics*

Ostomy

See Surgery, ostomy.

Overweight

See Weight control.

Oxygen

See also Respiratory system.

Branley, Franklyn M. *Oxygen Keeps You Alive*

Pain

See also Nervous system; Senses.

Adler, Irving, and Ruth Adler. *Taste, Touch and Smell*
Gelman, Rita Golden, and Susan Kovacs Buxbaum. *Ouch! All About Cuts and Other Hurts*
Harmin, Merrill. *Better Than Aspirin: How to Get Rid of Emotions That Give You a Pain in the Neck*
Jones, Rebecca C. *Angie and Me*
Kavaler, Lucy. *Cold Against Disease: The Wonders of Cold*
Lance, James W. *Headache: Understanding, Alleviation*
Marino, Barbara Pavis. *Eric Needs Stitches*
Mylander, Maureen. *The Great American Stomach Book: How Your Digestion Works and What to Do When It Doesn't*
Null, Gary, and Steve Null. *Why Your Stomach Hurts: A Handbook of Digestion and Nutrition*

Singer, Marilyn. *It Can't Hurt Forever*
Slote, Alfred. *Hang Tough, Paul Mather*
Touré, Halima. *Pain*

Paralysis

See also Bliss symbols; Nervous system; Wheelchair.

Bowe, Frank. *Comeback: Six Remarkable People Who Triumphed over Disability*
Bradbury, Bianca. *The Girl Who Wanted Out*
Brancato, Robin. *Winning*
Colman, Hila Crayder. *Accident*
Henriod, Lorraine. *Special Olympics and Paralympics*
Kingman, Lee. *Head over Wheels*
Lasker, Joe. *Nick Joins In*
Phipson, Joan. *A Tide Flowing*
Redpath, Ann. *Jim Boen: A Man of Opposites*
Rodowsky, Colby F. *P.S. Write Soon*
Savitz, Harriet May. *Run, Don't Walk*
Savitz, Harriet May. *Wheelchair Champions: A History of Wheelchair Sports*
Valens, E. G. *A Long Way Up: The Story of Jill Kinmont*

Paramedic

See also Emergency.

Keyes, Fenton. *Your Future in a Paramedic Career*
Steedman, Julie. *Emergency Room: An ABC Tour*
Wolfe, Bob, and Diane Wolfe. *Emergency Room*

Parapsychology

Akins, W. R. *ESP: Your Psychic Powers and How to Test Them*
Aylesworth, Thomas G. *ESP*
Cohen, Daniel. *ESP: The Search Beyond the Senses*
Hall, Elizabeth. *Possible Impossibilities: A Look at Parapsychology*
Kettelkamp, Larry. *Sixth Sense*

Pediatrician

See also Hospitalization; Physician.

Bell, David. *A Time to Be Born*
Lee, Mary Price. *A Future in Pediatrics: Medical and Non-Medical Careers in Child Health Care*

Perception

See also Brain.

Allington, Richard L., and Kathleen Cowles. *Looking*
Brown, Marcia. *Walk with Your Eyes*
Burns, Marilyn. *The Book of Think: Or How to Solve a Problem Twice Your Size*
Cobb, Vicki. *How to Really Fool Yourself: Illusions for All Your Senses*
Stanek, Muriel. *Left Right, Left Right*
Weiss, Malcolm E. *Seeing through the Dark: Blind and Sighted—A Vision Shared*

Phenylketonuria (PKU)

See also Nutrition.

Hyde, Margaret Oldroyd. *The New Genetics*

Physical Examination

See Doctor's Office; Doctor's office —animal; Hospitalization; Illness.

Physical Fitness

See also Disabled in sports; Exercise; Sports medicine.

Antonacci, Robert J., and Jene Barr. *Physical Fitness for Young Champions*
Neff, Fred. *Keeping Fit: A Handbook for Physical Conditioning and Better Health*
Schneider, Tom. *Everybody's a Winner: A Kid's Guide to New Sports and Fitness*

Physical Therapist

See also Hospitalization.

Lee, Robert C. *It's a Mile from Here to Glory*

Physician

See also Doctor's office; Doctor's office—animal; Hospitalization; Pediatrician.

Anckarsvärd, Karin. *Doctor's Boy*
Bluestone, Naomi. *"So You Want to Be a Doctor?": The Realities of Pursuing Medicine as a Career*
Freese, Arthur S. *The Bionic People Are Here*
Girion, Barbara. *A Handful of Stars*
Greene, Carla. *Doctors and Nurses: What Do They Do?*

Hayden, Robert C., and Jacqueline Harris. *Nine Black American Doctors*

Sobol, Harriet Langsam. *The Interns*

Thypin, Marilyn, and Lynne Glasner. *Health Care for the Wongs: Health Insurance, Choosing a Doctor*

Poisoning

See also Emergency.

Haines, Gail Kay. *Natural and Synthetic Poisons*

Tichy, William. *Poisons, Antidotes and Anecdotes*

Pregnancy

See also Adolescent, single pregnant; Reproductive system.

Banish, Roslyn. *I Want to Tell You About My Baby*

Dragonwagon, Crescent. *Wind Rose*

Gruenberg, Sidonie M. *The Wonderful Story of How You Were Born*

McCoy, Kathy. *The Teenage Body Book Guide to Sexuality*

Pursell, Margaret Sanford. *A Look at Birth*

Showers, Paul, and Kay Sperry Showers. *Before You Were a Baby*

Psychiatrist

Blume, Judy Sussman. *Then Again, Maybe I Won't*

Colman, Hila Crayder. *Diary of a Frantic Kid Sister*

Dengler, Marianna. *A Pebble in Newcomb's Pond*

Hermes, Patricia. *Nobody's Fault!*

Kelley, Sally. *Trouble with Explosives*

Platt, Kin. *The Boy Who Could Make Himself Disappear*

Psychologist

Cavallaro, Ann. *Blimp*

Pfeffer, Susan Beth. *What Do You Do When Your Mouth Won't Open!*

Psychology

Carlson, Dale Bick. *Where's Your Head! Psychology for Teenagers*

Hall, Elizabeth. *From Pigeons to People: A Look at Behavior Shaping*

Weinstein, Grace W. *People Study People: The Story of Psychology*

Psychosomatic Illness

See also Illness.

Blume, Judy Sussman. *Then Again, Maybe I Won't*

Colman, Hila Crayder. *Diary of a Frantic Kid Sister*

Danziger, Paula. *The Pistachio Prescription*

Harmin, Merrill. *Better Than Aspirin: How to Get Rid of Emotions That Give You a Pain in the Neck*

Laiken, Deidre S., and Alan J. Schneider. *Listen to Me, I'm Angry*

Langone, John. *Goodby to Bedlam: Understanding Mental Illness and Retardation*

Stiller, Richard. *Your Body Is*

*Trying to Tell You
Something: How to Under-
stand Its Signals and Re-
spond to Its Needs*
Touré, Halima. *Pain*

Psychotherapy

Anderson, Mary Quirk. *Step on a
Crack*
Carlson, Dale Bick. *Where's Your
Head? Psychology for
Teenagers*
Gilbert, Sara D. *What Happens in
Therapy?*
Green, Hannah. *I Never Promised
You a Rose Garden*
Greenberg, Harvey R. *Hanging In:
What You Should Know
About Psychotherapy*
Marks, Jane. *Help: A Guide to
Counseling and Therapy
Without a Hassle*
Neufield, John. *Lisa, Bright and
Dark*

Radiation Therapy

See also Cancer; Hair loss; Leukemia; X ray.

Baker, Lynn S., in collaboration
with Charles G. Roland and
Gerald Gilchrist. *You and
Leukemia: A Day at a Time*
Haines, Gail Kay. *Cancer*
Halacy, Daniel S., Jr. *X-Rays and
Gamma Rays*
Pringle, Laurence. *Radiation:
Waves and Particles, Benefits
and Risks*
Warmbier, Jenene, and Ellen
Vassy. *Hospital Days, Treat-
ment Ways*

Rape

See also Emergency; Sexual abuse/
Molestation; Sexual assault.

Bode, Janet. *Rape: Preventing
It, Dealing with the Legal,
Medical, and Emotional
Aftermath*
Booher, Dianna D. *Rape: What
Would You Do If . . . ?*
Dizenzo, Patricia. *Why Me? The
Story of Jenny*
Horos, Carol V. *Rape*
Peck, Richard. *Are You in the
House Alone?*
Scoppettone, Sandra. *Happy
Endings Are All Alike*
Shreve, Susan Richards. *Love-
letters*

Recreation Therapist

Brady, Mari. *Please Remember
Me: A Young Woman's Story
of Her Friendship with an
Unforgettable Fifteen-Year-
Old Boy*
Howe, James. *The Hospital Book*
Singer, Marilyn. *It Can't Hurt
Forever*

Reproductive System

See also Adolescent, single pregnant; Birth; Conception; Pregnancy; Sexuality.

Althea. *A Baby in the Family*
Banish, Roslyn. *I Want to Tell
You About My Baby*
Dragonwagon, Crescent. *Wind
Rose*
Fagerstrom, Grethe, and Gunilla
Hansson. *Our New Baby: A
Picture Story for Parents and
Children*

Gruenberg, Sidonie M. *The Wonderful Story of How You Were Born*

Johnson, Corinne Benson, and Eric W. Johnson. *Love and Sex and Growing Up*

Lerner, Marguerite Rush. *Twins: The Story of Twins*

Lipke, Jean Coryllel. *Conception and Contraception*

Loebl, Suzanne. *Conception, Contraception: A New Look*

Showers, Paul, and Kay Sperry Showers. *Before You Were a Baby*

Snyder, Gerald S. *Test-Tube Life: Scientific Advance and Moral Dilemma*

Voelckers, Ellen. *Girls' Guide to Menstruation*

Ward, Brian R. *Birth and Growth*

Respiratory System

See also Oxygen.

Marr, John S. *A Breath of Air and a Breath of Smoke*

Silverstein, Alvin, and Virginia B. Silverstein. *The Respiratory System: How Living Creatures Breathe*

Ward, Brian R. *The Lungs and Breathing*

Weart, Edith Lucie. *The Story of Your Respiratory System*

Retardation

Albert, Louise. *But I'm Ready to Go*

Anders, Rebecca. *A Look at Mental Retardation*

Antonacci, Robert J., and Jene Barr. *Physical Fitness for Young Champions*

Baldwin, Anne Norris. *A Little Time*

Bowe, Frank. *Comeback: Six Remarkable People Who Triumphed over Disability*

Branscum, Robbie. *For Love of Jody*

Brightman, Alan. *Like Me*

Brown, Roy. *Find Debbie!*

Byars, Betsy. *The Summer of the Swans*

Canada, Lena. *To Elvis, with Love*

Cleaver, Vera, and Bill Cleaver. *Me Too*

Clifton, Lucille. *My Friend Jacob*

Crane, Caroline. *A Girl Like Tracy*

Dunbar, Robert E. *Mental Retardation*

Fassler, Joan. *One Little Girl*

Garrigue, Sheila. *Between Friends*

Glazzard, Margaret H. *Meet Lance, He's a Special Person: Trainable Mentally Retarded*

Hanlon, Emily. *It's Too Late for Sorry*

Henriod, Lorraine. *Special Olympics and Paralympics*

Hirsch, Karen. *My Sister*

Hull, Eleanor. *Alice with Golden Hair*

Hunter, Edith Fisher. *Sue Ellen*

Klein, Gerda Weissmann. *The Blue Rose*

Langone, John. *Goodbye to Bedlam: Understanding Mental Illness and Retardation*

Larsen, Hanne. *Don't Forget Tom*

Little, Jean. *Take Wing*

Mazer, Harry. *The War on Villa Street*

Melton, David. *A Boy Called Hopeless*

Meyers, Robert. *Like Normal People*

Ominsky, Elaine. *Jon O.: A Special Boy*
Shyer, Marlene F. *Welcome Home, Jellybean*
Slepian, Jan. *The Alfred Summer*
Slepian, Jan. *Lester's Turn*
Smith, Lucia B. *A Special Kind of Sister*
Sobol, Harriet Langsam. *My Brother Steven Is Retarded*
Stefanik, Alfred T. *Copycat Sam: Developing Ties with a Special Child*
Thrasher, Crystal. *The Dark Didn't Catch Me*
Wartski, Maureen Crane. *My Brother Is Special*
Whitney, Phyllis. *Nobody Likes Trina*
Wright, Betty Ren. *My Sister Is Different*
Young, John Sacret. *Special Olympics*
Wolff, Ruth. *A Crack in the Sidewalk*

Rights

Agostinelli, Maria E. *On Wings of Love: The United Nations' Declaration of the Rights of the Child*
Archer, Jules. *Who's Running Your Life? A Look at Young People's Rights*
Dunbar, Robert E. *Mental Retardation*
Englebardt, Leland S. *You Have a Right: A Guide for Minors*
Haskins, James, and J. M. Stifle. *The Quiet Revolution: The Struggle for the Rights of Disabled Americans*
Simon, Nissa. *Don't Worry, You're Normal: A Teenager's*

Guide to Self-Health
Snyder, Gerald S. *Human Rights*
Sussman, Alan. *The Rights of Young People: The Basic ACLU Guide to a Young Person's Rights*

Schizophrenia

See also Emotional illness.

Dengler, Marianna. *A Pebble in Newcomb's Pond*
Langone, John. *Goodby to Bedlam: Understanding Mental Illness and Retardation*
Platt, Kin. *The Boy Who Could Make Himself Disappear*
Rothenberg, Mira. *Children with Emerald Eyes: Histories of Extraordinary Boys and Girls*

School, disabled in

See Disabled in school; Special education.

School Nurse

See Nurse, school.

Scientist

See also Laboratory test; Physician.

Archer, Jules. *Epidemic! The Story of the Disease Detectives*
Berger, Melvin. *Disease Detectives*
Berger, Melvin. *Medical Center Lab*
Facklam, Margery, and Howard Facklam. *The Brain: Magnificent Mind Machine*
Freese, Arthur S. *The Bionic*

People Are Here

Hayden, Robert C. *Seven Black American Scientists*

Reid, Robert. *Marie Curie*

Reynolds, Moira Davison. *Aim for a Job in a Medical Laboratory*

Scoliosis

Blume, Judy Sussman. *Deenie*

Sachs, Elizabeth-Ann. *Just Like Always*

Seeing Eye Dog

See also Guide Dog.

Holmes, Burnham. *The First Seeing Eye Dog*

Wolf, Bernard. *Connie's New Eyes*

Self-care

Bennett, Hal Zina. *The Doctor Within*

Boston Women's Health Book Collective. *Our Bodies, Ourselves: A Book by and for Women*

Cobb, Vicki. *How the Doctor Knows You're Fine*

Covelli, Pat. *Borrowing Time: Growing Up with Juvenile Diabetes*

Donahue, Parnell. *Sports Doc: Medical Advice, Diet, Fitness, Tips, and Other Essential Hints for Young Athletes*

Duncan, Theodore G. *The Diabetes Fact Book*

Gibbons, Thomas B. *How Doctors Diagnose You and How You Can Help*

Gilbert, Sara D. *Feeling Good: A Book About You and Your Body*

Goodbody, Slim. *The Force Inside You*

Goodbody, Slim. *The Healthy Habits Handbook*

Larsen, Hanne. *Don't Forget Tom*

Lipke, Jean Coryllel. *Puberty and Adolescence*

Nourse, Alan Edward. *Clear Skin, Healthy Skin*

Olshan, Neal H., and Julie Dreyer Wang. *Fears and Phobias: Fighting Back*

Plaut, Martin E. *The Doctor's Guide to You and Your Colon: A Candid, Helpful Guide to Our #1 Hidden Health Complaint*

Simon, Nissa. *Don't Worry, You're Normal: A Teenager's Guide to Self-Health*

Self-esteem

Ayrault, Evelyn West. *Sex, Love, and the Physically Handicapped*

Bauer, Marion Dane. *Tangled Butterfly*

Blue, Rose. *Me and Einstein: Breaking Through the Barrier*

Bottner, Barbara. *Dumb Old Casey Is a Fat Tree*

Cohen, Barbara. *Fat Jack*

Fassler, Joan. *One Little Girl*

Greene, Laura. *I Am Somebody*

Hazen, Barbara Shook. *To Be Me*

Kalb, Jonah, and David Viscott. *What Every Kid Should Know*

Kottler, Dorothy, and Eleanor Willis. *I Really Like Myself*

Lee, H. Alton. *Seven Feet Four and Growing*
Lee, Mildred Scudder. *The Skating Rink*
London, Kathy, and Frank Caparulo. *Who Am I? Who Are You?: Coping with Friends, Feelings, and Other Teenage Dilemmas*
McKillip, Patricia. *The Night Gift*
Mazer, Harry. *The War on Villa Street*
Mihaly, Mary E. *Getting Your Own Way: A Guide to Growing Up Assertively*
Moncure, Jane Belk. *About Me*
Orgel, Doris. *Next Door to Xanadu*
Richter, Betts. *Something Special Within*
Riskind, Mary. *Apple Is My Sign*
Robinson, Jean. *The Strange but Wonderful Cosmic Awareness of Duffy Moon*
Simon, Norma. *Why Am I Different?*
Sullivan, Mary Beth, Alan J. Brightman, and Joseph Blatt. *Feeling Free*
Thomas, William E. *The New Boy Is Blind*

Senses

Adler, Irving, and Ruth Adler. *Taste, Touch and Smell*
Aliki. *My Five Senses*
Allington, Richard L., and Kathleen Cowles. *Looking*
Allington, Richard L., and Kathleen Cowles. *Tasting*
Allington, Richard L., and Kathleen Cowles. *Touching*
Cobb, Vicki. *How to Really Fool Yourself: Illusions for All Your Senses*

Kettelkamp, Larry. *Sixth Sense*
Samson, Joan. *Watching the New Baby*
Showers, Paul. *Follow Your Nose*
Smith, Elwood H. *The See and Hear and Smell and Touch Book*
Ward, Brian R. *Touch, Taste and Smell*
Weiss, Malcolm E. *Seeing Through the Dark: Blind and Sighted—A Vision Shared*
White, Anne Terry, and Gerald S. Lietz. *Windows on the World*

Separation

Corey, Dorothy. *You Go Away*
Lisker, Sonia O. *Lost*

Sexual Abuse/Molestation

See also Child abuse/Neglect.

Dayee, Frances S. *Private Zone: A Book Teaching Children Sexual Assault Prevention Tools*
Dodson, Susan. *The Creep*
Dolan, Edward F., Jr. *Child Abuse*
Dunnahoo, Terry. *Who Cares About Espie Sanchez?*
Haskins, James, with Pat Connolly. *The Child Abuse Help Book*
Ruby, Lois. *What Do You Do in Quicksand?*
Winthrop, Elizabeth. *A Little Demonstration of Affection*

Sex Roles

See also Sexuality.

de Paola, Tomie. *Oliver Button Is a Sissy*

Greenwald, Sheila. *The Secret in Miranda's Closet*

Hall, Lynn. *Sticks and Stones*

Parkinson, Ethelyn M. *Rupert Piper and the Boy Who Could Knit*

Sullivan, Mary Beth, Alan J. Brightman, and Joseph Blatt. *Feeling Free*

Wandro, Mark, and Joani Blank. *My Daddy Is a Nurse*

Sexual Assault

See also Rape.

Dayee, Frances S. *Private Zone: A Book Teaching Children Sexual Assault Prevention Tools*

Sexuality

See also Contraception; Love; Reproductive system.

Ayrault, Evelyn West. *Sex, Love, and the Physically Handicapped*

Burgess-Kohn, Jane. *Straight Talk About Love and Sex for Teenagers*

Carlson, Dale Bick. *Boys Have Feelings Too*

Carlson, Dale Bick. *Loving Sex for Both Sexes: Straight Talk for Teenagers*

Garden, Nancy. *Annie on My Mind*

Hall, Lynn. *Sticks and Stones*

Hamilton, Eleanor. *Sex, with Love: A Guide for Young People*

Hanckel, Frances, and John Cunningham. *A Way of Love, a Way of Life: A Young Person's Introduction to What It Means to Be Gay*

Hass, Aaron. *Teenage Sexuality*

Hautzig, Deborah. *Hey Dollface*

Holland, Isabelle. *The Man Without a Face*

Hunt, Morton. *Gay: What You Should Know About Homosexuality*

Hunt, Morton. *The Young Person's Guide to Love*

Johnson, Corinne Benson, and Eric W. Johnson. *Love and Sex and Growing Up*

Johnson, Eric W. *Love and Sex in Plain Language*

Johnson, Eric W. *Sex: Telling It Straight*

Kaplan, Helen Singer. *Making Sense of Sex: The New Facts About Sex and Love for Young People*

Kelly, Gary F. *Learning About Sex: The Contemporary Guide for Young Adults*

Kerr, M. E. *I'll Love You When You're More Like Me*

Langone, John. *Like, Love, Lust: A View of Sex and Sexuality*

Lieberman, E. James, and Ellen Peck. *Sex and Birth Control: A Guide for the Young*

McCoy, Kathy. *The Teenage Body Book Guide to Sexuality*

Mayerson, Evelyn. *Sanjo*

Milgram, Gail G. *The Teenager and Sex*

Mintz, Thomas, and Lorelie Miller Mintz. *Threshold: Straight Answers to Teenagers' Questions About Sex*

Mitchell, Joyce Slayton. *Free to Choose: Decision Making for Young Men*

Oettinger, Katherine B., with

Elizabeth C. Mooney. *Not My Daughter: Facing Up to Adolescent Pregnancy*

Scoppettone, Sandra. *Happy Endings Are All Alike*

Scoppettone, Sandra. *Trying Hard to Hear You*

Spock, Benjamin McLane. *A Teenager's Guide to Life and Love*

Tensen, Gordon. *Youth and Sex: Pleasure and Responsibility*

Sexually Transmitted Disease

See also Venereal disease.

Lubowe, Irwin I., and Barbara Huss. *A Teen-Age Guide to Healthy Skin and Hair*

McCoy, Kathy. *The Teenage Body Book Guide to Sexuality*

Siblings of Ill, Disabled

Arthur, Catherine. *My Sister's Silent World*

Bach, Alice. *Waiting for Johnny Miracle*

Baldwin, Anne Norris. *A Little Time*

Baznik, Donna. *Becky's Story*

Brandenberg, Franz. *I Wish I Was Sick, Too!*

Branscum, Robbie. *For Love of Jody*

Brown, Roy. *Find Debbie!*

Burch, Robert. *D.J.'s Worst Enemy*

Byars, Betsy. *The Summer of the Swans*

Cleary, Beverly. *Mitch and Amy*

Cleaver, Vera, and Bill Cleaver. *Me Too*

Colman, Hila Crayder. *Diary of a Frantic Kid Sister*

Crane, Caroline. *A Girl Like Tracy*

Dunnahoo, Terry. *Who Cares About Espie Sanchez?*

Graber, Richard. *A Little Breathing Room*

Hall, Lynn. *Half the Battle*

Hirsch, Karen. *My Sister*

Lasker, Joe. *He's My Brother*

Little, Jean. *Listen for the Singing*

Little, Jean. *Take Wing*

Melton, David. *A Boy Called Hopeless*

Murray, Gloria, and Gerald G. Jampolsky, eds. *Straight from the Siblings: Another Look at the Rainbow*

Peter, Diana. *Claire and Emma*

Peterson, Jeanne Whitehouse. *I Have a Sister, My Sister Is Deaf*

Reynolds, Pamela. *Will the Real Monday Please Stand Up*

Robinson, Veronica. *David in Silence*

Smith, Lucia B. *A Special Kind of Sister*

Sobol, Harriet Langsam. *My Brother Steven Is Retarded*

Spence, Eleanor. *The Devil Hole*

Wartski, Maureen Crane. *My Brother Is Special*

Wojciechowska, Maia. *Tuned Out*

Wolde, Gunilla. *Betsy and the Chicken Pox*

Wolff, Ruth. *A Crack in the Sidewalk*

Wright, Betty Ren. *My Sister Is Different*

Sickle Cell Anemia

Hyde, Margaret Oldroyd. *The New Genetics*

Sign Language

See also Deafness; Hearing impairment.

Arthur, Catherine. *My Sister's Silent World*

Berger, Gilda, and Melvin Berger. *The Whole World of Hands*

Bove, Linda. *Sesame Street Sign Language Fun*

Charlip, Remy, and Mary Beth Sullivan. *Handtalk: An ABC of Finger Spelling and Sign Language*

Hirsch, Karen. *Becky*

Levine, Edna S. *Lisa and Her Soundless World*

Montgomery, Elizabeth Rider. *The Mystery of the Boy Next Door*

Neimark, Anne E. *A Deaf Child Listened: Thomas Gallaudet, Pioneer in American Education*

Pizer, Vernon. *You Don't Say: How People Communicate Without Speech*

Robinson, Veronica. *David in Silence*

Spradley, Thomas S., and James R. Spradley. *Deaf Like Me*

Sullivan, Mary Beth, and Linda Bourke. *A Show of Hands: Say It in Sign Language*

Yolen, Jane. *The Mermaid's Three Wisdoms*

Signed English

See also Deafness; Hearing impairment.

Collins-Ahlgren, Marianne. *Matthew's Accident*

Roy, Howard L. *Bobby Visits the Dentist*

Roy, Howard L. *We're Going to the Doctor*

Skeletal System

Balestrino, Philip. *The Skeleton Inside You*

Gross, Ruth Belov. *A Book About Your Skeleton*

Silverstein, Alvin, and Virginia B. Silverstein. *The Skeletal System: Frameworks for Life*

Thompson, Brenda, and Rosemary Giesen. *Bones and Skeletons*

Weart, Edith Lucie. *The Story of Your Bones*

Zim, Herbert S. *Bones*

Skin

Doss, Helen Grigsby. *Your Skin Holds You In*

Lerner, Marguerite Rush. *Color and People: The Story of Pigmentation*

Lubowe, Irwin I., and Barbara Huss. *A Teen-Age Guide to Healthy Skin and Hair*

Nourse, Alan Edward. *Clear Skin, Healthy Skin*

Showers, Paul. *Your Skin and Mine*

Silverstein, Alvin, and Virginia B. Silverstein. *The Skin: Coverings and Linings of Living Things*

Weart, Edith Lucie. *The Story of Your Skin*

Zim, Herbert S. *Your Skin*

Skin Conditions

Annexton, May, and Brent Schillinger. *Coping with Skin Care*

Doss, Helen Grigsby. *Your Skin Holds You In*

Dvorine, William. *A Dermatologist's Guide to Home Skin Treatment: An Up-to-Date Guide That Explains the Best Available Treatment for Every Common Skin Problem, from Acne to Warts*

Reeves, John R. T. *Questions and Answers About Acne*

Van Leeuwen, Jean. *I Was a 98-Pound Duckling*

Zizmor, Jonathan, and Diane English. *Doctor Zizmor's Guide to Clearer Skin*

Sleep

See also Dreams.

Goodbody, Slim. *The Healthy Habits Handbook*

Jacobsen, Karen. *Health*

Lindsay, Rae. *Sleep and Dreams*

Odor, Ruth S. *What's a Body to Do?*

Showers, Paul. *Sleep Is for Everyone*

Silverstein, Alvin, and Virginia B. Silverstein. *Sleep and Dreams*

Smell

See also Senses.

Adler, Irving, and Ruth Adler. *Taste, Touch and Smell*

Showers, Paul. *Follow Your Nose*

Ward, Brian R. *Touch, Taste and Smell*

Smoking

Berger, Gilda. *Addiction: Its Causes, Problems and Treatment*

Casewit, Curtis W. *The Stop Smoking Book for Teens*

Madison, Arnold. *Smoking and You*

Marr, John S. *A Breath of Air and a Breath of Smoke*

Sonnett, Sherry. *Smoking*

Terry, Luther L., and Daniel Horn. *To Smoke or Not to Smoke*

Tobias, Tobi. *The Quitting Deal*

Social Worker

Craig, Eleanor. *One, Two, Three . . . The Story of Matt, a Feral Child*

Keyes, Fenton. *Your Future in Social Work*

Peacock, Carol Antoinette. *Hand-Me-Down Dreams*

Special Education

See also Disabled in school.

Anker, Carol Teig. *Teaching Exceptional Children: A Special Career*

Canada, Lena. *To Elvis, with Love*

Fanshawe, Elizabeth. *Rachel*

Fassler, Joan. *Howie Helps Himself*

Frevert, Patricia Dendtler. *Patrick: Yes You Can*

Gilson, Jamie. *Do Bananas Chew Gum?*

Glazzard, Margaret H. *Meet Camille and Danille, They're Special Persons: Hearing Impaired*

Glazzard, Margaret H. *Meet Danny, He's a Special Person: Multiply Handicapped*

Glazzard, Margaret H. *Meet Lance, He's a Special Person: Trainable Mentally Retarded*

Glazzard, Margaret H. *Meet Scott, He's a Special Person: Learning Disabled*

Gollay, Elinor, and Alwina Bennett. *The College Guide for Students with Disabilities: A Detailed Directory of Higher Education Services, Programs, and Facilities Accessible to Handicapped Students in the United States*

Hawker, Frances, and Lee Withall. *Donna Finds Another Way*

Hawker, Frances, and Lee Withall. *With a Little Help from My Friends*

Heide, Florence Parry. *Secret Dreamer, Secret Dreams*

Hunter, Edith Fisher. *Sue Ellen*

Jones, Marilyn. *Exploring Careers in Special Education*

Levine, Edna S. *Lisa and Her Soundless World*

Litchfield, Ada Bassett. *A Cane in Her Hand*

Little, Jean. *From Anna*

MacCracken, Mary. *Lovey: A Very Special Child*

Neimark, Anne E. *A Deaf Child Listened: Thomas Gallaudet, Pioneer in American Education*

Neimark, Anne E. *Touch of Light: The Story of Louis Braille*

Special Olympics/ Paralympics

See also Disabled in sports; Paralysis; Retardation; Sports medicine.

Henriod, Lorraine. *Special Olympics and Paralympics*

Young, John Sacret. *Special Olympics*

Speech

See also Communication.

Bennett, Merilyn Brottman, and Sylvia Sanders. *How We Talk: The Story of Speech*

Showers, Paul. *How You Talk*

Speech Impairment

See also Communication disability; Stuttering.

Althea. *I Can't Talk Like You*

Bennett, Merilyn Brottman, and Sylvia Sanders. *How We Talk: The Story of Speech*

Berger, Gilda. *Speech and Language Disorders*

Burch, Robert. *D.J.'s Worst Enemy*

Fassler, Joan. *Don't Worry, Dear*

Holland, Isabelle. *Alan and the Animal Kingdom*

Lee, Mildred Scudder. *The Skating Rink*

Madison, Winifred. *Growing Up in a Hurry*

Platt, Kin. *The Boy Who Could Make Himself Disappear*

Rice, Eve. *Ebbie*

Stanek, Muriel. *Growl When You Say R*

Spina Bifida

See also Paralysis; Spinal disability; Wheelchair.

Frevert, Patricia Dendtler. *It's Okay to Look at Jamie*

Hawker, Frances, and Lee Withall.

With a Little Help from My Friends
White, Paul. *Janet at School*

Spinal Disability

See also Paralysis; Scoliosis; Spina bifida.

Blume, Judy Sussman. *Deenie*
Corcoran, Barbara. *A Row of Tigers*

Sports Medicine

See also Disabled in sports; Exercise; Nutrition; Physical fitness.

Berger, Melvin. *Sports Medicine*
Donahue, Parnell. *Sports Doc: Medical Advice, Diet, Fitness Tips, and Other Essential Hints for Young Athletes*

Stitches

See also Emergency; Surgery.

Marino, Barbara Pavis. *Eric Needs Stitches*
Vigna, Judith. *Gregory's Stitches*

Stomach

See also Digestion.

Zim, Herbert S. *Your Stomach and Digestive Tract*

Stomach Disorder

See also Digestion disorder.

Blume, Judy Sussman. *Then Again, Maybe I Won't*
Mylander, Maureen. *The Great American Stomach Book:*

How Your Digestion Works and What to Do When It Doesn't
Null, Gary, and Steve Null. *Why Your Stomach Hurts: A Handbook of Digestion and Nutrition*
Taylor, David M., and Maxine A. Rock. *Gut Reactions: How to Handle Stress and Your Stomach*

Stress

See also Psychosomatic illness.

Brown, Barbara B. *Stress and the Art of Biofeedback*
Buckalew, M. W., Jr. *Learning to Control Stress*
Cohen, Daniel. *Stress: Understanding the Tension You Feel at Home, at School and Among Your Friends*
Elkind, David. *The Hurried Child: Growing Up Too Fast Too Soon*
Kettelkamp, Larry. *A Partnership of Mind and Body: Biofeedback*
McQuade, Walter, and Ann Aikman. *Stress: What It Is, What It Can Do to Your Health, How to Fight Back*
Taylor, David M., and Maxine A. Rock. *Gut Reactions: How to Handle Stress and Your Stomach*

Stuttering

See also Speech impairment.

Christopher, Matt. *Glue Fingers*
Fassler, Joan. *Don't Worry, Dear*
Greene, Constance C. *The Unmaking of Rabbit*

Holland, Isabelle. *Alan and the Animal Kingdom*
Kelley, Sally. *Trouble with Explosives*
Lee, Mildred Scudder. *The Skating Rink*
Madison, Winifred. *Growing Up in a Hurry*

Suicide/Suicide Attempt

See also Death; Depression; Psychotherapy.

Bauer, Marion Dane. *Tangled Butterfly*
Culin, Charlotte. *Cages of Glass, Flowers of Time*
Ferris, Jean. *Amen, Moses Gardenia*
Gerson, Corinne. *Passing Through*
Guest, Judith. *Ordinary People*
Holland, Isabelle. *Heads You Win, Tails I Lose*
Hyde, Margaret Oldroyd, and Elizabeth Held Forsyth. *Suicide: The Hidden Epidemic*
Klagsbrun, Francine. *Too Young to Die: Youth and Suicide*
Langone, John. *Death Is a Noun: A View of the End of Life*
McKillip, Patricia. *The Night Gift*
Madison, Arnold. *Suicide and Young People*
Manes, Stephen. *I'll Live*
Oneal, Zibby. *The Language of Goldfish*

Surgery

See also Hospitalization.

Facklam, Margery, and Howard Facklam. *The Brain: Magnificent Mind Machine*

Freney, Rosemary, Lia Kapelis, and Peter Hicks. *Guess Where I've Been!*
Greenwald, Arthur, and Barry Head. *Having an Operation*
Haines, Gail Kay. *Cancer*
Howe, James. *The Hospital Book*
Kavaler, Lucy. *Cold Against Disease: The Wonders of Cold*
Penney, Peggy L. *Surgery: From Stone Scalpel to Laser Beam*

Surgery, appendectomy

Bemelmans, Ludwig. *Madeline*
Weber, Alfons. *Elizabeth Gets Well*

Surgery, cleft lip

See also Cleft lip/palate.

Weiss, Joan Talmage. *Home for a Stranger*

Surgery, eye

Althea. *Having an Eye Test*
Frevert, Patricia Dendtler. *Patrick: Yes You Can*
Hunt, Irene. *William*
National Association for Visually Handicapped. *Cathy*

Surgery, heart

See also Surgery, transplant.

Howe, James. *A Night Without Stars*
Limburg, Peter. *Story of Your Heart*
Nolen, William A. *Surgeon Under the Knife*
Poole, Victoria. *Thursday's Child*

Silverstein, Alvin, and Virginia B. Silverstein. *Heartbeats: Your Body, Your Heart*

Singer, Marilyn. *It Can't Hurt Forever*

Surgery, oral

Dunn, Graeme. *Benjamin Goes to the Dentist: An Introduction to the Dentist for Children and Parents*

Surgery, ostomy

Hawker, Frances, and Lee Withall. *With a Little Help from My Friends*

Jeter, Katherine F. *These Special Children: The Ostomy Book for Parents of Children with Colostomies, Ileostomies and Urostomies*

Trachtenberg, Irene. *My Daughter, My Son*

Surgery, plastic

See also Burns.

Cunningham, Glenn, with George X. Sand. *Never Quit*

Friis, Babbis. *Kristy's Courage*

Surgery, tonsillectomy

Anderson, Penny S. *The Operation*

Lipson, Tony, and the staff of the Royal Alexandra Hospital for Children. *Benjamin Goes to Hospital: An Introduction to Hospital for Children and Parents*

Snell, Nigel. *Lucy Loses Her Tonsils*

Stein, Sara Bonnett. *A Hospital Story: An Open Family Book for Parents and Children Together*

Ziegler, Sandra. *At the Hospital: A Surprise for Krissy*

Surgery, transplant

See also Artificial body parts.

Baker, Lynn S., in collaboration with Charles G. Roland and Gerald S. Gilchrist. *You and Leukemia: A Day at a Time*

Burton, Adrianne. *Your New Kidney*

The Coleman Family and Bill Davidson. *Gary Coleman: Medical Miracle*

Freese, Arthur S. *The Bionic People Are Here*

Nolen, William A. *Spare Parts for the Human Body*

Poole, Victoria. *Thursday's Child*

Surgery, tumor

See also Cancer.

Bach, Alice. *Waiting for Johnny Miracle*

Taste

See also Senses.

Adler, Irving, and Ruth Adler. *Taste, Touch and Smell*

Allington, Richard L., and Kathleen Cowles. *Tasting*

Ward, Brian R. *Touch, Taste and Smell*

Teeth

See also Dentist's office; Dentist's office—animal; Mouth.

Cooney, Nancy Evans. *The Wobbly Tooth*
Doss, Helen Grigsby, and Richard L. Wells. *All the Better to Bite With*
Fleege, Francis. *How to Eat: Chewing, Tooth Care, and Diet*
Hammond, Winifred G. *The Riddle of Teeth*
Nourse, Alan Edward. *The Tooth Book*
Pomerantz, Charlotte. *The Mango Tooth*
Rice, Eve. *Ebbie*
Ross, Pat. *Molly and the Slow Teeth*
Showers, Paul. *How Many Teeth?*

Teeth—Animal

McPhail, David. *The Bear's Toothache*

Teeth, braces

See Braces, teeth.

Thumbsucking

Ernst, Kathryn F. *Danny and His Thumb*
Fassler, Joan. *Don't Worry, Dear*
Tobias, Tobi. *The Quitting Deal*

Tonsillectomy

See Surgery, tonsillectomy.

Touch

See also Senses.

Adler, Irving, and Ruth Adler. *Taste, Touch and Smell*
Showers, Paul. *Find Out by Touching*
Ward, Brian R. *Touch, Taste and Smell*

Transplant

See Artificial body parts; Surgery, transplant.

Tumor

See Cancer; Surgery, tumor.

Twins

See also Reproductive system; Siblings of ill, disabled.

Bach, Alice. *Waiting for Johnny Miracle*
Cleary, Beverly. *Mitch and Amy*
Cleaver, Vera, and Bill Cleaver. *Me Too*
Cole, Joanna, and Madeleine Edmondson. *Twins: The Story of Multiple Births*
Lerner, Marguerite Rush. *Twins: The Story of Twins*

Ulcer

Eisenberg, Michael. *Ulcers*
Kerr, M. E. *I'll Love You When You're More Like Me*
Trachtenberg, Irene. *My Daughter, My Son*

Ultrasound

Knight, David C. *Silent Sound: The World of Ultrasonics*

Upper Respiratory Infection (URI)

See also Bacteria; Cold, common; Cold, common—animal; Infection; Virus.

Bennett, Hal Zina. *Cold Comfort*
Jessel, Camilla. *Going to the Doctor*
MacLachlan, Patricia. *The Sick Day*
Nourse, Alan Edward. *Viruses*
Numeroff, Laura Joffe. *Phoebe Dexter Has Harriet Peterson's Sniffles*

Vaccination

Nourse, Alan Edward. *Viruses*
Rosenberg, Nancy, and Louis Z. Cooper. *Vaccines and Viruses*
Showers, Paul. *No Measles, No Mumps for Me*

Venereal Disease

See also Contraception.

Blanzaco, Andre. *VD: Facts You Should Know*
Edwards, Gabrielle. *Coping with Venereal Disease*
Hyde, Margaret Oldroyd. *VD: The Silent Epidemic*
Johnson, Eric W. *V.D.: Venereal Disease and What You Should Do About It*
Sgroi, Suzanne M. *VD: A Doctor's Answers*

Virus

Knight, David C. *Viruses: Life's Smallest Enemies*
Nourse, Alan Edward. *Viruses*
Rosenberg, Nancy, and Louis Z. Cooper. *Vaccines and Viruses*

Vision

See also Eye.

Brindze, Ruth. *Look How Many People Wear Glasses: The Magic of Lenses*
Weiss, Malcolm E. *Seeing Through the Dark: Blind and Sighted—A Vision Shared*

Vision Aids

See also Blindness; Vision impairment.

Adler, Irving, and Ruth Adler. *Your Eyes*
Corn, Anne L. *Monocular Mac*
Frevert, Patricia Dendtler. *Patrick: Yes You Can*
Hall, Candace Catlin. *Shelley's Day: The Day of a Legally Blind Child*
Kelley, Alberta. *Lenses, Spectacles, Eyeglasses and Contacts: The Story of Vision Aids*
Litchfield, Ada Bassett. *A Cane in Her Hand*
National Association for Visually Handicapped. *Cathy*
National Association for Visually Handicapped. *Larry*
Neimark, Anne E. *Touch of Light: The Story of Louis Braille*
Petersen, Palle. *Sally Can't See*
Pizer, Vernon. *You Don't Say: How People Communicate Without Speech*

Thomas, William E. *The New Boy Is Blind*

Weiss, Malcolm E. *Blindness*

Vision Impairment

See also Blind; Contact lenses; Glasses.

Corn, Anne L. *Monocular Mac*

Goodsell, Jane. *Katie's Magic Glasses*

Hall, Candace Catlin. *Shelley's Day: The Day of a Legally Blind Child*

Kelley, Alberta. *Lenses, Spectacles, Eyeglasses and Contacts: The Story of Vision Aids*

Kropp, Paul. *Wilted*

Leggett, Linda Rodgers, and Linda Gambee Andrews. *The Rose-Colored Glasses: Melanie Adjusts to Poor Vision*

Litchfield, Ada Bassett. *A Cane in Her Hand*

Little, Jean. *Listen for the Singing*

Marcus, June Z. *Susan*

National Association for Visually Handicapped. *Cathy*

National Association for Visually Handicapped. *Larry*

Raskin, Ellen. *Spectacles*

Rosenberg, Maxine B. *My Friend Leslie: The Story of a Handicapped Child*

Snell, Nigel. *Johnny Gets Some Glasses*

Stanek, Muriel. *Left Right, Left Right*

Ward, Brian R. *The Eye and Seeing*

Wolff, Angelika. *Mom! I Need Glasses*

Vitamins

See also Nutrition.

Asimov, Isaac. *How Did We Find Out About Vitamins?*

Jones, Hettie. *How to Eat Your ABC's: A Book About Vitamins*

Nourse, Alan Edward. *Vitamins*

Weiss, Malcolm E., and Ann E. Weiss. *The Vitamin Puzzle*

Warts

See also Skin conditions.

Dvorine, William. *A Dermatologist's Guide to Home Skin Treatment: An Up-to-Date Guide That Explains the Best Available Treatment for Every Common Skin Problem, from Acne to Warts*

Simon, Norma. *Go Away, Warts!*

Weight Control

See also Exercise; Nutrition.

B., Bill. *Compulsive Overeater: The Basic Text for Compulsive Overeaters*

Balestrino, Philip. *Fat and Skinny*

Benziger, Barbara. *Controlling Your Weight*

Blume, Judy Sussman. *Blubber*

Bolian, Polly. *Growing Up Slim*

Bottner, Barbara. *Dumb Old Casey Is a Fat Tree*

Byars, Betsy. *After the Goat Man*

Cavallaro, Ann. *Blimp*

Cohen, Barbara. *Fat Jack*

Doss, Helen Grigsby. *Your Skin Holds You In*

Eagles, Douglas A. *Your Weight*

First, Julia. *Look Who's Beautiful!*

Gelinas, Paul J. *Coping with Weight Problems*

Gilbert, Nan. *The Unchosen*

Gilbert, Sara D. *Fat Free: Common Sense for Young Weight Worriers*
Greenberg, Jan. *The Pig-Out Blues*
Hall, Elizabeth. *From Pigeons to People: A Look at Behavior Shaping*
Hamilton, Virginia. *The Planet of Junior Brown*
Holland, Isabelle. *Dinah and the Fat Green Kingdom*
Holland, Isabelle. *Heads You Win, Tails I Lose*
Kerr, M. E. *Dinky Hocker Shoots Smack*
Lipsyte, Robert. *One Fat Summer*
Livingston, Carole. *I'll Never Be Fat Again!*
Mazer, Harry. *The Dollar Man*
Miles, Betty. *Looking On*
Orgel, Doris. *Next Door to Xanadu*
Perl, Lila. *Me and Fat Glenda*
Philips, Barbara. *Don't Call Me Fatso*
Pinkwater, Manus. *Fat Elliot and the Gorilla*
Rabinowich, Ellen. *Underneath I'm Different*
Savitz, Harriet May. *The Lionhearted*
Stolz, Mary. *In a Mirror*
Talbot, Charlene J. *The Great Rat Island Adventure*
Van Leeuwen, Jean. *I Was a 98-Pound Duckling*

Wheelchair

See also Disabled in school; Disabled in sports; Paralysis.

Althea. *I Use a Wheelchair*
Bradbury, Bianca. *The Girl Who Wanted Out*
Canada, Lena. *To Elvis, with Love*
Cook, Marjorie. *To Walk on Two Feet*
Fanshawe, Elizabeth. *Rachel*
Fassler, Joan. *Howie Helps Himself*
Greenfield, Eloise. *Darlene*
Hawker, Frances, and Lee Withall. *Donna Finds Another Way*
Henriod, Lorraine. *Special Olympics and Paralympics*
Lasker, Joe. *Nick Joins In*
Lee, Robert C. *It's a Mile from Here to Glory*
Payne, Sherry Newirth. *A Contest*
Phelan, Terry Wolfe. *The S.S. Valentine*
Pieper, Elizabeth. *A School for Tommy*
Rabe, Berniece. *The Balancing Girl*
Redpath, Ann. *Jim Boen: A Man of Opposites*
Savitz, Harriet May. *The Lionhearted*
Savitz, Harriet May. *Run, Don't Walk*
Savitz, Harriet May. *Wheelchair Champions: A History of Wheelchair Sports*
Southall, Ivan. *Head in the Clouds*
Valens, E.A. *A Long Way Up: The Story of Jill Kinmont*
White, Paul. *Janet at School*

X Ray

See also Cardiac catheterization; Dentist's office; Hospitalization.

Frevert, Patricia Dendtler. *It's Okay to Look at Jamie*
Greenwald, Arthur, and Barry Head. *Wearing a Cast*
Halacy, Daniel S., Jr. *X-Rays and Gamma Rays*
Hawker, Frances, and Lee Withall.

With a Little Help from My Friends

Klein, Aaron E. *Medical Tests and You*

NAWCH Research Team. *Andrew Goes for an X-Ray*

Pringle, Laurence. *Radiation: Waves and Particles, Benefits and Risks*

Reid, Robert. *Marie Curie*

Richter, Alice, and Laura Joffe Numeroff. *You Can't Put Braces on Spaces*

Rockwell, Harlow. *My Dentist*

Waidley, Ericka. *All About Your X-Ray: IVP*

Waidley, Ericka. *All About Your X-Ray: UGI*